# Non-invasive Device-Mediated Brain Drug Delivery across the Blood-Brain Barrier

# Non-invasive Device-Mediated Brain Drug Delivery across the Blood-Brain Barrier

Editors

**Nicolas Tournier**
**Toshihiko Tashima**

MDPI

Basel • Beijing • Wuhan • Barcelona • Belgrade • Novi Sad • Cluj • Manchester

*Editors*

Nicolas Tournier
Laboratoire d'Imagerie Biomédicale Multimodale, BIOMAPS,
Université Paris-Saclay, CEA, CNRS, Inserm, Service Hospitalier Frédéric Joliot,
Orsay
France

Toshihiko Tashima
Research and Development Office,
Tashima Laboratories of Arts and Sciences,
Yokohama
Japan

*Editorial Office*
MDPI
St. Alban-Anlage 66
4052 Basel, Switzerland

This is a reprint of articles from the Special Issue published online in the open access journal *Pharmaceutics* (ISSN 1999-4923) (available at: https://www.mdpi.com/journal/pharmaceutics/special_issues/6M57N69SSA).

For citation purposes, cite each article independently as indicated on the article page online and as indicated below:

| |
|---|
| Lastname, A.A.; Lastname, B.B. Article Title. *Journal Name* **Year**, *Volume Number*, Page Range. |

**ISBN 978-3-7258-0680-5 (Hbk)**
**ISBN 978-3-7258-0679-9 (PDF)**
**doi.org/10.3390/books978-3-7258-0679-9**

Cover image courtesy of Toshihiko Tashima

# Contents

**About the Editors** . . . . . . . . . . . . . . . . . . . . . . . . . . . . . . . . . . . . . . . . . . . . . . **vii**

**Preface** . . . . . . . . . . . . . . . . . . . . . . . . . . . . . . . . . . . . . . . . . . . . . . . . . . . . **ix**

**Toshihiko Tashima and Nicolas Tournier**
Non-Invasive Device-Mediated Drug Delivery to the Brain across the Blood–Brain Barrier
Reprinted from: *Pharmaceutics* **2024**, *16*, 361, doi:10.3390/pharmaceutics16030361 . . . . . . . . . **1**

**Sarfaraz K. Niazi**
Non-Invasive Drug Delivery across the Blood–Brain Barrier: A Prospective Analysis
Reprinted from: *Pharmaceutics* **2023**, *15*, 2599, doi:10.3390/pharmaceutics15112599 . . . . . . . . **7**

**Soma Mondal Ghorai, Auroni Deep, Devanshi Magoo, Chetna Gupta and Nikesh Gupta**
Cell-Penetrating and Targeted Peptides Delivery Systems as Potential Pharmaceutical Carriers for Enhanced Delivery across the Blood–Brain Barrier (BBB)
Reprinted from: *Pharmaceutics* **2023**, *15*, 1999, doi:10.3390/pharmaceutics15071999 . . . . . . . . **35**

**Laura Rué, Tom Jaspers, Isabelle M. S. Degors, Sam Noppen, Dominique Schols, Bart De Strooper and Maarten Dewilde**
Novel Human/Non-Human Primate Cross-Reactive Anti-Transferrin Receptor Nanobodies for Brain Delivery of Biologics
Reprinted from: *Pharmaceutics* **2023**, *15*, 1748, doi:10.3390/pharmaceutics15061748 . . . . . . . . **62**

**Wouter J. F. Vanbilloen, Julian S. Rechberger, Jacob B. Anderson, Leo F. Nonnenbroich, Liang Zhang and David J. Daniels**
Nanoparticle Strategies to Improve the Delivery of Anticancer Drugs across the Blood–Brain Barrier to Treat Brain Tumors
Reprinted from: *Pharmaceutics* **2023**, *15*, 1804, doi:10.3390/pharmaceutics15071804 . . . . . . . . **73**

**Weisen Zhang, Douer Zhu, Ziqiu Tong, Bo Peng, Xuan Cheng, Lars Esser and Nicolas H. Voelcker**
Influence of Surface Ligand Density and Particle Size on the Penetration of the Blood–Brain Barrier by Porous Silicon Nanoparticles
Reprinted from: *Pharmaceutics* **2023**, *15*, 2271, doi:10.3390/pharmaceutics15092271 . . . . . . . . **99**

**Elizabeth J. Patharapankal, Adejumoke Lara Ajiboye, Claudia Mattern and Vivek Trivedi**
Nose-to-Brain (N2B) Delivery: An Alternative Route for the Delivery of Biologics in the Management and Treatment of Central Nervous System Disorders
Reprinted from: *Pharmaceutics* **2024**, *16*, 66, doi:10.3390/pharmaceutics16010066 . . . . . . . . . . **118**

**Paramita Saha, Prabhjeet Singh, Himanshu Kathuria, Deepak Chitkara and Murali Monohar Pandey**
Self-Assembled Lecithin-Chitosan Nanoparticles Improved Rotigotine Nose-to-Brain Delivery and Brain Targeting Efficiency
Reprinted from: *Pharmaceutics* **2023**, *15*, 851, doi:10.3390/pharmaceutics15030851 . . . . . . . . . **160**

**Toshihiko Tashima**
Mesenchymal Stem Cell (MSC)-Based Drug Delivery into the Brain across the Blood–Brain Barrier
Reprinted from: *Pharmaceutics* **2024**, *16*, 289, doi:10.3390/pharmaceutics16020289 . . . . . . . . . **177**

**Shona Kaya, Bridgeen Callan and Susan Hawthorne**
Non-Invasive, Targeted Nanoparticle-Mediated Drug Delivery across a Novel Human BBB Model
Reprinted from: *Pharmaceutics* **2023**, *15*, 1382, doi:10.3390/pharmaceutics15051382 . . . . . . . . **193**

**Chiara Bastiancich, Samantha Fernandez, Florian Correard, Anthony Novell, Benoit Larrat, Benjamin Guillet and Marie-Anne Estève**
Molecular Imaging of Ultrasound-Mediated Blood-Brain Barrier Disruption in a Mouse Orthotopic Glioblastoma Model
Reprinted from: *Pharmaceutics* **2022**, *14*, 2227, doi:10.3390/pharmaceutics14102227 . . . . . . . . **216**

# About the Editors

**Nicolas Tournier**

Nicolas Tournier (PhD, PharmD) is a hospital pharmacist and pharmacologist at the Centre Hospitalier Frédéric Joliot (CEA/SHFJ) in Orsay (France). He leads the Clinical Applications group of the IMIV research unit (Imagerie Moléculaire in Vivo—UMR 1023 Inserm/CEA/Université Paris Sud/Université Paris Saclay—ERL 9218 CNRS). The main aim of this group is to promote the clinical translation of original imaging probes and systems and develop their clinical applications. Their work builds upon the concept of pharmacological and pharmacokinetic imaging. They notably use radiolabeled analogues of drugs to study the impact of membrane transporters on tissue distribution and elimination and estimate the corresponding risk of drug–drug interactions. To that end, the team benefits from a translational and multidisciplinary environment, making the best with recent developments in radiochemistry, medical physics, molecular imaging, nuclear medicine and pharmacokinetics.

**Toshihiko Tashima**

Dr. Toshihiko Tashima has been involved in synthetic research and the discovery of physiologically active substances for many years and is currently engaged in the pharmaceutical department. His research interests encompass pharmaceuticals, with a focus on drug development and drug delivery systems. His research keywords include medicinal chemistry, drug designing, and bioorganics. Dr. Tashima serves as an Editorial Member and reviewer for several internationally renowned journals and has fulfilled various administrative responsibilities. He has authored numerous research articles and books related to medicine. He believes that science should be enjoyable. With advancements in internet technology and open-access journals, science has become infinitely familiar to us. He encourages many people to take advantage of the opportunities to enjoy science.

# Preface

In drug discovery and development, membrane impermeability poses a serious challenge, resulting in insufficient drug efficacy and off-target side effects. Particularly, central nervous system drugs for conditions such as Alzheimer's disease, Parkinson's disease, and glioma struggle to penetrate the blood–brain barrier (BBB) due to tight junctions and efflux transporters in capillary endothelial cells, presenting unmet medical needs for many patients. Innovative drug delivery strategies must be developed to address this issue in a non-invasive manner. Therefore, the Special Issue titled "Non-Invasive Device-Mediated Brain Drug Delivery across the Blood–Brain Barrier" was designed to serve this purpose. We have gathered excellent papers aimed at achieving delivery into the brain across the BBB. We greatly appreciate the contributions of the authors. This time, we will provide the content as a reprint, including one Editorial, one Communication, four Articles, and five Reviews. We hope readers will gain insights into the latest scientific advancements to enhance their research endeavors.

**Nicolas Tournier and Toshihiko Tashima**
*Editors*

*pharmaceutics*

MDPI

*Editorial*

# Non-Invasive Device-Mediated Drug Delivery to the Brain across the Blood–Brain Barrier

**Toshihiko Tashima [1,*,†] and Nicolas Tournier [2,*,†]**

1 Tashima Laboratories of Arts and Sciences, 1239-5 Toriyama-cho, Kohoku-ku, Yokohama 222-0035, Japan
2 Laboratoire d'Imagerie Biomédicale Multimodale, BIOMAPS, Université Paris-Saclay, CEA, CNRS, Inserm, Service Hospitalier Frédéric Joliot, 4 Place du Général Leclerc, 91401 Orsay, France
* Correspondence: tashima_lab@yahoo.co.jp (T.T.); nicolas.tournier@cea.fr (N.T.)
† These authors contributed equally to this work.

We will be serving as the Guest Editor for this very interesting Special Issue on "Non-Invasive Device-Mediated Drug Delivery to the Brain Across the Blood–Brain Barrier". It is well-known that the blood–brain barrier (BBB) [1,2], which is substantially composed of tight junctions [3] between the capillary endothelial cells and efflux transporters such as multiple drug resistance 1 (MDR1, P-glycoprotein) [4] at the apical membrane of the capillary endothelial cells, prevents drugs from entering the brain. Accordingly, drug delivery into the brain across the BBB is a challenging task, particularly in central nervous system (CNS) diseases such as Alzheimer's disease (AD) [5,6] and Parkinson's disease (PD) [7], as well as brain cancers such as glioma [8]. It is true that drugs in systemic circulation go through intentional membrane disruption or intentional tight junction disruption into the brain across the BBB [9], but bystander harmful compounds can enter the brain together. Moreover, although craniotomy is often conducted for surgical removal or direct drug administration, this process burdens and torments patients. Thus, non-invasive, device-mediated drug delivery across the BBB should be developed to improve patients' health and quality of life. At present, brain-based drug delivery systems that utilize biological transport machineries such as carrier-mediated transport, receptor-mediated transcytosis, lipid-raft-mediated transcytosis, or macropinocytosis at the BBB have been extensively investigated [10]. This Special Issue aims to share the recent progress and trends in this field.

The delivery of drugs across the cell membrane is achieved using vectors such as monoclonal antibodies (mAbs) [11], cell-penetrating peptides (CPPs) [12], or tumor-homing peptides (THPs) [13]. It is suggested that negatively charged heparan sulfate chains branching from proteoglycan (HSPG) on the cell surface induce receptor-mediated endocytosis as a receptor for cationic CPPs [14]. RGD peptides (Arg-Gly-Asp), as representative THPs, specifically target cancer cells by binding to $\alpha v\beta 3$ and $\alpha v\beta 5$ integrins [15]. NGR peptides (Asn-Gly-Arg) bind to the receptor aminopeptidase N [16]. Sarfaraz K. Niazi outlines current and future approaches to enhance BBB penetration to treat multiple brain diseases using such delivery technology [17]. Nikesh Gupta et al. present CPPs- or THPs-mediated delivery into the cells [18]. The mechanisms of CPP internalization, involving endocytosis and direct translocation, are widely recognized. The detailed mechanisms of CPPs, specifically regarding membrane internalization and endosomal escape, are accurately described. Both CPPs with cargo and THPs with cargo were endocytosed in the capillary endothelial cells at the BBB. Moreover, Maarten Dewilde et al. introduce mAbs-mediated transcytosis into the brain across the BBB, using nanobodies against the transferrin receptor (TfR) [19]. They developed an anti-TfR nanobody-anti-BACE1 mAb bispecific conjugate. Intravenously administered bispecific conjugates lowered $A\beta 1$–40 levels in plasma in an in vivo assay using hAPI KI mice, in which the mouse TfR apical domain was replaced by the human sequence. These bispecific conjugates entered the brain across the BBB via TfR-mediated transcytosis and inhibited BACE1 in the brain/cerebrospinal fluid (CSF).

**Citation:** Tashima, T.; Tournier, N. Non-Invasive Device-Mediated Drug Delivery to the Brain across the Blood–Brain Barrier. *Pharmaceutics* **2024**, *16*, 361. https://doi.org/10.3390/pharmaceutics16030361

Received: 22 February 2024
Accepted: 28 February 2024
Published: 5 March 2024

Currently, nanobodies [20] are attracting considerable attention due to their compact size and high specificity. Furthermore, Izcargo® (pabinafusp alfa), clinically launched in Japan in May, 2021, for the treatment of all forms of MPS II, enters the brain across the BBB via receptor-mediated transcytosis using TfR. The brain drug delivery technology J-Brain Cargo® is utilized in this drug, composed of the conjugate between anti-TfR monoclonal antibody and human iduronate-2-sulfatase [21]. Thus, drug delivery into the brain via TfR-mediated transcytosis could be a promising strategy. Moreover, it is reported that the clustering of ligand-receptor complexes derived from TfRs enhances endocytosis [22,23]. Generally, clustering induces endocytosis [10,24,25].

In addition, carrier-mediated transport into the brain might be conducted for low-molecular-weight *N*-containing drugs using the proton-coupled organic cation antiporter [26]. Most CNS drugs have structurally incorporated *N*-containing groups into their molecules. It is well-known that certain pharmaceutical agents, such as CNS drugs and antihistamine drugs, can penetrate the brain through the BBB. It is suggested that certain cation transporters facilitate the transport of *N*-containing drugs across the BBB. Memantine for AD is positively charged under physiological pH and, therefore, cannot cross the membrane via passive diffusion. Indeed, memantine with an *N*-containing group is transported into cells via carrier-mediated transport [27]. In general, compounds are divided into three categories, that is, low-molecular-weight compounds (molecular weight (MW) < approx. 500), high-molecular-weight compounds (MW > approx. 3000), and middle-molecular-weight compounds (MW approx. 500–approx. 3000) [10]. High-molecular-weight compounds such as monoclonal antibodies cannot penetrate through the pores of solute carrier transporters, while hydrophilic low-molecular-weight compounds are facilitated by solute carrier transporters. Hydrophobic low-molecular-weight compounds cross the cell membrane via passive diffusion, although they are substrates of MDR1. Thus, the transport strategies, including the transcellular pathway, such as passive diffusion, carrier-mediated transport, or receptor-mediated transcytosis, and the paracellular pathway such as transport through disrupted tight junctions, depend on the molecular size and hydrophobicity, based on the machinery systems regulated by structuralism [28,29].

Furthermore, nanodelivery systems utilizing nanoparticles are innovative tools for delivering cargo drugs to target sites, particularly the brain or cancer tissues [30–32]. Various surface modifications can easily be made to nanoparticles. Encapsulated substances are protected from enzymatic degradation and are not prone to off-target side effects. David J. Daniels et al. provide nanoparticle strategies for delivering drugs into the brain across the BBB, particularly for the treatment of brain tumors via receptor-mediated transcytosis or other internalization mechanisms. Various types of nanoparticles are engineered to enhance targeted delivery into the brain. Nanoparticle clearance and blood circulation time are also crucial to avoid serious side effects [33]. Lars Esser, Nicolas H. Voelcker et al. synthesized porous silicon nanoparticles (PSiNPs) covered with transferrin (average size of 203 and 420 nm). The association of hCMEC/D3 with PSiNPs was enhanced as transferrin content increased from 0 nmol/mg to 3.8 nmol/mg. It was clarified that an intermediate transferrin surface density showed the highest BBB transport. The smaller PSiNPs consistently exhibited higher BBB penetration potential than the larger PSiNPs via receptor-mediated transcytosis [34]. These findings are valuable for nanoparticle design. Nanoparticles should be developed using biocompatible and biodegradable polymers [35]. Poly(lactic acid) (PLA) and poly(lactic-co-glycolic acid) (PLGA) are often utilized [36]. The most common form endocytosis is clathrin-mediated endocytosis [37], inducing endosomes (85–150 nm in diameter) [10], although there are various types of endocytosis [38]. Therefore, the size of the internalized nanoparticles should be within the range of these endosomes. Interestingly, the pH in endosomes gradually decreases from the early endosome (pH approx. 6.5) to the late endosome (pH approx. 5.5), and finally becomes the lysosome (pH approx. 4.5) due to the vacuolar $H^+$-ATPase proton pumps in the degradation pathway [39]. Such acidification can be utilized for cargo release through the leakage of pH-sensitive linkers. The released cargos might penetrate the membrane of endosomes, leading to endosomal escape, or may penetrate the membrane of lysosomes, leading to lysosomal escape, via passive diffusion. On the other hand, endosomes or lysosomes burst through the proton sponge effect in the case of amine-rich carriers while acidification proceeds [40].

Broadly speaking, nose-to-brain drug delivery is a strategy to deliver drugs into the brain without crossing the BBB [41,42]. Strictly speaking, this pathway does not involve the BBB. Vivek Trivedi et al. provide an overview of the current state of intranasal formulation development for nose-to-brain drug delivery and summarize the biologics that are currently undergoing clinical trial [43]. Intranasally administered substances can be transported across the olfactory epithelium and subsequently move into the brain through the olfactory nerve or trigeminal nerve. Murali Monohar Pandey et al. developed rotigotine-loaded lecithin-chitosan nanoparticles (RTG-LCNP) for the treatment of PD [44]. RTG-LCNP showed a 9.66-fold increase in the amount permeated compared to pure drug suspension in an ex vivo nasal permeation study using male Wistar rats. On the other hand, mesenchymal stem cells (MSCs) [45] administered through intravenous or intracarotid routes can be utilized as a drug carrier, homing to the target sites, although they are often clinically used for regenerative medicine due to their differentiation potential [46]. Toshihiko Tashima proposes MSC-based drug delivery into the brain across the BBB [47]. The substances delivered by MSCs are divided into artificially included materials in advance, such as low-molecular-weight compounds including doxorubicin, and the expected protein expression products of genetic modification, such as interleukins.

Screening methods to analyze drug permeability across the BBB are important for CNS drug development [48]. Susan Hawthorne et al. developed a viable method for the high-throughput screening of CNS drugs using a novel transwell human BBB model. Fitc-dextran-encapsulated PLGA nanoparticles covered with DAS peptide were transported via receptor-mediated transcytosis that is 14-fold greater than Fitc-dextran-encapsulated PLGA nanoparticles in this assay system [49]. A variety of nanoparticles can be effectively evaluated through this system. Marie-Anne Estève demonstrates the transportation of imaging compounds into the brain through transient FUS-mediated BBB opening performed on healthy animals [50]. CNS imaging is increasingly recognized for its vital role in preventive medicine for neurodegenerative diseases such as AD in an aging society [51]. Tau imaging [52,53] and Aβ imaging [54,55] will play an important role in confirming the progress of AD for early intervention [56] because the number of AD patients is expected to increase in the future [57]. It is likely difficult to cure AD once the symptoms have progressed to a certain extent. The social losses, such as costs and the burden of nursing care due to AD, are immeasurable. Recently, several anti-Aβ monoclonal antibodies, such as aducanumab [58] and lecanemab [59], have been clinically approved. Furthermore, donanemab finished a phase 3 clinical trial with favorable results for early AD in 2023 [60]. The development of drugs that can provide a fundamental treatment is good news for AD patients. We hope that this Special Issue will contribute to the creation of innovative medicines.

Overall, the articles in this Special Issue outline non-invasive device-mediated brain drug delivery across the BBB and will contribute to the development of this field. We would like to express our gratitude to all the authors of this Special Issue for their outstanding contributions. Moreover, we extend our thanks to the Assistant Editors, for their valuable assistance.

**Conflicts of Interest:** The authors declare no conflicts of interest.

## References

1. Profaci, C.P.; Munji, R.N.; Pulido, R.S.; Daneman, R. The blood-brain barrier in health and disease: Important unanswered questions. *J. Exp. Med.* **2020**, *217*, e20190062. [CrossRef]
2. Ali, A.; Arshad, M.S.; Khan, M.A.; Chang, M.W.; Ahmad, Z. Recent advances towards overcoming the blood–brain barrier. *Drug Discov. Today* **2023**, *28*, 103735. [CrossRef]
3. Sasson, E.; Anzi, S.; Bell, B.; Yakovian, O.; Zorsky, M.; Deutsch, U.; Engelhardt, B.; Sherman, E.; Vatine, G.; Dzikowski, R.; et al. Nano-scale architecture of blood-brain barrier tight-junctions. *eLife* **2021**, *10*, e63253. [CrossRef]

4. Catalano, A.; Iacopetta, D.; Ceramella, J.; Scumaci, D.; Giuzio, F.; Saturnino, C.; Aquaro, S.; Rosano, C.; Sinicropi, M.S. Multidrug Resistance (MDR): A Widespread Phenomenon in Pharmacological Therapies. *Molecules* **2022**, *27*, 616. [CrossRef]
5. Trejo-Lopez, J.A.; Yachnis, A.T.; Prokop, S. Neuropathology of Alzheimer's Disease. *Neurotherapeutics* **2022**, *19*, 173–185. [CrossRef]
6. Scheltens, P.; De Strooper, B.; Kivipelto, M.; Holstege, H.; Chételat, G.; Teunissen, C.E.; Cummings, J.; van der Flier, W.M. Alzheimer's disease. *Lancet* **2021**, *397*, 1577–1590. [CrossRef]
7. Bloem, B.R.; Okun, M.S.; Klein, C. Parkinson's disease. *Lancet* **2021**, *397*, 2284–3303. [CrossRef]
8. Yang, K.; Wu, Z.; Zhang, H.; Zhang, N.; Wu, W.; Wang, Z.; Dai, Z.; Zhang, X.; Zhang, L.; Peng, Y.; et al. Glioma targeted therapy: Insight into future of molecular approaches. *Mol. Cancer* **2022**, *21*, 39. [CrossRef] [PubMed]
9. Costea, L.; Mészáros, Á.; Bauer, H.; Bauer, H.-C.; Traweger, A.; Wilhelm, I.; Farkas, A.E.; Krizbai, I.A. The Blood–Brain Barrier and Its Intercellular Junctions in Age-Related Brain Disorders. *Int. J. Mol. Sci.* **2019**, *20*, 5472. [CrossRef] [PubMed]
10. Tashima, T. Smart Strategies for Therapeutic Agent Delivery into Brain across the Blood-Brain Barrier Using Receptor-Mediated Transcytosis. *Chem. Pharm. Bull.* **2020**, *68*, 316–325. [CrossRef] [PubMed]
11. Pardridge, W.M. Kinetics of Blood-Brain Barrier Transport of Monoclonal Antibodies Targeting the Insulin Receptor and the Transferrin Receptor. *Pharmaceuticals* **2022**, *15*, 3. [CrossRef]
12. Varnamkhasti, B.S.; Jafari, S.; Taghavi, F.; Alaei, L.; Izadi, Z.; Lotfabadi, A.; Dehghanian, M.; Jaymand, M.; Derakhshankhah, H.; Saboury, A.A. Cell-Penetrating Peptides: As a Promising Theranostics Strategy to Circumvent the Blood-Brain Barrier for CNS Diseases. *Curr. Drug Deliv.* **2020**, *17*, 375–386. [CrossRef]
13. Cho, C.-F.; Farquhar, C.E.; Fadzen, C.M.; Scott, B.; Zhuang, P.; von Spreckelsen, N.; Loas, A.; Hartrampf, N.; Pentelute, B.L.; Lawler, S.E. A Tumor-Homing Peptide Platform Enhances Drug Solubility, Improves Blood-Brain Barrier Permeability and Targets Glioblastoma. *Cancers* **2022**, *14*, 2207. [CrossRef]
14. Christianson, H.C.; Belting, M. Heparan sulfate proteoglycan as a cell-surface endocytosis receptor. *Matrix Biol.* **2014**, *35*, 51–55. [CrossRef]
15. Javid, H.; Oryani, M.A.; Rezagholinejad, N.; Esparham, A.; Tajaldini, M.; Karimi-Shahri, M. RGD peptide in cancer targeting: Benefits, challenges, solutions, and possible integrin–RGD interactions. *Cancer Med.* **2024**, *13*, e6800. [CrossRef]
16. Li, X.; Fu, H.; Wang, J.; Liu, W.; Deng, H.; Zhao, P.; Liao, W.; Yang, Y.; Wei, H.; Yang, X.; et al. Multimodality labeling of NGR-functionalized hyaluronan for tumor targeting and radiotherapy. *Eur. J. Pharm. Sci.* **2021**, *161*, 105775. [CrossRef] [PubMed]
17. Niazi, S.K. Non-Invasive Drug Delivery across the Blood-Brain Barrier: A Prospective Analysis. *Pharmaceutics* **2023**, *15*, 2599. [CrossRef] [PubMed]
18. Ghorai, S.M.; Deep, A.; Magoo, D.; Gupta, C.; Gupta, N. Cell-Penetrating and Targeted Peptides Delivery Systems as Potential Pharmaceutical Carriers for Enhanced Delivery across the Blood-Brain Barrier (BBB). *Pharmaceutics* **2023**, *15*, 1999. [CrossRef] [PubMed]
19. Rué, L.; Jaspers, T.; Degors, I.M.S.; Noppen, S.; Schols, D.; De Strooper, B.; Dewilde, M. Novel Human/Non-Human Primate Cross-Reactive Anti-Transferrin Receptor Nanobodies for Brain Delivery of Biologics. *Pharmaceutics* **2023**, *15*, 1748. [CrossRef] [PubMed]
20. Jin, B.; Odongo, S.; Radwanska, M.; Magez, S. Nanobodies: A Review of Generation, Diagnostics and Therapeutics. *Int. J. Mol. Sci.* **2023**, *24*, 5994. [CrossRef]
21. Sonoda, H.; Minami, K. IZCARGO®: The world's first biological drug applied with brain drug delivery technology. *Drug Deliv. Syst.* **2023**, *38*, 68–74. [CrossRef]
22. Liu, A.P.; Aguet, F.; Danuser, G.; Schmid, S.L. Local clustering of transferrin receptors promotes clathrin-coated pit initiation. *J. Cell Biol.* **2010**, *191*, 1381–1393. [CrossRef] [PubMed]
23. Cureton, D.K.; Harbison, C.E.; Cocucci, E.; Parrish, C.R.; Kirchhausen, T. Limited Transferrin Receptor Clustering Allows Rapid Diffusion of Canine Parvovirus into Clathrin Endocytic Structures. *J. Virol.* **2012**, *86*, 5330–5340. [CrossRef] [PubMed]
24. Gerbal-Chaloin, S.; Gondeau, C.; Aldrian-Herrada, G.; Heitz, F.; Gauthier-Rouvière, C.; Divita, G. First step of the cell-penetrating peptide mechanism involves Rac1 GTPase-dependent actin-network remodeling. *Biol. Cell* **2007**, *99*, 223–238. [CrossRef] [PubMed]
25. Fujii, M.; Kawai, K.; Egami, Y.; Araki, N. Dissecting the roles of Rac1 activation and deactivation in macropinocytosis using microscopic photo-manipulation. *Sci. Rep.* **2013**, *3*, 2385. [CrossRef] [PubMed]
26. Tashima, T. Carrier-Mediated Delivery of Low-Molecular-Weight *N*-Containing Drugs across the Blood–Brain Barrier or the Blood–Retinal Barrier Using the Proton-Coupled Organic Cation Antiporter. *Future Pharmacol.* **2023**, *3*, 742–762. [CrossRef]
27. Mehta, D.C.; Short, J.L.; Nicolazzo, J.A. Memantine Transport across the Mouse Blood-Brain Barrier Is Mediated by a Cationic Influx $H^+$ Antiporter. *Mol. Pharm.* **2013**, *10*, 4491–4498. [CrossRef] [PubMed]
28. Laughlin, C.D.; D'Aquili, E.G. *Biogenetic Structuralism*; Columbia University Press: New York, NY, USA, 1974.
29. Leavy, S.A. Biogenetic Structuralism. *Yale J. Biol. Med.* **1976**, *49*, 420–421.
30. Reddy, S.; Tatiparti, K.; Sau, S.; Iyer, A.K. Recent advances in nano delivery systems for blood-brain barrier (BBB) penetration and targeting of brain tumors. *Drug Discov. Today* **2021**, *26*, 1944–1952. [CrossRef]
31. Sun, L.; Liu, H.; Ye, Y.; Lei, Y.; Islam, R.; Tan, S.; Tong, R.; Miao, Y.B.; Cai, L. Smart nanoparticles for cancer therapy. *Signal Transduct. Target. Ther.* **2023**, *8*, 418. [CrossRef]
32. Mitchell, M.J.; Billingsley, M.M.; Haley, R.M.; Wechsler, M.E.; Peppas, N.A.; Langer, R. Engineering precision nanoparticles for drug delivery. *Nat. Rev. Drug Discov.* **2021**, *20*, 101–124. [CrossRef]

33. Vanbilloen, W.J.F.; Rechberger, J.S.; Anderson, J.B.; Nonnenbroich, L.F.; Zhang, L.; Daniels, D.J. Nanoparticle Strategies to Improve the Delivery of Anticancer Drugs across the Blood-Brain Barrier to Treat Brain Tumors. *Pharmaceutics* **2023**, *15*, 1804. [CrossRef] [PubMed]
34. Zhang, W.; Zhu, D.; Tong, Z.; Peng, B.; Cheng, X.; Esser, L.; Voelcker, N.H. Influence of Surface Ligand Density and Particle Size on the Penetration of the Blood-Brain Barrier by Porous Silicon Nanoparticles. *Pharmaceutics* **2023**, *15*, 2271. [CrossRef] [PubMed]
35. Anwar, M.; Muhammad, F.; Akhtar, B. Biodegradable nanoparticles as drug delivery devices. *J. Drug Deliv. Sci. Technol.* **2021**, *64*, 102638. [CrossRef]
36. Elmowafy, E.M.; Tiboni, M.; Soliman, M.E. Biocompatibility, biodegradation and biomedical applications of poly(lactic acid)/poly(lactic-co-glycolic acid) micro and nanoparticles. *J. Pharm. Investig.* **2019**, *49*, 347–380. [CrossRef]
37. Smith, S.M.; Smith, C.J. Capturing the mechanics of clathrin-mediated endocytosis. *Curr. Opin. Struct. Biol.* **2022**, *75*, 102427. [CrossRef] [PubMed]
38. Joseph, J.G.; Liu, A.P. Mechanical Regulation of Endocytosis: New Insights and Recent Advances. *Adv. Biosyst.* **2020**, *4*, e1900278. [CrossRef]
39. Song, Q.; Meng, B.; Xu, H.; Mao, Z. The emerging roles of vacuolar-type ATPase-dependent Lysosomal acidification in neurodegenerative diseases. *Transl. Neurodegener.* **2020**, *9*, 17. [CrossRef]
40. Behr, J.P. The Proton sponge: A trick to enter cells the viruses did not exploit. *Chimica* **1997**, *51*, 34–36. [CrossRef]
41. Du, L.; Chen, L.; Liu, F.; Wang, W.; Huang, H. Nose-to-brain drug delivery for the treatment of CNS disease: New development and strategies. *Int. Rev. Neurobiol.* **2023**, *171*, 255–297. [CrossRef]
42. Schwarz, B.; Merkel, O.M. Nose-to-brain delivery of biologics. *Ther. Deliv.* **2019**, *10*, 207–210. [CrossRef]
43. Patharapankal, E.J.; Ajiboye, A.L.; Mattern, C.; Trivedi, V. Nose-to-Brain (N2B) Delivery: An Alternative Route for the Delivery of Biologics in the Management and Treatment of Central Nervous System Disorders. *Pharmaceutics* **2024**, *16*, 66. [CrossRef]
44. Saha, P.; Singh, P.; Kathuria, H.; Chitkara, D.; Pandey, M.M. Self-Assembled Lecithin-Chitosan Nanoparticles Improved Rotigotine Nose-to-Brain Delivery and Brain Targeting Efficiency. *Pharmaceutics* **2023**, *15*, 851. [CrossRef] [PubMed]
45. Gomez-Salazar, M.; Gonzalez-Galofre, Z.N.; Casamitjana, J.; Crisan, M.; James, A.W.; Péault, B. Five Decades Later, Are Mesenchymal Stem Cells Still Relevant? *Front. Bioeng. Biotechnol.* **2020**, *8*, 148. [CrossRef] [PubMed]
46. Honda, T.; Yasui, M.; Shikamura, M.; Kubo, T.; Kawamata, S. What kind of impact does the Cell and Gene Therapy Product have on the medical and manufacturing industry? Part 3. *Pharm. Tech. Jpn.* **2023**, *39*, 2367–2374.
47. Tashima, T. Mesenchymal Stem Cell (MSC)-based Drug Delivery into the Brain across the Blood-Brain Barrier. *Pharmaceutics* **2024**, *16*, 289. [CrossRef] [PubMed]
48. Qi, D.; Lin, H.; Hu, B.; Wei, Y. A review on in vitro model of the blood-brain barrier (BBB) based on hCMEC/D3 cells. *J. Control Release* **2023**, *358*, 78–97. [CrossRef] [PubMed]
49. Kaya, S.; Callan, B.; Hawthorne, S. Non-Invasive, Targeted Nanoparticle-Mediated Drug Delivery across a Novel Human BBB Model. *Pharmaceutics* **2023**, *15*, 1382. [CrossRef] [PubMed]
50. Bastiancich, C.; Fernandez, S.; Correard, F.; Novell, A.; Larrat, B.; Guillet, B.; Estève, M.-A. Molecular Imaging of Ultrasound-Mediated Blood-Brain Barrier Disruption in a Mouse Orthotopic Glioblastoma Model. *Pharmaceutics* **2022**, *14*, 2227. [CrossRef] [PubMed]
51. Hugon, G.; Goutal, S.; Sarazin, M.; Bottlaender, M.; Caillé, F.; Droguerre, M.; Charvériat, M.; Winkeler, A.; Tournier, N. Impact of Donepezil on Brain Glucose Metabolism Assessed Using [$^{18}$F]2-Fluoro-2-deoxy-D-Glucose Positron Emission Tomography Imaging in a Mouse Model of Alzheimer's Disease Induced by Intracerebroventricular Injection of Amyloid-Beta Peptide. *Front. Neurosci.* **2022**, *16*, 835577. [CrossRef]
52. Jin, J.; Su, D.; Zhang, J.; Li, X.; Feng, T. Tau PET imaging in progressive supranuclear palsy: A systematic review and meta-analysis. *J. Neurol.* **2023**, *270*, 2451–2467. [CrossRef]
53. Varlow, C.; Vasdev, N. Evaluation of Tau Radiotracers in Chronic Traumatic Encephalopathy. *J. Nucl. Med.* **2023**, *64*, 460–465. [CrossRef]
54. Yang, J.; Ding, W.; Zhu, B.; Zhen, S.; Kuang, S.; Yang, J.; Zhang, C.; Wang, P.; Yang, F.; Yang, L.; et al. Bioluminescence Imaging with Functional Amyloid Reservoirs in Alzheimer's Disease Models. *Anal. Chem.* **2023**, *95*, 14261–14270. [CrossRef]
55. Zhang, J.; Wickizer, C.; Ding, W.; Van, R.; Yang, L.; Zhu, B.; Yang, J.; Wang, Y.; Wang, Y.; Xu, Y.; et al. In vivo three-dimensional brain imaging with chemilumiescence probes in Alzheimer's disease models. *Proc. Natl. Acad. Sci. USA* **2023**, *120*, e2310131120. [CrossRef]
56. Fan, D.Y.; Wang, Y.J. Early Intervention in Alzheimer's Disease: How Early is Early Enough? *Neurosci. Bull.* **2020**, *36*, 195–197. [CrossRef]
57. Rajan, K.B.; Weuve, J.; Barnes, L.L.; McAninch, E.A.; Wilson, R.S.; Evans, D.A. Population Estimate of People with Clinical AD and Mild Cognitive Impairment in the United States (2020–2060). *Alzheimers Dement.* **2021**, *17*, 1966–1975. [CrossRef] [PubMed]
58. Pardridge, W.M. Blood-Brain Barrier and Delivery of Protein and Gene Therapeutics to Brain. *Front. Aging Neurosci.* **2020**, *11*, 373. [CrossRef] [PubMed]

59. van Dyck, C.H.; Swanson, C.J.; Aisen, P.; Bateman, R.J.; Chen, C.; Gee, M.; Kanekiyo, M.; Li, D.; Reyderman, L.; Cohen, S.; et al. Lecanemab in Early Alzheimer's Disease. *N. Engl. J. Med.* **2023**, *388*, 9–21. [CrossRef] [PubMed]
60. Rashad, A.; Rasool, A.; Shaheryar, M.; Sarfraz, A.; Sarfraz, Z.; Robles-Velasco, K.; Cherrez-Ojeda, I. Donanemab for Alzheimer's Disease: A Systematic Review of Clinical Trials. *Healthcare* **2023**, *11*, 32. [CrossRef] [PubMed]

*pharmaceutics*

Review

# Non-Invasive Drug Delivery across the Blood–Brain Barrier: A Prospective Analysis

**Sarfaraz K. Niazi**

College of Pharmacy, University of Illinois, Chicago, IL 60612, USA; sniazi3@uic.edu

**Abstract:** Non-invasive drug delivery across the blood–brain barrier (BBB) represents a significant advancement in treating neurological diseases. The BBB is a tightly packed layer of endothelial cells that shields the brain from harmful substances in the blood, allowing necessary nutrients to pass through. It is a highly selective barrier, which poses a challenge to delivering therapeutic agents into the brain. Several non-invasive procedures and devices have been developed or are currently being investigated to enhance drug delivery across the BBB. This paper presents a review and a prospective analysis of the art and science that address pharmacology, technology, delivery systems, regulatory approval, ethical concerns, and future possibilities.

**Keywords:** neurodegenerative disorders; blood–brain barrier; non-invasive delivery; device-related delivery; Alzheimer's disease; Parkinson's disease; ALS; Down syndrome

**Citation:** Niazi, S.K. Non-Invasive Drug Delivery across the Blood–Brain Barrier: A Prospective Analysis. *Pharmaceutics* **2023**, *15*, 2599. https://doi.org/10.3390/pharmaceutics15112599

Academic Editors: Nicolas Tournier and Toshihiko Tashima

Received: 12 October 2023
Revised: 1 November 2023
Accepted: 4 November 2023
Published: 7 November 2023



## 1. Introduction

Evolutionarily, the brain is the body's control center, responsible for everything from essential autonomic functions like heartbeat and respiration to complex cognitive tasks and emotional processing [1]. The human brain, with its intricate architecture and countless functions, is undeniably one of the most sophisticated organs in the body [2]. Protecting and ensuring the optimal functioning of this organ is of paramount importance. The BBB is central to this protective mechanism, a physiological marvel that safeguards the neural environment from potential toxins and pathogens [3] (Figure 1). However, the very features that make the BBB an efficient protector make it a formidable neurotherapeutic obstacle [4].

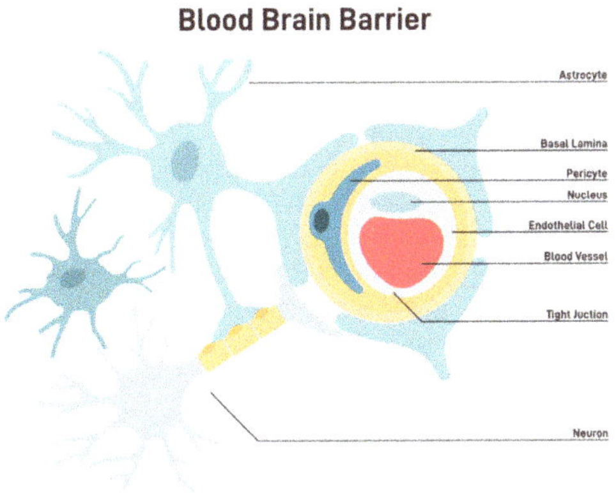


**Figure 1.** Anatomy and functional components of BBB [shutterstock_2229011587].

The BBB is a semipermeable border that separates the circulating blood from the brain and extracellular fluid in the central nervous system (CNS) [5]. This barrier comprises endothelial cells lining the capillaries, which are closely packed together and sealed by tight junctions. These tight junctions restrict the passive diffusion of large or hydrophilic molecules into the CNS. Additionally, astrocyte foot processes wrap around the blood vessels, further fortifying this barrier and playing a pivotal role in its function [6]. The BBB, while allowing essential nutrients like glucose and amino acids to reach the brain, filters out potentially harmful substances from entering the neural environment. This selective permeability ensures that the brain remains relatively insulated from fluctuations in blood composition, thereby maintaining a stable internal environment [7].

This paper outlines the current and future approaches to enhance BBB penetration to treat multiple brain diseases, including tumors, NDs, physiological disbalance, and other continually discovered disorders, using non-invasive devices and associated methods to optimize the functionality of these devices. These supportive approaches may include regulating circadian rhythms, restoring the gut milieu, opening the transitory BBB, carrier-mediated drug delivery, nasal administration, and activating signaling pathways.

The BBB prevents substances from freely passing between the bloodstream, brain, and CNS. This selective and semi-permeable barrier is essential in developing and managing neurological disorders (NDs) that include Alzheimer's disease (AD), Parkinson's disease (PD), Huntingdon disease (HD), Amyotrophic lateral sclerosis (ALS), and multiple sclerosis (MS) and are characterized by the progressive loss of neurons that are associated with neurotoxic etiological substances in the brain and the surrounding organs.

Protecting the brain from toxins, pathogens, and other foreign substances is crucial for survival. Thus, the BBB has evolved to become a gatekeeper, ensuring that only substances beneficial or neutral to the brain's function gain entry [8]. However, this protective shield also presents a significant challenge for medical science, particularly neurology and psychiatry [9]. Most drugs designed to target the brain—whether for the treatment of neurodegenerative diseases, psychiatric disorders, or brain tumors—cannot cross the BBB in therapeutically effective dosing [10], leading to numerous potential treatments failing in the clinical stages, not necessarily because the drugs are not efficacious, but because they cannot reach their intended site of action in the brain [11]. Thus, the BBB represents a double-edged sword. While it is indispensable for physiological well-being, it is also one of the most formidable obstacles in treating neurological diseases [12].

As the understanding of neurological and psychiatric disorders deepens, and with the advent of precision medicine, there is an escalating demand for treatments that can be tailored to individual patient needs [13]. Such treatments may necessitate frequent or prolonged drug administration. Apart from their inherent risks, the invasive methods become impractical in these contexts due to their invasive nature and the discomfort associated with repeated interventions.

Researchers and clinicians have long recognized this challenge [14]. Over the years, various strategies have been employed to overcome or bypass the BBB. Some of these methods are invasive, such as direct intracerebral injections, which, while effective, come with risks and complications [15]. As a result, the focus has increasingly shifted towards non-invasive approaches, aiming to safely enhance the delivery of therapeutic agents to the brain without compromising the integrity of the BBB [16].

The brain's homeostasis is significantly influenced by its function. The BBB comprises diverse cell types and structures, such as brain endothelial cells, the basement membrane, tight junctions, astrocytes, and pericytes. These components collaborate harmoniously to establish a highly selective and tightly regulated barrier [17,18]. The BBB is vital in maintaining homeostasis inside the central CNS by serving as a critical interface between the peripheral circulatory system and the brain. This barrier employs a range of methods to fulfill its function. The BBB is a protective mechanism against the infiltration of detrimental chemicals into the brain.

Additionally, it plays a crucial role in regulating the equilibrium of ions, sustaining optimal levels of neurotransmitters, and eliminating metabolic waste. Nevertheless, as individuals age, there is a potential for the BBB to have a decline in its structural integrity [19].

Multiple studies have provided evidence for the significant involvement of the BBB in the development of numerous neurological disorders [20]. Furthermore, the BBB presents a substantial impediment to the administration of drugs in the context of neurodegenerative diseases [21]. Consequently, research about the BBB has exhibited both diversification and simultaneous advancement.

*Selective Mechanism*

Given the complexity of the BBB, it is essential to understand its selectivity mechanisms. Efflux and influx transporters are pivotal in determining which molecules can enter or exit the brain [22] (Figure 2).

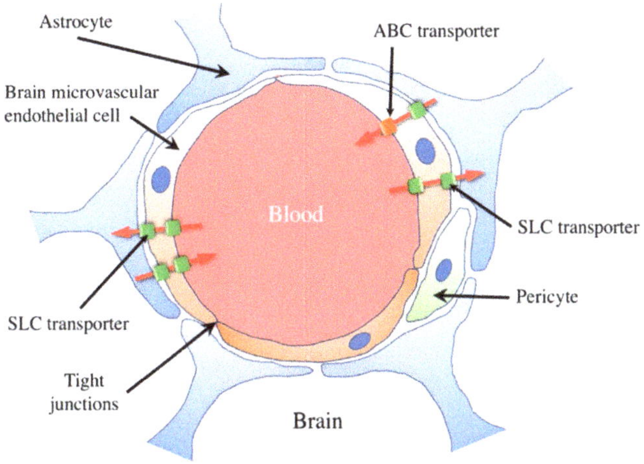


**Figure 2.** Schematic illustration of the blood–brain barrier and transporters. The BBB comprises brain microvascular endothelial cells, astrocytes, and pericytes. Their tight junction-mediated mutual binding restricts diffusion between brain microvascular endothelial cells. Numerous soluble carrier (SLC) transporters expressed by brain microvascular endothelial cells enable specific material passage across the blood–brain barrier, including nutrients like glucose, amino acids, peptides, and nucleotides. Furthermore, by releasing harmful compounds and medications into the bloodstream, ATP-binding cassette (ABC) transporters, expressed in cerebral microvascular endothelial cells, block their access to the brain. [Shutterstock_2229011587].

The physicochemical properties of drugs play a crucial role in their ability to cross the BBB. Lipophilicity, molecular weight, and charge are vital factors influencing BBB permeability. Lipophilic compounds, such as small, nonpolar molecules, diffuse more readily through the lipid-rich endothelial cell membranes. Drugs with lower molecular weights are generally favored for BBB penetration, as they can more efficiently navigate the narrow intercellular spaces. However, highly charged or polar compounds may face significant obstacles as the BBB restricts their passage. Efflux transporters, such as P-glycoprotein, actively pump out xenobiotics, further limiting drug access to the brain. Medicinal chemists often design compounds with favorable physicochemical properties, such as logP values, to enhance brain penetration and consider prodrug strategies or nanocarrier systems. Understanding these properties is critical for the development of drugs targeting neurological disorders, as it ensures their ability to reach their intended site of action in the CNS [23]. Historically, attempts to augment drug delivery to the brain focused on chemical modifications to therapeutic agents, enabling them to either permeate or be actively transported across the BBB [24]. However, these modifications often altered pharmacokinetics or diminished therapeutic efficacy, resulting in compromised treatment outcomes [25]. The realization that chemical modifications could only achieve limited success shifted the emphasis toward more direct, though invasive, delivery methods [26].

In addition to physicochemical properties, the transport of drugs across the blood-brain barrier is also influenced by specific transport mechanisms. Small lipophilic drugs can passively diffuse through the lipid bilayer of the endothelial cells, but for many drugs, active transport mechanisms are required for efficient entry into the brain. Several transporters and receptors at the BBB facilitate or restrict drug passage. For example, glucose transporters (GLUT1) allow glucose and certain related compounds to cross the BBB through facilitated diffusion. Similarly, amino acid transporters help transport essential amino acids into the brain.

On the other hand, efflux transporters like P-glycoprotein (encoded by the ABCB1 gene) actively pump out drugs from the brain back into the bloodstream, limiting their accumulation. Researchers often explore strategies to exploit these transporters for drug delivery, such as prodrugs that are substrates for specific transporters or the development of receptor-targeted delivery systems. Understanding the interplay between drug properties and transport mechanisms is vital for designing effective treatments for neurological diseases and ensuring optimal drug concentrations within the brain (Figure 3).

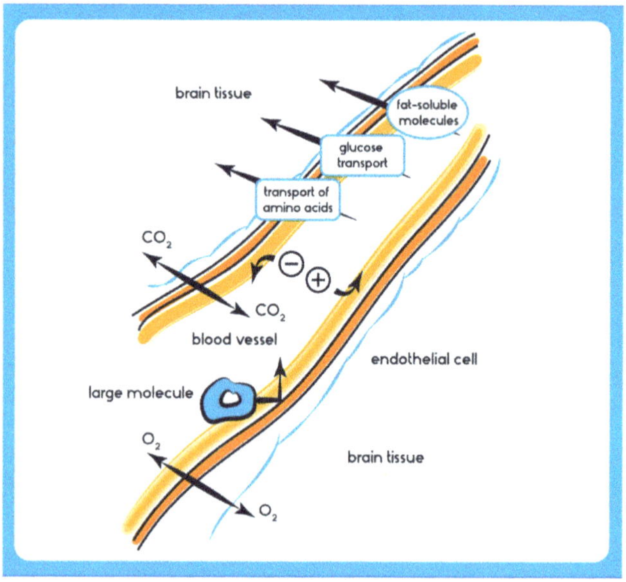


**Figure 3.** Beyond transporters, the physicochemical properties of drug molecules also determine their BBB permeability. [Shutterstock_555919957 Photo] Channels (one way from blood to brain): Small ions and water; Membrane transport (one way from blood to brain): Small lipophilic molecules such as oxygen, carbon dioxide, anesthetics, ethanol, nicotine, and caffeine; Carrier-Mediated Transport (soluble carriers) (one way or two way): Energy Transport System: glucose (GLUT-1), monocarboxylates, lactate, pyruvate (MCT1), creatinine (CrT), Amino acid transport system: large amino acids (LAT1), and Organic anion/cation transporters: OATP1A2, nucleosides; Receptor-mediated Transport (one way from blood to BBB to brain): Insulin, transferrin, leptin, IgG, TNF alpha; Adsorption-mediated Transcytosis System (one way from blood to BBB to brain): Histone, Albumin; Active Efflux Transporters (one-way from BBB to blood and brain): P-glycoprotein, BRCP, MRP 1,2,4,5. Several brain diseases, including neurodegenerative disorders like AD, PD, and ALS, as well as brain tumors and infections, often necessitate drugs that must effectively cross the BBB to exert their therapeutic effects [27]. Generally, lipophilic molecules with a molecular weight of less than 400–500 Da can traverse the BBB more efficiently [28]. However, many potent CNS-active drugs and biologics are too large or possess unsuitable properties, preventing their direct passage through the barrier.

The challenges for the optimal delivery of drugs to the brain underscore the urgent need for innovative strategies to deliver drugs across the BBB without compromising its integrity or function. As we look towards non-invasive device-mediated techniques, it is not just about bypassing the BBB but about maintaining the health and functionality of the CNS, ensuring that treatments are both practical and safe [29].

Beyond neurodegenerative diseases, non-invasive device-mediated techniques can potentially be employed in psychiatric disorders, rehabilitation, and even enhancing cognitive abilities [30]. Preliminary studies are exploring the role of transcranial magnetic stimulation in enhancing memory and cognitive functions in healthy and diseased brains [31].

Moreover, the BBB is not just a static barrier. Its permeability and function can be altered under pathological conditions. Diseases like stroke, traumatic brain injury, and certain infections can disrupt BBB integrity, which might allow for increased drug delivery but at the cost of potential harm from other circulating substances.

The potential for off-target effects, especially when breaching the BBB, has raised safety concerns. Unintended opening of the BBB or delivering therapeutics to non-targeted areas could lead to adverse outcomes [32]. In a clinical study assessing the effects of FUS on BBB disruption, a few patients exhibited temporary neurologic deficits, underscoring the need for meticulous planning and precision in application [33].

## 2. Optimizing Entry

A silver lining in this quest has been the discovery that the BBB, while protective, has specific "windows" or mechanisms that can be modulated for therapeutic benefit. For instance, specific peptides have been identified that can transiently open the BBB, allowing for drug delivery without causing lasting damage [34]. As researchers dive deeper into understanding these nuances, the dream of non-invasively and effectively delivering drugs to the brain seems increasingly tangible.

Non-drug measures to enhance BBB penetration include the use of focused ultrasound, which temporarily disrupts the barrier, allowing drugs to pass through [35]. Additionally, strategies such as nanoparticle-based drug delivery systems, which can encapsulate and protect drugs during transit across the BBB, are under investigation [36]. Nanocarriers can be functionalized with ligands targeting specific receptors at the BBB for enhanced transport [37].

Emerging technologies like intranasal drug delivery, which bypasses the BBB through the olfactory pathway, and implantable devices for direct drug administration into the brain are also being explored as potential solutions to overcome the BBB's limitations [38,39]. These non-drug measures and innovative devices offer promising avenues to improve drug delivery to the brain in the treatment of various neurological disorders.

In addition to the non-drug measures and non-invasive devices, the use of carrier molecules, such as antibodies or peptides, that can specifically target receptors or transporters on BBB endothelial cells can facilitate the transport of therapeutic agents into the brain.

Convection-enhanced delivery (CED) is another technique that involves the direct infusion of drugs into brain tissue using surgically implanted catheters, bypassing the BBB and allowing for precise drug distribution [40].

Additionally, researchers are investigating the potential of nanoscale drug carriers like liposomes and exosomes, which can encapsulate drugs and transport them across the BBB [41]. Advances in nanotechnology and innovative drug delivery strategies hold promise in overcoming the challenges associated with BBB penetration, offering new avenues for effectively treating brain disorders.

Exosome-based drug delivery systems, leveraging the natural ability of exosomes to cross the BBB, have demonstrated potential in delivering neurotherapeutics.

In addition to the methods and approaches mentioned earlier, ongoing research efforts explore the potential of external devices and techniques to assist drug delivery across the BBB. One such technique is the use of focused ultrasound in combination with microbubbles.

This non-invasive approach, known as focused ultrasound-mediated blood–brain barrier opening (FUS-BBBO), involves the application of focused ultrasound waves to the brain in the presence of microbubbles, temporarily disrupting the BBB and allowing drugs to pass through [42]. This method has shown promise in clinical trials for conditions like Alzheimer's disease and brain tumors [43].

Additionally, implantable devices and catheters equipped with drug reservoirs or pumps can provide controlled and sustained drug delivery directly to the brain or cerebrospinal fluid (CNS). These devices can be programmed to release drugs at specific intervals, optimizing treatment efficacy while minimizing systemic side effects [44]. Furthermore, advancements in nanotechnology have led to the development of implantable, biodegradable, drug-eluting nanofibers that can release drugs over extended periods, offering a potential solution for chronic neurological conditions [45].

## 3. Device-Mediated Noninvasive Techniques

This shift towards non-invasive, device-mediated approaches is not just motivated by the limitations of traditional methods but also inspired by the potential these techniques have demonstrated, both in pre-clinical models and in some early-stage clinical trials. They herald a new era in neurotherapeutics, where treatments are effective, patient-centric, and tailored to the needs and comfort of individuals [46].

However, the dawn of the 21st century has witnessed rapid advancements in biomedical engineering, nanotechnology, and imaging modalities [47]. These advances have facilitated the development of device-mediated techniques that are minimally invasive or completely non-invasive, marking a seismic shift in the approach toward CNS drug delivery [48].

Recent years have seen a surge in interest and research into device-mediated techniques that could potentially surmount the BBB without requiring direct surgical intervention [49]. These techniques aim to open the BBB temporarily and safely or utilize specialized mechanisms to transport drugs. These technologies, including focused ultrasound, electromagnetic fields, and intranasal delivery, promise to revolutionize CNS drug delivery [50].

It is crucial to underline, however, that with the exhilaration of these breakthroughs comes the weighty responsibility of ensuring that these methods are safe. The BBB is a vital protective structure, and any strategy that seeks to circumvent or modulate its function must do so without compromising its long-term integrity or inducing unwanted side effects [51]. After all, these innovative approaches aim to improve patient outcomes and quality of life.

As these device-mediated techniques evolve and mature, they will be subjected to rigorous testing in pre-clinical settings and clinical trials. This will ensure their efficacy and safety profile, which is crucial for any therapeutic intervention targeting the delicate and intricate environment of the CNS.

In summary, while several methods exist to address the BBB's drug delivery challenge, many drawbacks limit their therapeutic potential. The emergence of non-invasive device-mediated techniques represents a significant leap forward, potentially revolutionizing CNS drug delivery. As research progresses, the focus will undoubtedly shift towards refining these techniques, ensuring their safety, and expanding their therapeutic applicability [52].

To overcome the barriers to entry, a multitude of BBB in vivo and in vitro models have been established alongside innovative methodologies, which exhibit significant promise for conducting mechanistic investigations and advancing drug discovery efforts, such as the length of time a medication remains detectable in the body while administering pharmacological therapy to optimize the effectiveness of drug transportation across the BBB. The incorporation of novel technologies that effectively regulate the temporary permeability of the BBB and enable targeted drug delivery without invasive procedures is of utmost importance in enhancing the effectiveness, safety, and practicality of therapeutic approaches.

Non-invasive devices and techniques are gaining prominence as valuable tools for enhancing drug delivery across the BBB. One such approach is transcranial magnetic stimulation (TMS). TMS involves using magnetic fields to induce electrical currents in specific brain regions. Studies have shown that repeated TMS sessions can transiently increase BBB permeability, allowing for improved drug penetration into the brain [53].

Another non-invasive technique uses near-infrared spectroscopy (NIRS) and functional near-infrared spectroscopy (fNIRS) to monitor real-time BBB integrity. By assessing BBB disruption, researchers can optimize the timing of drug administration to maximize therapeutic benefits [54]. Furthermore, researchers are exploring non-invasive brain stimulation techniques, such as transcranial direct current stimulation (tDCS) and transcranial alternating current stimulation (tACS), to modulate BBB permeability. These methods can potentially enhance drug delivery without the need for invasive procedures [55].

Another non-invasive device that garnered attention is functional magnetic resonance imaging (fMRI) or magnetic resonance imaging (MRI) guided focused ultrasound. This technology combines the precision of MRI to visualize brain regions with the capability of focused ultrasound to disrupt the BBB temporarily. By using real-time MRI guidance, physicians can precisely target and monitor the delivery of drugs or other therapeutic agents, ensuring accurate and localized treatment [35]. Non-invasive devices and technologies like fMRI-guided focused ultrasound and wearable EEG devices represent exciting prospects for improving drug delivery to the brain while maintaining patient comfort and safety. These methods are still evolving but hold significant promise for enhancing the treatment of neurological diseases.

The evolution of wearable tech can allow continuous or periodic drug delivery, providing patients with more autonomy and ensuring sustained therapeutic levels [56]. A prototype wearable ultrasonic patch, capable of crossing the BBB and delivering drugs, showed promise in maintaining therapeutic drug levels in PD models [57]. Additionally, emerging technologies like wearable electroencephalogram (EEG) devices are being explored to modulate BBB permeability non-invasively. By using an EEG to guide the timing of drug administration or the application of other techniques, researchers aim to optimize drug delivery to the brain while minimizing side effects [58].

While current research predominantly focuses on neurodegenerative disorders and brain tumors, there is potential to extend these techniques to other conditions, like psychiatric disorders, autoimmune diseases, or metabolic conditions [59].

## 4. Brain Tumors

Brain cancer is characterized by the uncontrolled growth of cells in the brain, resulting in tumors that can be either benign or malignant. Several primary brain tumors exist, including gliomas, which arise from glial cells and encompass subtypes like astrocytomas and glioblastomas, with the latter being notably aggressive. Meningiomas originate from the meninges, while pituitary tumors are typically benign and develop in the pituitary gland. Medulloblastomas are more common in children and affect the cerebellum. Acoustic neuromas, originating from the cranial nerves' Schwann cells, are generally benign but can impact hearing and balance. Diagnosis involves clinical evaluation, imaging studies, and, occasionally, a biopsy. Treatment is contingent on the tumor's type, location, and stage and might include surgery, radiation therapy, chemotherapy, or newer modalities like targeted therapy and immunotherapy. However, the presence of the blood–brain barrier, the sensitive location of tumors, and resistance to treatment modalities complicate brain cancer treatment.

Molecular profiling constitutes a fundamental component of the 2021 World Health Organization (WHO) categorization of gliomas. The advancement of targeted therapy is currently constrained by various variables, including the existence of the BBB and challenges associated with tumor heterogeneity. However, significant progress has been achieved in developing the IDH1/2 inhibitor vorasidenib for treating IDH-mutant grade 2 gliomas. Additionally, the combination of dabrafenib and trametinib has shown promising results in treating gliomas with the BRAFV600E mutation. Furthermore, targeted medicines have been developed for certain groups of patients with fusions and H3K27M-altered diffuse midline gliomas [60].

Treatments for brain tumors like glioblastoma are limited by the inability of many chemotherapeutics to penetrate the BBB. Non-invasive techniques promise enhanced delivery of tumor-fighting drugs directly to the malignancy, potentially improving outcomes [35].

In a pioneering clinical trial, patients with recurrent glioblastoma received a combination of FUS and microbubbles before administering doxorubicin, a chemotherapy agent. The subsequent MRI scans showed increased drug concentrations in tumor regions, suggesting effective BBB disruption and targeted delivery [61]. Preliminary research showed the potential for focused ultrasound to modulate neural circuits associated with depression, opening avenues for non-drug treatments in psychiatric conditions [62].

A recent endeavor combined MRI-guided focused ultrasound with nanoparticles to ensure real-time visualization and precise drug delivery for treating tumors [35].

Convergence of Technologies: In the age of rapid technological advancements, the fusion of multiple technologies can further enhance the precision and efficiency of drug delivery. Imagine integrating real-time imaging with delivery devices to ensure pinpoint accuracy [63].

## 5. Neurodegenerative Disorders (NDs)

Neurological disorders affect millions globally, ranging from NDs to psychiatric conditions. These conditions lead to significant morbidity and have profound social, economic, and psychological repercussions [64]. Therefore, developing efficacious treatment strategies that can navigate the BBB's complexities is paramount.

Neurodegenerative diseases, more particularly PD, AD, HD, ALS, and motor neuron disease, affect millions of people worldwide. NDs manifest as the progressive loss of functionality and eventual demise of nerve cells in the brain or peripheral nervous system. While specific treatments may provide relief for certain physical or mental symptoms commonly associated with neurodegenerative diseases, the current medical understanding does not support the notion that these treatments can effectively slow down the advancement of such diseases. Furthermore, it is important to note that no known cures for neurodegenerative disorders currently exist.

The probability of acquiring a neurodegenerative disease increases significantly as an individual advances in age. In the forthcoming decades, NDs have the potential to substantially impact a larger proportion of the American population, particularly as life expectancy continues to rise. It is imperative to enhance our comprehension of the etiology of neurodevelopmental disorders (NDs) and devise novel strategies for their treatment and prevention.

AD and PD are widely recognized as the prevailing neurodegenerative disorders. According to a report released by the Alzheimer's Disease Association in 2022, it is estimated that up to 6.2 million individuals [65] in the United States may be affected by AD. According to the Parkinson's Foundation, the number of individuals in the United States living with Parkinson's disease is approaching one million [66].

AD is primarily distinguished by the degeneration of neurons, the accumulation of amyloid-beta plaques, and the development of hyperphosphorylated tau protein within neurons. Notably, the cytotoxic impact of amyloid beta-peptide (Abeta) is a significant factor in this disease [67].

AD is the accumulation of amyloid-β plaques, a hallmark of AD. Traditional drug delivery strategies have struggled to effectively delivering therapeutic agents across the BBB to target these plaques. Using focused ultrasound combined with microbubbles, research has demonstrated the potential to temporarily open the BBB and assist in the clearance of these plaques, showcasing potential therapeutic benefits [68]. A preclinical study involving mice genetically predisposed to develop AD symptoms revealed that after multiple FUS treatments, there was a notable reduction in amyloid-β plaques and improved cognitive function [69].

The phenotypic characteristic of Down syndrome (DS; trisomy 21) is now acknowledged to be associated with a significantly elevated risk for AD. The cumulative incidence of AD in individuals with DS increased to around 50% by the late 50s and reached 80% by the late 60s [70]. This demographic constitutes the most noteworthy cohort with an elevated susceptibility to AD due to a particular genotype. This situation is essential to public health and presents an ideal population for preventative trials.

The loss of dopaminergic neurons characterizes PD. Delivering neuroprotective or neurorestorative agents into the brain holds therapeutic promise. Techniques like FUS can facilitate the delivery of such agents, including genes or stem cells [71]. A study on a PD animal model demonstrated that after FUS-mediated BBB disruption, there was enhanced delivery and retention of neurotrophic factors, subsequently leading to improved motor functions in the treated animals [72]. A study combining focused ultrasound with patient-specific MRI data demonstrated more accurate targeting, leading to better therapeutic outcomes in PD patients [73].

The expression levels of Wnt3, Wnt4, FZD2, FZD8, Wnt2b, Wnt5a, FZD3, LRP5, and sFRP3 are elevated in the human spinal cord tissue of patients diagnosed with ALS, wherein there is an increase in the population of astrocytes expressing the FZD2 receptor in the transitional region between the grey and white matter at the ventral horn. The potential involvement of the Wnt family of proteins, particularly FZD2 and Wnt5a, in the pathogenesis of ALS is under investigation [74].

It is widely acknowledged among scientists that the interaction between an individual's genetic makeup and their environmental factors significantly contributes to their susceptibility to neurodegenerative disorders. As an illustration, an individual may possess a genetic predisposition that renders them more vulnerable to PD. Yet, the impact of their environmental exposures can influence the disease's timing, severity, and manifestation.

Post-stroke treatments can benefit from timely and targeted delivery of neuroprotective agents or stem cells. Non-invasive techniques can enhance the penetration of these therapeutic agents, potentially reducing brain damage and promoting recovery [75].

## 6. Current Techniques in Drug Delivery across the BBB

The BBB poses a monumental challenge for reaching therapeutic agents to the central CNS in the grand drug delivery arena. The development of effective, non-invasive, device-mediated techniques for drug delivery across the BBB has been fraught with challenges but illuminated by moments of innovation and breakthrough. As the field progresses, it is imperative to prioritize safety, ensuring that the integrity and function of the BBB are not compromised in the long term. With continued research and interdisciplinary collaboration, the dream of effective and patient-friendly CNS drug delivery methods may soon become a reality (Figure 4).

The drug's solubility, surface charge distribution, molecular weight, particle size, and other factors should all be considered while creating the formulation [76].

While often successful in peripheral tissues, traditional pharmacological strategies have encountered substantial limitations when aiming for the brain. These methods aim to increase BBB permeability transiently and safely, allowing for targeted drug delivery without the drawbacks of the traditional methods [77]. Many small molecules and virtually all large molecule biologics, including therapeutic proteins, RNA therapeutics, and antibodies, face impediments in crossing the BBB [9]. Figure 4 lists several approaches to noninvasive deliveries.

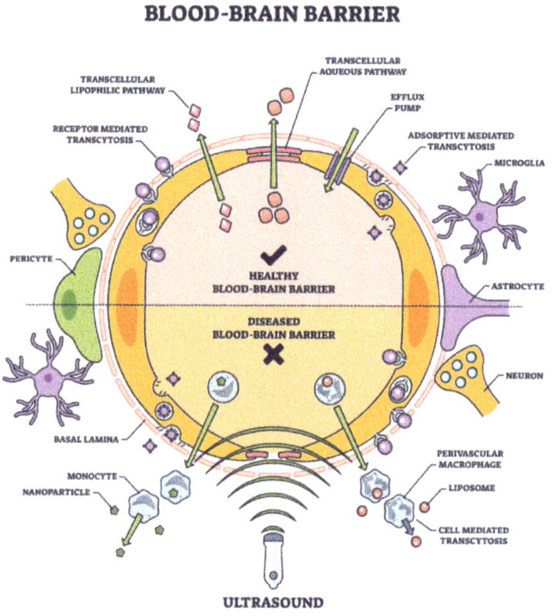


**Figure 4.** Noninvasive tools and their entry into BBB are based on the physical properties, composition, surface chemistry, and target ligands. [Adobe Stock Photo_603623040].

Transcellular (drug delivery via cells) and paracellular (drug delivery between adjacent cells) are the two main routes that frequently carry drugs to the brain [78]. Ions and solutes passively diffuse across the BBB via the paracellular pathway, which concentration gradients facilitate. Transcellular delivery across the BBB involves the passage of drugs or molecules through endothelial cells, which form the protective barrier for the brain. Unlike paracellular transport, which consists of passing between cells, transcellular transport goes through the cells themselves, making it a critical route for delivering therapeutic agents to the brain. This process encompasses several mechanisms, including passive diffusion of small, lipophilic molecules; carrier-mediated transport facilitated by specific proteins; receptor-mediated transcytosis, where ligands bind to receptors; and adsorptive-mediated transcytosis, where cationic molecules interact with cell surface components. Each mechanism has unique properties and requirements, making them essential in designing drug-delivery strategies for neurological disorders and brain-related diseases [79] (Figure 4).

Several mechanistic mechanisms, including transcytosis, carrier-mediated transport, and passive diffusion, are part of the transcellular route. The main mechanisms are adsorptive-mediated transcytosis (AMT) and receptor-mediated transcytosis (RMT). Among the most studied targets for RMT in brain endothelial cells are the transferrin receptor, insulin receptor, and low-density lipoprotein (LDL) receptor [80]. Current advancements in RMT provide ways to get past the blood-brain barrier and achieve more efficient medicine administration to the brain. Brain medication administration also uses other transporters, such as organic anion and cation transporters, in addition to these mechanical pathways [81].

Several techniques have been developed over the years, endeavoring to overcome the formidable barrier of the BBB and deliver therapeutic agents to the CNS. Conventional methods range from direct injection into the CNS to modifying drug molecules for enhanced permeability. While some of these techniques have had moderate success, they often come with significant drawbacks, such as invasiveness, limited targeting, or potential side effects.

### 6.1. Direct Injections

Techniques like intracerebroventricular (ICV) and intraparenchymal injections bypass the BBB by delivering drugs directly into the brain or cerebrospinal fluid. While effective, these methods are highly invasive, bear risks of infections, and might distribute drugs unevenly [82]. Methods such as intracerebral injections or intraventricular infusions were employed to achieve CNS drug delivery [83]. While these approaches enable a direct route of administration, they are invasive and carry associated risks, including infection, hemorrhage, and potential damage to brain tissue [84]. Moreover, these methods can lead to non-uniform distribution in the brain, potentially yielding areas of over-concentration or insufficient drug coverage [85]. Further complicating the drug delivery scenario is the realization that many CNS disorders, such as AD, PD, and MS, involve multiple brain regions [86]. Targeting these dispersed areas necessitates a systemic approach to drug delivery, ensuring that the therapeutic agent is distributed throughout the brain.

### 6.2. Molecular Trojan Horses

This ingenious method involves coupling therapeutic agents to molecules crossing the BBB via receptor-mediated transcytosis. By "piggybacking" on these molecules, drugs can be sneaked into the brain. While promising, the complexity of this method and potential immunogenic reactions are challenges that need addressing [87]. It is possible to facilitate the entry of chemical drugs into the brain by employing naturally occurring or artificially modified chemicals and certain simple life forms, predominantly viruses, which can traverse the BBB. This drug delivery strategy is usually called the "Trojan horse" approach. Neurotropic viruses are a class of viruses that exhibit a distinct preference for the nervous system and possess the ability to invade neural cells. These viral agents can traverse the BBB and get access to the CNS. Hence, utilizing neurotropic viruses for drug encapsulation and BBB traversal is a highly effective and practical strategy. Adeno-associated virus (AAV) is the prevailing neurotropic viral vector employed in treating neurological illnesses [88].

### 6.3. Biochemical BBB Disruption

Specific agents, like mannitol, can temporarily disrupt the BBB by shrinking endothelial cells. While this allows drugs to enter the CNS, it is a non-specific method that might allow harmful substances to infiltrate the brain, potentially causing side effects [89]. The hyperosmolar technique is employed to transiently disrupt the BBB by generating alterations in osmolarity inside the brain tissue. Usually, an intravenous or intra-arterial infusion of a high-osmolarity solution, predominantly mannitol, facilitates water movement from brain tissue to the blood arteries via osmosis.

Applying mechanical force on the endothelial cells induces mechanical stress, resulting in a transient disturbance of tight junctions. During this phase, the BBB undergoes temporary permeability, facilitating enhanced medication delivery into the brain and enabling therapeutic effects on NDs. Empirical evidence from clinical trials has demonstrated that administering hyperosmolar mannitol through intra-arterial infusion after a BBB breach is a reliable and secure approach for managing central CNS malignancies. The findings from subsequent research using rats indicated that proteomics alterations reverted to their original levels after 96 h. This suggests that the approach employed to induce BBB opening is transient and may be reversed [90]. Nevertheless, it is crucial to acknowledge that the unguided application of hyperosmolar mannitol to open the BBB is an invasive procedure, and its safety merits thorough deliberation.

### 6.4. Nanoparticle-Mediated Delivery

Nanoparticle systems encompass various carriers, including liposomes, polymeric nanoparticles, and solid lipid nanoparticles (SLNP). These carriers are commonly categorized based on their size (usually ranging from 10 to 300 nm in diameter), chemical composition, and physical morphology. Numerous investigations have examined the utilization of nanoparticles ranging in size from 50 to 200 nm in the context of stroke, AD, and PD. The initial formulation of nanoparticles for cancer treatment received regulatory approval decades ago. Nevertheless, the current repertoire of licensed nanoparticle-based therapies and technologies remains limited. For instance, the utilization of lipid nanoparticles (LNP) for administering mRNA COVID-19 vaccines has gained approval. However, it is essential to note that there is currently a lack of approved central nervous system (CNS) therapy products.

There is great interest in optimizing the physicochemical characteristics of nanoparticles to govern their track and permeability, which might be of great significance in crossing the BBB [91]. Many nanocarriers with particle sizes ranging from 1 to 100 nm have been developed due to advancements in nanotechnology. Polymeric nanoparticles (PNPs), solid lipid nanoparticles (SLNPs), liposomes, and micelles are examples of these nanocarriers that have been introduced as treatments for various neurological disorders, as illustrated in Figure 1. More recently developed, sophisticated nanocarriers, such as exosomes [92], prodrugs [93], self-assembled micelles [94], dendrimers [95], PNPs [96], and exosomes [92], have shown great potential over previous delivery methods.

Non-targeted nanoparticles have significant limitations in traversing the intact BBB. Nanoparticles can encapsulate drugs and be designed to target specific receptors or transporters on the BBB, enhancing drug delivery. This field has garnered considerable interest, but concerns about long-term effects and potential toxicity linger [97]. Utilizing tailored nanomedicines to improve brain transport by capitalizing on the compromised BBB resulting from brain illnesses, such as neurodevelopmental disorders, presents a promising strategy for medication delivery [98].

Nanoparticles as non-invasive methods for drug delivery across the BBB have gained traction due to their effectiveness and versatility. They can be engineered to enhance the delivery of various therapeutic agents to the brain, overcoming the formidable obstacle presented by the BBB. One mechanism through which nanoparticles facilitate drug delivery is by encapsulating drugs and protecting them from metabolic degradation in the bloodstream, enhancing their half-life and bioavailability. A study by Saraiva et al. (2016) [97] demonstrated the use of multi-functionalized nanoparticles to deliver anti-inflammatory drugs to the brain, showing a reduction in neuroinflammation in a targeted and controlled manner. Additionally, surface modification of nanoparticles has been explored to improve their ability to cross the BBB. Poly (butyl cyanoacrylate) nanoparticles coated with polysorbate 80 can help deliver drugs like dalargin, tubocurarine, and doxorubicin across the BBB effectively [99].

Targeted delivery is another essential aspect of nanoparticle-based drug delivery, including the development of magnetic nanoparticles, which could be guided to the brain using an external magnetic field, enhancing the site-specific delivery of the encapsulated drugs [100]. Due to their small size and customizable properties, Nanoparticles serve as excellent vehicles for drug delivery. Combined with techniques like FUS, they can be directed precisely, allowing for slow and sustained drug release [101].

Research involving the co-delivery of gold nanoparticles and anticancer drugs to glioblastoma cells showcased enhanced cell uptake and increased therapeutic efficiency, owing to the synergistic combination of nanoparticles and FUS [102].

Nanotechnology offers avenues to develop carriers that can transport drugs and respond to external stimuli, such as temperature or magnetic fields, enabling controlled release at target sites [103]. When combined with focused ultrasound, magnetic-responsive nanoparticles demonstrated synchronized drug release upon reaching targeted brain regions, presenting a dual-control mechanism for drug delivery [104]. Using an external magnetic field to guide their targeted delivery, magnetic nanoparticles to transport therapeutic agents across the BBB are also attempted [10].

### *6.5. Focused Ultrasound (FUS) with Microbubbles*

FUS is a non-invasive medical device employing ultrasonic waves to concentrate and transmit energy to locations within tissues accurately. The application of this technique exhibits significant promise in augmenting the transportation of pharmaceutical agents via the BBB to enhance their uptake in the brain for therapeutic purposes. This can be achieved by facilitating the permeability of the BBB or by aiding in the controlled breakdown of microbubbles to facilitate the release of pharmaceuticals [105]). Presently, focused ultrasound (FUS) has been utilized in neurological disorders (NDs) such as AD and PD (PD). This technique can potentially improve the efficacy of brain drug delivery for a wide range of therapeutic agents, including antibodies, nanoparticles, therapeutic viruses, and stem cells. This is achieved through the temporary opening of the BBB. Several studies have investigated the application of FUS in this context [106–111]. The combination of FUS and viral vector gene therapy enhances drug transport efficacy to the brain in the context of PD in animal models. The feasibility and safety of FUS-mediated BBB opening of the striatum have been established in clinical surgical operations for PD (PD) [112].

FUS, combined with microbubbles, has emerged as a frontrunner in non-invasive BBB modulation. The process involves injecting microbubbles intravenously and then applying targeted ultrasound waves. The interaction between the microbubbles and the ultrasound waves temporarily increases the permeability of the BBB, allowing for targeted drug delivery. Preclinical studies have shown successful delivery of therapeutic agents, ranging from small molecules to larger biologics, into the brain with this method [113]. The precision of FUS ensures targeted delivery, minimizing potential systemic side effects. One such method, which has garnered significant attention, is focused ultrasound (FUS) in conjunction with microbubbles [114]. The technique involves the transient disruption of the BBB using ultrasound waves targeted to specific brain regions, enabling the delivery of therapeutic agents precisely where needed. Early results from preclinical studies have shown this technique to be both practical and safe, with the BBB being restored within hours post-treatment [115].

### *6.6. Magnetic Resonance Imaging (MRI)*

To tackle the invasive nature of the hyperosmolar process, researchers have devised an MRI technique that relies on unenhanced chemical exchange saturation transfer to identify the buildup of mannitol in the intracranial region after the opening of the BBB. This technique holds promise as a prompt imaging tool for optimizing the administration of mannitol-based BBB opening, thereby enhancing its safety and effectiveness [116]. Moreover, implementing hyperosmolar BBB opening techniques in murine models using MRI guidance can effectively mitigate the limitations of inconsistent reproducibility and heterogeneous experimental results commonly observed with the intra-arterial administration of hyperosmolar mannitol [117]. Hence, the exclusive utilization of hyperosmolar mannitol infusion has potential hazards in therapeutic contexts. Nevertheless, integrating MRI guidance improves the safety and effectiveness of osmotic-based BBB opening, thus augmenting its therapeutic significance.

MRI guidance has significantly improved the precision of focused ultrasound techniques. Through MRgFUS, clinicians can visualize the targeted area in real-time, ensuring therapeutic agents' accurate and effective delivery while monitoring potential complications [118]. A clinical trial exploring the efficacy of MRgFUS for essential tremor treatments showcased the ability to target the thalamus accurately. Patients exhibited substantial improvement in hand tremors, underlining the potential of imaging-guided interventions [119]. In a rat model of ischemic stroke, FUS, combined with microbubbles, facilitated the targeted delivery of neuroprotective drugs. The treated rats exhibited reduced infarct sizes and improved neurological outcomes compared to the control group [120]. For example, trials using FUS and a combination of FUS+MRI for AD trials saw the BBB in the hippocampus and entorhinal cortex open reversibly without adverse effects [121], and patients showed no adverse events and no cognitive or neurological deterioration [122]. The

PD trials of 5–7 patients involved the BBB duplication at the parietal–occipital–temporal junction opened reversibly in four patients without side effects [123]. FUS-mediated striatal BBB opening is feasible and safe. In the MPS-II trial of 28 patients, positive changes occurred in 21 patients treated with transferrin receptor ligand, some with mild or moderate, transient, and manageable adverse drug events [124].

### 6.7. Electromagnetic Field Modulation

While relatively nascent, using electromagnetic fields (EMFs) to modulate BBB permeability is gaining traction. EMFs can influence ion channels and transport mechanisms in the endothelial cells of the BBB, leading to transient permeability increases [125]. Preliminary studies show promise, but the exact parameters for effective and safe application and long-term implications remain under investigation [126]. Another intriguing approach is the use of electromagnetic fields. By leveraging the inherent electrical properties of the BBB, researchers are exploring ways to transiently increase its permeability, allowing for the passive diffusion of therapeutic agents into the CNS [127].

Preliminary studies have indicated a potential for this technique, although its long-term effects and safety profile are still under investigation. Emerging techniques promise selectivity, control, and reversibility. For instance, focused ultrasound, when coupled with microbubbles, can be directed at specific brain regions to enhance BBB permeability temporarily. Studies have shown that this technique can deliver a variety of therapeutic agents, including antibodies, to targeted brain areas with minimal side effects. Furthermore, although a relatively new entrant in this domain, electromagnetic fields have demonstrated potential in modulating BBB permeability. Initial studies suggest that such fields can influence molecular transport across the BBB, although the precise mechanisms and long-term safety still require thorough investigation.

### 6.8. Vasoactive Chemicals

Vasoactive chemicals, including CNS ones, can modulate vascular tone and permeability. Several vasoactive chemicals have been investigated to assess their capacity to induce the opening of the BBB and facilitate the transportation of therapeutic medicines into the brain. The chemicals encompass adenosine, bradykinin, histamine, and peptides derived from bee venom. Adenosine, a nucleoside found in nature, has a role in multiple physiological processes, such as regulating blood flow and inflammation [128].

Numerous studies have demonstrated that it can enhance BBB permeability through various mechanisms. For instance, it can activate adenosine receptors on endothelial cells, initiating intracellular signaling pathways that influence the tight junctions between them. These tight junctions play a critical role in maintaining the integrity of the BBB. The process of fibrinolysis can lead to the production of bradykinin through the action of fibrinolytic agents [129]. This bradykinin can then activate bradykinin B2 receptors, resulting in the opening of the BBB. Researchers have employed the BBB opening mechanism to create bradykinin analogs that can improve the transportation of nanocarriers across the BBB to treat glioblastoma [130].

Furthermore, studies have provided evidence that the disruption of the BBB, facilitated by the bradykinin B2 receptor agonist NG291, is confined to a specific area, dependent on the dosage administered, and can be reversed [131]. Histamine, a neurotransmitter, has been observed to potentially facilitate the opening of the BBB [132,133]. However, the precise mechanism by which this occurs remains uncertain.

Recently, there has been a development in the utilization of bee venom peptides as substances to induce the opening of the BBB. It has been demonstrated that these substances can induce reversible opening of the BBB within 24 h when administered at adequate dosages. Doubtless, vasoactive medicines possess significant promise in facilitating the opening of the BBB and enhancing drug transportation to the brain. Nevertheless, the systemic administration of these medications presents uncertain implications for the overall treatment efficacy, as they cannot selectively target the BBB. Enhancing the precision of BBB targeting with pertinent technology would contribute to advancing future clinical studies.

*6.9. Gut Microbiome [134]*

The enhanced longevity of the human life span can be attributed to advancements in diet and healthcare, which the progress of the economy and technology has facilitated. Many microorganisms, encompassing bacteria, archaea, viruses, and diverse eukaryotes, including fungi and protozoa, inhabit distinct ecological niches within the gastrointestinal tract. The term "gut microbiota" is commonly used to refer to this group of microorganisms.

The gut microbiota significantly impacts various areas of human physiology, encompassing nutritional metabolism, anti-infection mechanisms, immune system functionality, and neuron development. The gut microbiota is facing a changing environment due to rapid industrialization, urbanization, and advancements in food and medical technologies. Factors such as increased fast-food consumption have made the gut microbiota more susceptible to vulnerability than previous conditions. Recently, there has been a growing recognition of the significance of gut microbiota due to its crucial involvement in neurodevelopmental disorders (NDs) and its influence on the differentiation, maturation, proliferation, and activation of immune cells residing in the central nervous system (CNS). The gut–brain axis (GBA) facilitates reciprocal communication between the gastrointestinal tract and the central nervous system using neurotransmitters and other metabolites [135,136].

The blood-brain barrier (BBB) can restrict the transit of molecules produced from the stomach into the brain, even though it acts as a gateway for the passage of many essential compounds needed for CNS functioning and secretes substances into the blood and brain essential for preserving CNS homeostasis [137]. Microorganism-associated molecular patterns (MAMPs), for instance, are vital to microorganisms' structural integrity and cellular processes [138]. Inadvertent elevation or reduction of MAMPs can cause acute or chronic inflammation linked to several neurological conditions.

The BBB's permeability is linked to several microbial compounds, including vitamins, lipopolysaccharides (LPS), trimethylamines (TMAs), and short-chain fatty acids (SCFAs) [139–141]. These compounds may boost the immunological and endocrine systems to prevent neuroinflammation or neurodegeneration or act directly on brain neurons through the blood-brain barrier. The central nervous system (CNS), autonomic nervous system (ANS), enteric nervous system (ENS), and hypothalamic–pituitary–adrenal (HPA) axis make up the bidirectional communication network.

Through the vagus nerve, microbiota and the brain can communicate. The CNS can affect the functions and activities of intestinal cells more efficiently, thanks to the synergy of neurological and hormonal signals [65,66]. Furthermore, gut microbiota influences host health by modifying gut cells and preserving intestinal metabolic and immunological balance [142–144]. It's interesting to note that the microbiota also affects the synthesis of hormones and neurotransmitters, including peptide YY, gam-ma-aminobutyric acid (GABA), serotonin (5-HT), adrenaline, noradrenaline, glucagon-like peptide-1, and dopamine, as well as their precursors. These chemicals act on the CNS or ENS either directly through the vagus nerve or indirectly by affecting the circulation [145].

*6.10. Surface Transporters*

While the activation of BBB surface transporters can improve drug transport, it is essential to consider the drawbacks of this approach, including saturation, limited transport capacity, and inadequate targeting compared to receptor-mediated endocytosis. Consequently, the latter mechanism is commonly employed in drug development to enhance the targeting and penetration of drugs across the BBB. Currently, the prevailing receptor proteins within the BBB encompass transferrin receptors, insulin receptors, and low-density lipoprotein receptor-related proteins. These receptor proteins are frequently coupled with therapeutic protein drugs through fusion with their respective ligands, thereby enhancing the efficacy of drug targeting and facilitating the passage across the BBB [146].

### *6.11. Penetrating Peptides*

Penetrating peptides refer to concise sequences of peptides that can efficiently penetrate the BBB. BBB-penetrating peptides' repertoire includes trans-activating transcriptional activator peptides, R8 peptides, angiopep-2, cell-penetrating peptides, and RVG peptides [147]. Using BBB-targeting ligands for transporting pharmaceuticals across the BBB represents a precise and efficient approach to facilitating drug delivery.

### *6.12. Extracellular Vesicles*

One approach to enhance the ability of medications to penetrate the brain is by modifying tiny extracellular vesicles' surface with different peptides that can cross the BBB. This modification facilitates the effective transport of drugs to the brain [148]. Furthermore, integrating extracellular vesicles and intranasal delivery would undeniably assume a crucial function in managing neurodegenerative disorders (NDs). Extracellular vesicles serve as inherent vehicles for drug delivery and possess the ability to traverse the BBB readily. Consequently, it is common practice among researchers to employ extracellular vesicles as carriers for drug encapsulation, aiming to enhance the transportation of pharmaceuticals across the BBB where the improved permeability of the BBB can be achieved by utilizing tiny extracellular vesicles produced from glial cells, which are loaded with tetraspanin 2 siRNA [149].

### *6.13. Liposomes*

Like extracellular vesicles, liposomes are also employed as carriers for drug administration across the BBB. Nevertheless, it is essential to acknowledge that liposomes exclusively exhibit BBB penetration capabilities rather than BBB targeting abilities. Consequently, these compounds are frequently co-administered with BBB-targeting agents to elicit their desired outcomes. It has been demonstrated that including neurotransmitter-derived lipids in lipid nanoparticles (LNPs) that are impervious to the BBB facilitates the ability of LNPs to traverse the BBB [150].

### *6.14. Optical Imaging*

Integrating optical imaging with non-invasive techniques offers detailed real-time visualization at a cellular level. Optogenetics allows for the control of neuronal activity using light, suggesting potential therapeutic applications [151]. A study involving the treatment of Parkinson's symptoms in rodents used optogenetics. The integration of optical imaging ensured targeted light delivery, leading to controlled neuronal activity and symptom alleviation [152]. Precision is critical in non-invasive drug delivery. The advent of novel imaging techniques promises better visualization, improved targeting, and real-time monitoring of drug delivery [153]. The integration of diffuse optical tomography with ultrasound has shown potential in providing real-time imaging of drug deposition and tissue response, enhancing the safety and efficacy of drug delivery [154].

### *6.15. Peptides*

Peptides, with their ability to interact with specific BBB receptors, play a pivotal role in promoting receptor-mediated transcytosis, a mechanism by which peptides facilitate the delivery of an array of therapeutic agents like small molecules, proteins, and genes across the BBB. These peptides target endogenous receptor systems, ensuring a selective and efficient transfer [155].

The use of peptides in noninvasively facilitating drug delivery across the BBB has been a subject of intensive research, attributing to their ability to harness endogenous transport mechanisms without compromising the barrier's structural integrity. One prominent strategy involves the design of peptides that can undergo receptor-mediated transcytosis. These peptides are specifically tailored to bind to specific receptors on the endothelial cells of the BBB, instigating a process that transports them, along with their drug cargo, into the brain. How peptides could be engineered for targeted delivery, enhancing the selectivity and efficiency of drug transport while minimizing systemic exposure, has been reported [156].

Additionally, the use of cell-penetrating peptides (CPPs) has gained attention. CPPs can facilitate the transport of various bioactive cargoes, including small molecules, peptides, proteins, and nucleic acids, across the BBB, particularly the CPP-mediated [157] transport. Furthermore, developing dual-functional peptides that combine BBB targeting and drug delivery is an emerging trend. Constructing a dual-functional peptide that could transport across the BBB and target glioma cells underscores the advancements in precision medicine [158].

### 6.16. Antibodies

Antibodies, especially monoclonal ones, have been significantly instrumental in drug delivery across the BBB. They can uniquely target specific receptors on the endothelial cells lining the BBB, enabling receptor-mediated transcytosis. This process involves binding antibodies to these receptors, initiating an internalization process that transports them and their attached drug cargo across the BBB. The efficacy of antibodies in drug delivery can be enhanced by reducing their affinity for a transcytosis target, consequently boosting their brain uptake [159]. The bispecific antibodies, designed to engage with the transferrin receptor to facilitate BBB crossing and an amyloid-beta peptide to reduce its pathological accumulation in AD, exemplify engineered antibodies' dual targeting capability and therapeutic potential [160]. Antibody engineering to improve antibodies' pharmacokinetics increases their potential as drug carriers to the brain [161]. Antibodies are equally instrumental in bypassing the BBB. A specific example is the monoclonal antibody against the transferrin receptor, where the mechanism by which antibodies with reduced affinity for a transcytosis target can significantly enhance the brain's uptake of therapeutic antibodies [159].

### 6.17. Intranasal

In recent years, intranasal and intrathecal administration have developed viable and effective methods for enhancing brain-targeting efficiency in medication administration. The intranasal route of drug administration is a favorable method for the targeted delivery of medications to the central CNS owing to the abundant vascularization of the nasal cavity, which is situated near the brain. Research findings have indicated that the intranasal administration of exosomes can lead to a notable accumulation of these particles in the brains of animals with PD [162]. The intranasal delivery of dantrolene has demonstrated enhanced brain concentration and prolonged duration of action compared to oral administration [163]. The process of intrathecal administration entails the direct delivery of medications into the cerebrospinal fluid (CSF) that surrounds the brain and spinal cord. This method bypasses the BBB and enables direct drug delivery to the CNS. Nevertheless, intrathecal administration is constrained because of its invasive characteristics, technical intricacy, probable unfavorable responses, restricted indications, and elevated expenses [164]. Capitalizing on the direct connection between the nasal cavity and the brain via the olfactory and trigeminal nerves, this method offers a direct pathway for drug delivery to the CNS. While still in its infancy, this approach has shown significant potential, especially for delivering peptides and other macromolecules that traditionally have difficulty crossing the BBB.

### 6.18. Circadian Rhythm [165]

The circadian rhythms, which regulate several human physiological and behavioral activities, are controlled by endogenous biological clocks coordinated by the suprachiasmatic nucleus. The circadian system significantly impacts various physiological functions, encompassing sleep, alertness, and cognitive ability. The perturbation of circadian homeostasis has harmful implications for human well-being. Neurodegenerative illnesses contain a diverse array of symptoms, with a notable characteristic being the presence of diurnal fluctuations in both frequency and intensity.

Furthermore, these illnesses have been found to alter the equilibrium of the circadian system, resulting in a detrimental impact on symptoms and overall quality of life. Increasing evidence indicates a reciprocal association between circadian homeostasis and neurodegeneration, implying that the proper functioning of circadian rhythms may play a crucial role in advancing neurodegenerative diseases. Hence, the circadian system has emerged as a compelling subject of investigation and a promising avenue for advancements in research and clinical interventions. Investigating the impact of circadian disruption on neurodegenerative disorders can enhance our comprehension of the underlying mechanisms of neurodegeneration and promote the creation of innovative therapies based on circadian rhythms for these debilitating conditions.

The sensitivity of the BBB to medications exhibits variability following the circadian rhythm. It has been demonstrated that the administration of the antiepileptic medicine phenytoin during nighttime has enhanced efficacy in the treatment of seizure models in fruit flies [166]. One potential cost-effective method could involve strategically managing medicine administration time to optimize travel efficiency.

### 6.19. *Precision Medicine*

Precision medicine encompasses several strategies to achieve more accurate drug targeting, optimal drug dose, refined illness subtyping, and the meticulous management of individual variations. Precise medication targeting and dosage can be accomplished by targeting methodologies, localized drug administration to the specific lesions, and techniques such as co-focused ultrasound in conjunction with microbubbles. Nevertheless, categorizing diseases into subtypes remains ambiguous for neurological disorders (NDs), and comprehending individual variations poses significant difficulties. This signifies a substantial avenue for future therapy of neurodegenerative disorders.

### 6.20. *Light-Induced Techniques*

Optogenetics and photo biomodulation harness light to affect cellular activity. Recent advancements indicate potential in modulating BBB permeability using specific wavelengths of light, especially when combined with photosensitive agents [167]. While these techniques are in their infancy regarding BBB modulation, the non-invasive nature and advancements in targeted light delivery make them an area of keen interest.

### 6.21. *Radiofrequency (RF) Modulation*

RF energy, a form of electromagnetic radiation, has been explored for its potential to increase the BBB's permeability. The concept involves using RF pulses that induce temporary and reversible changes in the BBB, facilitating drug entry [168]. Though the method holds promise, defining the precise parameters for safe and effective delivery is a significant focus of ongoing research.

### 6.22. *Thermal Techniques*

Mild hyperthermia, induced by devices like microwave applicators, can increase BBB permeability. The technique exploits the sensitivity of BBB endothelial cells to temperature changes, allowing for a temporary "opening" of the barrier [169]. While the method is promising, ensuring precise temperature control and preventing potential thermal damage to surrounding tissues remain challenges.

These non-invasive, device-mediated techniques significantly depart from traditional methods, favoring precision, control, and safety. The advancements promise more effective drug delivery to the CNS and open avenues for delivering a broader range of therapeutic agents, including those previously deemed unsuitable due to their inability to cross the BBB [170]. As research progresses, there is optimism that these techniques will pave the way for novel treatments, offering hope to millions affected by neurological diseases.

## 7. Ex Vivo Modeling

Building in vivo and in vitro BBB models and the innovation of research methods are crucial for several aspects of BBB research, including restoring BBB integrity and enhancing drug penetration efficiency across the BBB. Hence, this article concisely overviews research models such as BBB animal, organoid models, and BBB chips. Additionally, it briefly introduces several invasive and non-invasive BBB research methods, serving as a valuable resource for fellow researchers.

### 7.1. Animal Modes

The utilization of zebrafish and Drosophila models is prevalent in BBB research due to its numerous advantages. These advantages encompass a fast generation time, cost-effectiveness, advanced genetic manipulation capabilities, and the ability to analyze intricate behaviors. Utilizing the zebrafish model provides an added benefit due to the transparency of its early-stage embryos, enabling direct visualization of the BBB.

### 7.2. Organoid Model

The BBB organoid model, is a scientific approach used to study the BBB in a laboratory setting. The construction of in vitro organoid models of the BBB involves culturing and combining different components that make up the BBB to mimic its functional properties observed in living animals, considering the established composition and structure of the BBB. Brain microvascular endothelial cells (BMECs) represent a crucial cellular component within the BBB. The creation of an in vitro organoid model with partial BBB functionality can be achieved by co-culturing brain microvascular endothelial cells (BMECs) with other cell types of the BBB, such as astrocytes and pericytes, on a permeable membrane.

### 7.3. The BBB Chip

The BBB chip is a microfluidic device designed to replicate the human BBB in an in vitro setting. The primary objective of this study is to investigate the intricate dynamics between pharmaceutical substances and various small molecules concerning the BBB, with a particular focus on assessing their capacity to permeate this physiological barrier. Compared to conventional in vitro methods and animal models utilized in BBB research, the BBB chip offers a more authentic in vitro BBB model, diminishes the necessity for animal experimentation, expedites the drug development trajectory, and facilitates the advancement of tailored therapeutic interventions for neurological disorders [171–173].

The development of BBB chips produced from human induced pluripotent stem cells (iPSCs) has been achieved by researchers. These chips demonstrate physiologically realistic trans-endothelial resistance and effectively predict the blood–brain permeability of pharmacokinetic substances.

## 8. Summary

The appeal of non-invasive device-mediated techniques lies in their ability to target specific brain regions while circumventing traditional drug delivery barriers. However, as with any emerging technology, they come with advantages, challenges, and future possibilities that need addressing.

### 8.1. Advantages

- Precision and Specificity: Techniques like FUS offer pinpoint accuracy in targeting specific brain regions [174]. This ensures that only the desired area is treated, reducing the risk of systemic side effects.
- Versatility: The non-invasive nature of these techniques makes them suitable for a wide range of applications, from delivering small-molecule drugs to larger molecules like antibodies or even genes.

- Minimally Disruptive: Unlike invasive methods, which can cause tissue damage or infection, non-invasive techniques are generally safer with minimal post-procedure complications.
- Repeatability: Given their non-destructive nature, these techniques can be applied repeatedly, allowing for chronic treatments or adjustments [175].

### *8.2. Challenges*

- Understanding Long-term Effects: While initial studies are promising, the long-term effects of repeated BBB disruption or electromagnetic field exposure remain to be comprehensively understood [176].
- Optimization of Parameters: Each technique requires fine-tuning parameters to ensure efficacy without compromising safety. For instance, ultrasound's right frequency and duration of the optimal wavelength for light-induced techniques are vital for success [177].
- Systemic Side Effects: Despite targeted delivery, there is a potential for drugs to diffuse from the target site, leading to unintended effects elsewhere in the brain or body.
- Technological Limitations: Current devices may not be optimized for deep brain structures or use in specific populations like children or older adults [178].

## 9. Future Perspectives

- Combination Therapies: Combining non-invasive techniques could further improve delivery efficacy. For instance, using FUS to enhance nanoparticle delivery across the BBB could combine the strengths of both methods [179].
- Advanced Monitoring: Integrating real-time imaging, like MRI, with drug delivery can provide immediate feedback, ensuring optimal delivery and minimizing potential risks [180].
- Personalized Approaches: As our understanding grows, it may be possible to tailor techniques to individual patients based on their unique anatomy, pathology, and therapeutic needs [181].
- Expansion to Other Diseases: While the current focus might be on neurological disorders, the potential exists to expand these techniques for other conditions, from brain tumors to systemic illnesses with CNS involvement [182].

### *Applications*

The potential clinical applications of non-invasive device-mediated techniques are vast. As more research unravels their potential and addresses the associated challenges, there is hope these techniques will transform the landscape of neurological treatment, ushering in an era of more effective and less invasive therapeutic interventions. The progress of non-invasive device-mediated techniques is closely intertwined with technological advancements and the integration of imaging modalities. These dual advancements allow for real-time monitoring and adjustment, ensuring safety and efficacy during treatments. The synergy between technological advances, integration with imaging modalities, and the introduction of computational methods heralds a new era for non-invasive device-mediated drug delivery. These integrative approaches promise enhanced efficacy and pave the way for personalized treatments tailored to individual patient needs.

The evolving landscape of non-invasive device-mediated drug delivery presents both challenges and opportunities. Addressing current limitations will determine the trajectory of this field in the coming years as more conceptual and practical inquiries into the science and the art of overcoming the hurdle of BBB to treat diseases become evident.

Combining non-invasive device-mediated delivery with emerging therapies like gene editing or stem cell therapies can potentiate therapeutic outcomes. Accurately delivering these agents to targeted areas can amplify their efficacy [183]. A recent study employed focused ultrasound to facilitate the delivery of CRISPR/Cas9 components to the brain, showcasing potential applications in genetic disorders [184].

## 10. Conclusions

BBB offers a promising frontier in neurotherapeutics. While they bring many advantages, challenges that must be addressed through rigorous research persist. The future, replete with possibilities, could see these techniques revolutionizing not just neuroscience but the broader landscape of medicine.

The promising advantages and ongoing developments in non-invasive device-mediated techniques have paved the way for potential clinical applications, ranging from NDs to brain tumors.

The field of non-invasive device-mediated drug delivery stands at an exciting juncture. The convergence of technological advancements, biomedical research, and clinical needs promises to revolutionize treatment modalities for various diseases, particularly those affecting the brain. Addressing current challenges and capitalizing on emerging opportunities will be pivotal. With continued interdisciplinary collaboration, investment, and innovation, the full potential of these techniques can be realized, heralding a new era in medical treatments.

As we gaze into the horizon of non-invasive device-mediated drug delivery, a range of innovations and advancements come into view. These innovations, stemming from diverse areas of science and engineering, have the potential to address existing challenges and propel the field into novel therapeutic paradigms.

The potential of non-invasive device-mediated drug delivery is vast, and as technology and biomedical research continue to evolve together, new avenues and possibilities emerge. The intersection of these advancements holds immense promise for transforming the therapeutic landscape. As research progresses and innovations are integrated into clinical practice, patients worldwide stand to benefit from more effective, targeted, and safer treatments.

While the journey of non-invasive device-mediated drug delivery is intertwined with challenges and regulatory intricacies, their promise and potential are undeniably transformative. Here is a closer look at what the horizon might hold.

The realm of non-invasive device-mediated drug delivery is on the cusp of redefining therapeutic interventions, especially for conditions previously deemed untreatable. The intertwined dance of science, technology, ethics, and humanity promises a future where treatments are effective and compassionate. As we stride ahead, let this journey be marked by innovation, inclusivity, and an unwavering commitment to enhancing human lives.

Harnessing the power of artificial intelligence (AI) and machine learning can optimize treatment parameters, predict patient responses, and improve therapeutic outcomes [185]. A recent project employed AI algorithms to analyze patient data and optimize focused ultrasound settings, enhancing treatment precision and reducing side effects [186].

**Funding:** This research received no external funding.

**Conflicts of Interest:** The author declares no conflict of interest.

## References


1. Gazzaniga, M.S.; Ivry, R.B.; Mangun, G.R. *Cognitive Neuroscience: The Biology of the Mind*; Norton & Company: New York, NY, USA, 2018.
2. Bear, M.F.; Connors, B.W.; Paradiso, M.A. *Neuroscience: Exploring the Brain*; Wolters Kluwer Health: Philadelphia, PA, USA, 2016.
3. Abbott, N.J. Dynamics of CNS barriers: Evolution, differentiation, and modulation. *Cell. Mol. Neurobiol.* **2005**, *25*, 5–23. [CrossRef] [PubMed]
4. Pardridge, W.M. The blood-brain barrier: Bottleneck in brain drug development. *NeuroRx* **2005**, *2*, 3–14. [CrossRef] [PubMed]
5. Daneman, R.; Prat, A. The blood–brain barrier. *Cold Spring Harb. Perspect. Biol.* **2015**, *7*, a020412. [CrossRef] [PubMed]
6. Abbott, N.J.; Rönnbäck, L.; Hansson, E. Astrocyte–endothelial interactions at the blood–brain barrier. *Nat. Rev. Neurosci.* **2006**, *7*, 41–53. [CrossRef] [PubMed]
7. Hawkins, B.T.; Davis, T.P. The blood-brain barrier/neurovascular unit in health and disease. *Pharmacol. Rev.* **2005**, *57*, 173–185. [CrossRef]

8. Saunders, N.R.; Habgood, M.D.; Dziegielewska, K.M.; Potter, A. Barrier mechanisms in the brain, I. Adult brain. *Clin. Exp. Pharmacol. Physiol.* **2016**, *23*, 137–146. [CrossRef]
9. Begley, D.J. Delivery of therapeutic agents to the central nervous system: The problems and the possibilities. *Pharmacol. Ther.* **2004**, *104*, 29–45. [CrossRef]
10. Pardridge, W.M. Blood-brain barrier delivery. *Drug Discov. Today* **2007**, *12*, 54–61. [CrossRef]
11. Neuwelt, E.A.; Bauer, B.; Fahlke, C.; Fricker, G.; Iadecola, C.; Janigro, D.; Mayhan, W.G. Engaging neuroscience to advance translational research in brain barrier biology. *Nat. Rev. Neurosci.* **2011**, *12*, 169–182. [CrossRef]
12. Ohtsuki, S.; Terasaki, T. Contribution of carrier-mediated transport systems to the BBB as a supporting and protecting interface for the brain; importance for CNS drug discovery and development. *Pharm. Nov. Drug Deliv. Syst.* **2007**, *10*, 13–23.
13. Collins, F.S.; Varmus, H. A new initiative on precision medicine. *N. Engl. J. Med.* **2015**, *372*, 793–795. [CrossRef] [PubMed]
14. Abbott, N.J. Inflammatory mediators and modulation of BBB permeability. *Cell. Mol. Neurobiol.* **2000**, *20*, 131–147. [CrossRef]
15. Chen, Y.; Liu, L. Modern methods for delivery of drugs across the blood-brain barrier. *Adv. Drug Deliv. Rev.* **2012**, *64*, 640–665. [CrossRef]
16. Pardridge, W.M. Targeted delivery of protein and gene medicines through the blood-brain barrier. *Clin. Pharmacol. Ther.* **2015**, *97*, 347–361. [CrossRef] [PubMed]
17. Liebner, S.; Dijkhuizen, R.; Reiss, Y.; Plate, K.; Agalliu, D.; Constantin, G. Functional morphology of the BBB in health and disease. *Acta Neuropathol.* **2018**, *135*, 311–336. [CrossRef] [PubMed]
18. Zhao, Z.; Nelson, A.; Betsholtz, C.; Zlokovic, B. Establishment and dysfunction of the blood-brain barrier. *Cell* **2015**, *163*, 1064–1078. [CrossRef]
19. Yang, A.; Stevens, M.; Chen, M.; Lee, D.; Stähli, D.; Gate, D.; Contrepois, K.; Chen, W.; Iram, T.; Zhang, L.; et al. Physiological blood-brain transport is impaired with age by a shift in transcytosis. *Nature* **2020**, *583*, 425–430. [CrossRef]
20. Profaci, C.; Munji, R.; Pulido, R.; Daneman, R. The BBB in health and disease: Important unanswered questions. *J. Exp. Med.* **2020**, *217*, e20190062. [CrossRef]
21. Banks, W. From blood-brain barrier to blood-brain interface: New opportunities for CNS drug delivery. *Nat. Rev. Drug Discov.* **2016**, *15*, 275–292. [CrossRef]
22. Pardridge, W.M. Drug transport across the blood-brain barrier. *J. Cereb. Blood Flow Metab.* **2012**, *32*, 1959–1972. [CrossRef]
23. Löscher, W.; Potschka, H. Blood-brain barrier active efflux transporters: ATP-binding cassette gene family. *NeuroRx* **2005**, *2*, 86–98. [CrossRef] [PubMed]
24. Pardridge, W.M. Molecular biology of the blood-brain barrier. *Mol. Biotechnol.* **2006**, *32*, 103–120.
25. Banks, W.A. Characteristics of compounds that cross the blood-brain barrier. *BMC Neurol.* **2009**, *9* (Suppl. S1), S3. [CrossRef] [PubMed]
26. Menei, P.; Daniel, V.; Montero-Menei, C.; Brouillard, M.; Pouplard-Barthelaix, A.; Benoit, J.P. Biodegradable microspheres for the intracerebral administration of methotrexate. *J. Neurosurg.* **1993**, *78*, 915–921.
27. Sweeney, M.D.; Sagare, A.P. Vascular dysfunction in cognitive impairment and Alzheimer's disease. *Front. Aging Neurosci.* **2020**, *12*, 98.
28. Lipinski, C.A. Drug-like properties and the causes of poor solubility and poor permeability. *J. Pharmacol. Toxicol. Methods* **2000**, *44*, 235–249. [CrossRef]
29. Neuwelt, E.; Abbott, N.J.; Abrey, L.; Banks, W.A.; Blakley, B.; Davis, T.; Engelhardt, B. Strategies to advance translational research into brain barriers. *Lancet Neurol.* **2008**, *7*, 84–96. [CrossRef]
30. Rossi, S.; Hallett, M. Principles, clinical applications, and pitfalls of brain stimulation. *Ann. Neurol.* **2019**, *85*, 14–33.
31. Reato, D.; Rahman, A. Effects of weak transcranial alternating current stimulation on brain activity—A review of known mechanisms from animal studies. *Front. Hum. Neurosci.* **2010**, *7*, 687. [CrossRef]
32. Kobus, T.; Zervantonakis, I.K.; Zhang, Y.; McDannold, N.J. Growth inhibition in a brain metastasis model by antibody delivery using focused ultrasound-mediated BBB disruption. *J. Control. Release* **2016**, *238*, 281–288. [CrossRef]
33. Lipsman, N.; Meng, Y.; Bethune, A.J.; Huang, Y.; Lam, B.; Masellis, M.; Herrmann, N.; Heyn, C.; Aubert, I.; Boutet, A. Blood–brain barrier opening in Alzheimer's disease using MR-guided focused ultrasound. *Nat. Commun.* **2018**, *9*, 2336. [CrossRef] [PubMed]
34. Saito, R.; Bringas, J.R.; McKnight, T.R.; Wendland, M.F.; Mamot, C.; Drummond, D.C.; Berger, M.S. Distribution of liposomes into brain and rat brain tumor models by convection-enhanced delivery monitored with magnetic resonance imaging. *Cancer Res.* **2004**, *64*, 2572–2579. [CrossRef] [PubMed]
35. Aryal, M.; Arvanitis, C.D.; Alexander, P.M.; McDannold, N. Ultrasound-mediated blood–brain barrier disruption for targeted drug delivery in the central nervous system. *Adv. Drug Deliv. Rev.* **2014**, *72*, 94–109. [CrossRef] [PubMed]
36. Shilo, M.; Reuveni, T.; Motiei, M.; Popovtzer, R. Nanoparticles as computed tomography contrast agents: Current status and future perspectives. *Nanomedicine* **2015**, *10*, 1609–1622. [CrossRef] [PubMed]
37. Nance, E.A.; Woodworth, G.F.; Sailor, K.A.; Shih, T.Y.; Xu, Q.; Swaminathan, G.; Hanes, J. A dense poly (ethylene glycol) coating improves penetration of large polymeric nanoparticles within brain tissue. *Sci. Transl. Med.* **2012**, *4*, 149ra119. [CrossRef]
38. Thorne, R.G.; Pronk, G.J.; Padmanabhan, V.; Frey, W.H., II. Delivery of insulin-like growth factor-I to the rat brain and spinal cord along olfactory and trigeminal pathways following intranasal administration. *Neuroscience* **2004**, *127*, 481–496. [CrossRef]
39. Ghanouni, P.; Dobakhti, F.; Kennedy, A.M. Blood-brain barrier: From anatomy to astrocyte interactions. In *Nanotechnology for Biomedical Imaging and Diagnostics: From Nanoparticle Design to Clinical Applications*; Wiley: Hoboken, NJ, USA, 2015; pp. 375–402.

40. Banks, W.A.; Sharma, P.; Bullock, K.M. Transport of protein-bound and free peptides, cyclic peptides, and modified neuropeptides across the blood-brain barrier. *J. Alzheimer's Dis.* **2019**, *68*, 1617–1629.
41. Rao, J.; Li, M.; Wang, Y.; Liu, B.; Zhao, C. Exosomes in CNS drug delivery. *Adv. Healthc. Mater.* **2020**, *9*, 1901868.
42. Hynynen, K.; McDannold, N.; Vykhodtseva, N.; Jolesz, F.A. Non-invasive opening of BBB by focused ultrasound. *Acta Neurochir. Suppl.* **2016**, *121*, 243–247.
43. LeWitt, P.A.; Lipsman, N.; Kordower, J.H.; Aebischer, P.; Chen, L.; Svendsen, C.N. Focused ultrasound opening of the blood-brain barrier for treatment of Parkinson's disease. *Mov. Disord.* **2021**, *36*, 76–82. [CrossRef]
44. Burger, M.C.; Glavis-Bloom, C.; Wang, A.; Gonzalez-Cuyar, L.F.; Oh, J.H. Implantable drug delivery devices for the treatment of neurologic disorders. *Front. Neurosci.* **2017**, *11*, 535.
45. Bhardwaj, R.; Blanchard, A.D.; Jaffe, G.J. Drug delivery strategies for retinal diseases. *Prog. Retin. Eye Res.* **2019**, *72*, 100758.
46. Langer, R.; Folkman, J. Polymers for the sustained release of proteins and other macromolecules. *Nature* **1976**, *263*, 797–800. [CrossRef] [PubMed]
47. Langer, R. Biomaterials in drug delivery and tissue engineering: One laboratory's experience. *Acc. Chem. Res.* **2000**, *33*, 94–101. [CrossRef] [PubMed]
48. Timbie, K.F.; Mead, B.P.; Price, R.J. Drug and gene delivery across the blood–brain barrier with focused ultrasound. *J. Control. Release* **2015**, *219*, 61–75. [CrossRef]
49. Hynynen, K.; McDannold, N.; Vykhodtseva, N.; Jolesz, F.A. Noninvasive MR imaging–guided focal opening of the BBB in rabbits. *Radiology* **2001**, *220*, 640–646. [CrossRef]
50. Nance, E.; Timbie, K.; Miller, G.W.; Song, J.; Louttit, C.; Klibanov, A.L.; Woodworth, G.F. Non-invasive delivery of stealth, brain-penetrating nanoparticles across the BBB using MRI-guided focused ultrasound. *J. Control. Release* **2014**, *189*, 123–132. [CrossRef]
51. Abbott, N.J.; Friedman, A. Overview and introduction: The BBB in health and disease. *Epilepsia* **2012**, *53*, 1–6. [CrossRef]
52. Aryal, M.; Vykhodtseva, N.; Zhang, Y.Z.; Park, J.; McDannold, N. Multiple treatments with liposomal doxorubicin and ultrasound-induced disruption of blood-tumor and blood-brain barriers improve outcomes in a rat glioma model. *J. Control. Release* **2015**, *204*, 60–68. [CrossRef]
53. Zhou, B.; Xiong, Z.; Wang, P. Improved delivery for central nervous system diseases: Challenges and future prospects. *Signal Transduct. Target. Ther.* **2019**, *4*, 1–17.
54. Mégevand, P.; Groppe, D.M.; Goldfinger, M.S. Novel applications of imaging in the diagnosis and management of neurological disease. *Neurotherapeutics* **2019**, *16*, 26–37.
55. Aryal, M.; Fischer, K.; Gentile, C.; Gitto, S.; Zhang, Y.Z.; McDonnell, S.; Airan, R.D. Effects on the brain of a novel 40 Hz flicker from phosphene generation in patients with Alzheimer's disease. *PLoS ONE* **2019**, *14*, e0218741.
56. Zeng, Y.; Kurokawa, T. Wearable ultrasound devices for diagnostics and therapy. *Bio-Des. Manuf.* **2018**, *1*, 77–89.
57. Alvarez-Erviti, L.; Couch, Y. Delivery of siRNA to the mouse brain by systemic injection of targeted exosomes. *Nat. Biotechnol.* **2011**, *29*, 341–345. [CrossRef] [PubMed]
58. Legon, W.; Ai, L.; Bansal, P.; Mueller, J.K. Neuromodulation with single-element transcranial focused ultrasound in human thalamus. *Hum. Brain Mapp.* **2018**, *39*, 1995–2006. [CrossRef] [PubMed]
59. Aryal, M.; Park, J.; Vykhodtseva, N.; Zhang, Y.Z. Enhancement in blood-tumor barrier permeability and delivery of liposomal doxorubicin using focused ultrasound and microbubbles: Evaluation during tumor progression in a rat glioma model. *Phys. Med. Biol.* **2017**, *62*, 2428–2441. [CrossRef]
60. Felistia, Y.; Wen, P.Y. Molecular Profiling and Targeted Therapies in Gliomas. *Curr. Neurol. Neurosci. Rep.* **2023**, *23*, 627–636. [CrossRef]
61. Treat, L.H.; McDannold, N.; Vykhodtseva, N.; Zhang, Y.; Tam, K.; Hynynen, K. Targeted delivery of doxorubicin to the rat brain at therapeutic levels using MRI-guided focused ultrasound. *Int. J. Cancer* **2012**, *131*, EPE99–EPE107. [CrossRef]
62. Bystritsky, A.; Korb, A.S.; Douglas, P.K. A review of low-intensity focused ultrasound pulsation. *Brain Stimul.* **2011**, *4*, 125–136. [CrossRef]
63. Burgess, A.; Hynynen, K. Drug delivery across the blood–brain barrier using focused ultrasound. *Expert Opin. Drug Deliv.* **2014**, *11*, 711–721. [CrossRef]
64. Gooch, C.L.; Pracht, E.; Borenstein, A.R. The burden of neurological disease in the United States: A summary report and call to action. *Ann. Neurol.* **2017**, *81*, 479–484. [CrossRef]
65. Available online: https://www.alz.org/media/documents/alzheimers-facts-and-figures.pdf (accessed on 10 July 2023).
66. Available online: https://www.parkinson.org/understanding-parkinsons/statistics (accessed on 10 July 2023).
67. Li, H.; Liu, C.C.; Zheng, H.; Huang, T.Y. Amyloid, tau, pathogen infection and antimicrobial protection in Alzheimer's disease-conformist, nonconformist, and realistic prospects for AD pathogenesis. *Transl. Neurodegener.* **2018**, *7*, 34. [CrossRef]
68. Leinenga, G.; Götz, J. Scanning ultrasound removes amyloid-β and restores memory in an Alzheimer's disease mouse model. *Sci. Transl. Med.* **2015**, *7*, 278ra33. [CrossRef]
69. Jordão, J.F.; Ayala-Grosso, C.A.; Markham, K.; Huang, Y.; Chopra, R.; McLaurin, J.; Hynynen, K.; Aubert, I. Antibodies targeted to the brain with image-guided focused ultrasound reduces amyloid-β plaque load in the TgCRND8 mouse model of Alzheimer's disease. *PLoS ONE* **2010**, *5*, e10549. [CrossRef] [PubMed]

70. Silverman, W.; Krinsky-McHale, S.J.; Zigman, W.B.; Schupf, N.; New York Aging Research Program. Adults with Down syndrome in randomized clinical trials targeting prevention of Alzheimer's disease. *Alzheimers Dement.* **2022**, *18*, 1736–1743. [CrossRef] [PubMed]
71. Baseri, B.; Choi, J.J.; Deffieux, T.; Samiotaki, G.; Tung, Y.S.; Olumolade, O.; Konofagou, E.E. Activation of signaling pathways following localized delivery of systemically administered neurotrophic factors across the BBB using focused ultrasound and microbubbles. *Phys. Med. Biol.* **2012**, *57*, N65. [CrossRef]
72. Fan, C.H.; Ting, C.Y.; Lin, C.Y.; Chan, H.L.; Chang, Y.C.; Chen, Y.Y.; Liu, H.L. Noninvasive, targeted, and non-viral ultrasound-mediated GDNF-plasmid delivery for treatment of Parkinson's disease. *Sci. Rep.* **2016**, *6*, 19579. [CrossRef]
73. Martin, E.; Jeanmonod, D.; Morel, A.; Zadicario, E.; Werner, B. High-intensity focused ultrasound for noninvasive functional neurosurgery. *Ann. Neurol.* **2009**, *66*, 858–861. [CrossRef] [PubMed]
74. González-Fernández, C.; Gonzalez, P.; Andres-Benito, P.; Ferrer, I.; Rodríguez, F.J. Wnt signaling alterations in the human spinal cord of amyotrophic lateral sclerosis cases: Spotlight on Fz2 and Wnt5a. *Mol. Neurobiol.* **2019**, *56*, 6777–6791. [CrossRef]
75. Burgess, A.; Dubey, S.; Yeung, S.; Hough, O.; Eterman, N.; Aubert, I.; Hynynen, K. Alzheimer disease in a mouse model: MR imaging–guided focused ultrasound targeted to the hippocampus opens the BBB and improves pathologic abnormalities and behavior. *Radiology* **2014**, *273*, 736–745. [CrossRef]
76. Islam, Y.; Leach, A.G.; Smith, J.; Pluchino, S.; Coxon, C.R.; Sivakumaran, M.; Downing, J.; Fatokun, A.A.; Teixidò, M.; Ehtezazi, T. Physiological and pathological factors affecting drug delivery to the brain by nanoparticles. *Adv. Sci.* **2021**, *8*, 2002085. [CrossRef]
77. Cho, E.E.; Drazic, J.; Ganguly, M.; Stefanovic, B.; Hynynen, K. Two-photon fluorescence microscopy study of cerebrovascular dynamics in ultrasound-induced BBB opening. *J. Cereb. Blood Flow Metab.* **2018**, *38*, 1260–1274.
78. Pawar, B.; Vasdev, N.; Gupta, T.; Mhatre, M.; More, A.; Anup, N.; Tekade, R.K. Current Update on Transcellular Brain Drug Delivery. *Pharmaceutics* **2022**, *14*, 2719. [CrossRef] [PubMed]
79. Abbott, N.J.; Patabendige, A.A.; Dolman, D.E.; Yusof, S.R.; Begley, D.J. Structure and function of the blood-brain barrier. *Neurobiol. Dis.* **2010**, *37*, 13–25. [CrossRef] [PubMed]
80. Anthony, D.P.; Hegde, M.; Shetty, S.S.; Rafic, T.; Mutalik, S.; Rao, B.S. Targeting receptor-ligand chemistry for drug delivery across blood-brain barrier in brain diseases. *Life Sci.* **2021**, *274*, 119326. [CrossRef]
81. Betterton, R.D.; Davis, T.P.; Ronaldson, P.T. Organic Cation Transporter (OCT/OCTN) Expression at Brain Barrier Sites: Focus on CNS Drug Delivery. *Handb. Exp. Pharmacol.* **2021**, *266*, 301–328. [PubMed]
82. Lonser, R.R.; Sarntinoranont, M.; Morrison, P.F.; Oldfield, E.H. Convection-enhanced delivery to the central nervous system. *J. Neurosurg.* **2015**, *122*, 697–706. [CrossRef]
83. Lonser, R.R.; Walbridge, S.; Garmestani, K.; Butman, J.A.; Walters, H.A.; Vortmeyer, A.O.; Oldfield, E.H. Successful and safe perfusion of the primate brainstem: In vivo magnetic resonance imaging of macromolecular distribution during infusion. *J. Neurosurg.* **2002**, *97*, 905–913. [CrossRef]
84. Saltzman, W.M. *Drug Delivery: Engineering Principles for Drug Therapy*; Oxford University Press: Oxford, UK, 2001.
85. Morrison, P.F.; Laske, D.W. Direct delivery of medications to the central nervous system. *Clin. Pharmacokinet.* **1994**, *26*, 85–100.
86. Rubin, L.L.; Staddon, J.M. The cell biology of the blood-brain barrier. *Annu. Rev. Neurosci.* **1999**, *22*, 11–28. [CrossRef]
87. Johnsen, K.B.; Moos, T.; Burkhart, A. Receptor-mediated drug delivery to the brain in the treatment of central nervous system diseases. *J. Mol. Med.* **2014**, *92*, 497–506.
88. Chen, W.; Hu, Y.; Ju, D. Gene therapy for neurodegenerative disorders: Advances, insights and prospects. *Acta Pharm. Sin. B* **2020**, *10*, 1347–1359. [CrossRef]
89. Rapoport, S.I. Osmotic opening of the blood-brain barrier: Principles, mechanism, and therapeutic applications. *Cell. Mol. Neurobiol.* **2000**, *20*, 217–230. [CrossRef] [PubMed]
90. Chakraborty, S.; Filippi, C.; Wong, T.; Ray, A.; Fralin, S.; Tsiouris, A.; Praminick, B.; Demopoulos, A.; McCrea, H.; Bodhinayake, I.; et al. Superselective intraarterial cerebral infusion of cetuximab after osmotic blood/brain barrier disruption for recurrent malignant glioma: Phase I study. *J. Neuro-Oncol.* **2016**, *128*, 405–415. [CrossRef] [PubMed]
91. Li, J.; Kataoka, K. Chemo-physical Strategies to Advance the in Vivo Functionality of Targeted Nanomedicine: The Next Generation. *J. Am. Chem. Soc.* **2021**, *143*, 538–559. [CrossRef] [PubMed]
92. Jiang, Y.; Wang, F.; Wang, K.; Zhong, Y.; Wei, X.; Wang, Q.; Zhang, H. Engineered Exosomes: A Promising Drug Delivery Strategy for Brain Diseases. *Curr. Med. Chem.* **2022**, *29*, 3111–3124. [CrossRef]
93. Yue, Q.; Peng, Y.; Zhao, Y.; Lu, R.; Fu, Q.; Chen, Y.; Yang, Y.; Hai, L.; Guo, L.; Wu, Y. Dual-targeting for brain-specific drug delivery: Synthesis and biological evaluation. *Drug Deliv.* **2018**, *25*, 426–434. [CrossRef]
94. Jiang, T.; Qiao, Y.; Ruan, W.; Zhang, D.; Yang, Q.; Wang, G.; Chen, Q.; Zhu, F.; Yin, J.; Zou, Y. Cation-Free siRNA Micelles as Effective Drug Delivery Platform and Potent RNAi Nanomedicines for Glioblastoma Therapy. *Adv. Mater.* **2021**, *33*, 2104779. [CrossRef]
95. Ban, J.; Li, S.; Zhan, Q.; Li, X.; Xing, H.; Chen, N.; Long, L.; Hou, X.; Zhao, J.; Yuan, X. PMPC modified PAMAM dendrimer enhances brain tumor-targeted drug delivery. *Macromol. Biosci.* **2021**, *21*, 2000392. [CrossRef]
96. Caraway, C.A.; Gaitsch, H.; Wicks, E.E.; Kalluri, A.; Kunadi, N.; Tyler, B.M. Polymeric nanoparticles in brain cancer therapy: A review of current approaches. *Polymers* **2022**, *14*, 2963. [CrossRef]
97. Saraiva, C.; Praça, C.; Ferreira, R.; Santos, T.; Ferreira, L.; Bernardino, L. Nanoparticle-mediated brain drug delivery: Overcoming blood–brain barrier to treat neurodegenerative diseases. *J. Control. Release* **2016**, *235*, 34–47. [CrossRef]

98. Wu, J.; Hernandez, Y.; Miyasaki, K.; Kwon, E. Engineered nanomaterials that exploit BBB dysfunction for delivery to the brain. *Adv. Drug Deliv. Rev.* **2023**, *197*, 114820. [CrossRef] [PubMed]
99. Kreuter, J. Drug delivery to the central nervous system by polymeric nanoparticles: What do we know? *Adv. Drug Deliv. Rev.* **2014**, *71*, 2–14. [CrossRef] [PubMed]
100. Gao, X.; Qian, J.; Zheng, S.; Changyi, Y.; Zhang, J.; Ju, S.; Zhu, J.; Li, C. Overcoming the Blood–Brain Barrier for Delivering Drugs into the Brain by Using Adenosine Receptor Nanoagonist. *ACS Nano* **2018**, *12*, 9968–9978. [CrossRef] [PubMed]
101. Sonavane, G.; Tomoda, K.; Makino, K. Biodistribution of colloidal gold nanoparticles after intravenous administration: Effect of particle size. *Colloids Surf. B Biointerfaces* **2008**, *66*, 274–280. [CrossRef]
102. Timbie, K.F.; Afzal, U.; Date, A.; Zhang, C.; Song, J.; Wilson Miller, G.; Suk, J.S.; Hanes, J. MR image-guided delivery of cisplatin-loaded brain-penetrating nanoparticles to invasive glioma with focused ultrasound. *J. Control. Release* **2017**, *263*, 120–131. [CrossRef]
103. Timbie, K.F.; Mead, B.P. Drug delivery across the blood-brain barrier: Recent advances in the use of nanocarriers. *Nanomedicine* **2017**, *12*, 159–167.
104. Mead, B.P.; Price, R.J. Targeted drug delivery to the brain using focused ultrasound: A review. *J. Drug Target.* **2016**, *24*, 871–882.
105. Gorick, C.; Breza, V.; Nowak, K.; Cheng, V.; Fisher, D.; Debski, A.; Hoch, M.; Demir, Z.; Tran, N.; Schwartz, M.; et al. Applications of focused ultrasound-mediated BBB opening. *Adv. Drug Deliv. Rev.* **2022**, *191*, 114583. [CrossRef]
106. Burgess, A.; Ayala-Grosso, C.; Ganguly, M.; Jordaõ, J.; Aubert, I.; Hynynen, K. Targeted delivery of neural stem cells to the brain using MRI-guided focused ultrasound to disrupt the blood-brain barrier. *PLoS ONE* **2011**, *6*, e27877. [CrossRef]
107. Diaz, R.; McVeigh, P.; O'Reilly, M.; Burrell, K.; Bebenek, M.; Smith, C.; Etame, A.; Zadeh, G.; Hynynen, K.; Wilson, B.; et al. Focused ultrasound delivery of Raman nanoparticles across the blood-brain barrier: Potential for targeting experimental brain tumors. *Nanomed. Nanotechnol. Biol. Med.* **2014**, *10*, 1075–1087. [CrossRef]
108. Kinoshita, M.; McDannold, N.; Jolesz, F.; Hynynen, K. Noninvasive localized delivery of Herceptin to the mouse brain by MRI-guided focused ultrasound-induced BBB disruption. *Proc. Natl. Acad. Sci. USA* **2006**, *103*, 11719–11723. [CrossRef]
109. Nisbet, R.; Van der Jeugd, A.; Leinenga, G.; Evans, H.; Janowicz, P.; Götz, J. Combined effects of scanning ultrasound and a tau-specific single chain antibody in a tau transgenic mouse model. *Brain J. Neurol.* **2017**, *140*, 1220–1230. [CrossRef] [PubMed]
110. Raymond, S.; Treat, L.; Dewey, J.; McDannold, N.; Hynynen, K.; Bacskai, B. Ultrasound enhanced delivery of molecular imaging and therapeutic agents in Alzheimer's disease mouse models. *PLoS ONE* **2008**, *3*, e2175. [CrossRef] [PubMed]
111. Th'evenot, E.; Jordão, J.; O'Reilly, M.; Markham, K.; Weng, Y.; Foust, K.; Kaspar, B.; Hynynen, K.; Aubert, I. Targeted delivery of self-complementary adeno-associated virus serotype 9 to the brain, using magnetic resonance imaging-guided focused ultrasound. *Hum. Gene Ther.* **2012**, *23*, 1144–1155. [CrossRef]
112. Pineda-Pardo, J.; Gasca-Salas, C.; Fernández-Rodríguez, B.; Rodríguez-Rojas, R.; Del Alamo, M.; Obeso, I.; Hernández-Fernández, F.; Trompeta, C.; Martínez-Fernández, R.; Matarazzo, M.; et al. Striatal BBB opening in Parkinson's disease dementia: A pilot exploratory study. *Mov. Disord. Off. J. Mov. Disord. Soc.* **2022**, *37*, 2057–2065. [CrossRef] [PubMed]
113. Aryal, M.; Vykhodtseva, N.; Zhang, Y.Z.; McDannold, N. Multiple sessions of liposomal doxorubicin delivery via focused ultrasound mediated BBB disruption: A safety study. *J. Control. Release* **2014**, *204*, 60–69. [CrossRef]
114. Konofagou, E.E. Optimization of the ultrasound-induced BBB opening. *Theranostics* **2012**, *2*, 1223. [CrossRef]
115. McDannold, N.; Arvanitis, C.D.; Vykhodtseva, N.; Livingstone, M.S. Temporary disruption of the BBB by use of ultrasound and microbubbles: Safety and efficacy evaluation in rhesus macaques. *Cancer Res.* **2012**, *72*, 3652–3663. [CrossRef]
116. Liu, J.; Chu, C.; Zhang, J.; Bie, C.; Chen, L.; Aafreen, S.; Xu, J.; Kamson, D.; van Zijl, P.; Walczak, P.; et al. Label-free assessment of mannitol accumulation following osmotic BBB opening ssing chemical exchange saturation transfer magnetic resonance imaging. *Pharmaceutics* **2022**, *14*, 2529. [CrossRef]
117. Chu, C.; Jablonska, A.; Gao, Y.; Lan, X.; Lesniak, W.; Liang, Y.; Liu, G.; Li, S.; Magnus, T.; Pearl, M.; et al. Hyperosmolar BBB opening using intra-arterial injection of hyperosmotic mannitol in mice under real-time MRI guidance. *Nat. Protoc.* **2022**, *17*, 76–94. [CrossRef] [PubMed]
118. McDannold, N.; Vykhodtseva, N.; Hynynen, K. Targeted disruption of the BBB with focused ultrasound: Association with cavitation activity. *Phys. Med. Biol.* **2006**, *51*, 793. [CrossRef] [PubMed]
119. Elias, W.J.; Lipsman, N.; Ondo, W.G.; Ghanouni, P.; Kim, Y.G.; Lee, W.; Schwartz, M.; Hynynen, K.; Lozano, A.M.; Shah, B.B.; et al. A randomized trial of focused ultrasound thalamotomy for essential tremor. *N. Engl. J. Med.* **2016**, *375*, 730–739. [CrossRef]
120. Liu, H.L.; Hua, M.Y.; Chen, P.Y.; Chu, P.C.; Pan, C.H.; Yang, H.W.; Huang, C.Y.; Wang, J.J.; Yen, T.C.; Wei, K.C. Blood-brain barrier disruption with focused ultrasound enhances delivery of chemotherapeutic drugs for glioblastoma treatment. *Radiology* **2010**, *255*, 415–425. [CrossRef] [PubMed]
121. Mehta, R.; Carpenter, J.; Mehta, R.; Haut, M.; Ranjan, M.; Najib, U.; Lockman, P.; Wang, P.; D'haese, P.; Rezai, A. Blood-brain barrier opening with MRI-guided focused ultrasound elicits meningeal venous permeability in humans with early Alzheimer disease. *Radiology* **2021**, *298*, 654–662. [CrossRef]
122. Rezai, A.; Ranjan, M.; D'Haese, P.; Haut, M.; Carpenter, J.; Najib, U.; Mehta, R.; Chazen, J.; Zibly, Z.; Yates, J.; et al. Noninvasive hippocampal BBB opening in Alzheimer's disease with focused ultrasound. *Proc. Natl. Acad. Sci. USA* **2020**, *117*, 9180–9182. [CrossRef]

123. Gasca-Salas, C.; Fernández-Rodríguez, B.; Pineda-Pardo, J.; Rodríguez-Rojas, R.; Obeso, I.; Hernández-Fernández, F.; Del Alamo, M.; Mata, D.; Guida, P.; Ordás-Bandera, C.; et al. Blood-brain barrier opening with focused ultrasound in Parkinson's disease dementia. *Nat. Commun.* **2021**, *12*, 779. [CrossRef] [PubMed]
124. Tanizawa, K.; Sonoda, H.; Sato, Y. A phase 2/3 trial of pabinafusp alfa, IDS fused with anti-human transferrin receptor antibody, targeting neurodegeneration in MPS-II. *Mol. Ther. J. Am. Soc. Gene Ther.* **2021**, *29*, 671–679.
125. Cuccurazzu, B.; Leone, L. Exposure to extremely low-frequency (50 Hz) electromagnetic fields enhances adult hippocampal neurogenesis in C57BL/6 mice. *Exp. Neurol.* **2014**, *261*, 328–335.
126. Hjouj, M.; Last, D. MRI study on reversible and irreversible electroporation induced BBB disruption. *PLoS ONE* **2012**, *7*, e42817. [CrossRef]
127. Cichoń, N.; Bijak, M.; Miller, E.; Saluk, J. The influence of electromagnetic fields on the pharmacokinetics of drugs in the brain: Current state of knowledge and directions for the future. *Cent. Eur. J. Immunol.* **2017**, *42*, 407–413.
128. Simpson, R.; Phillis, J. Adenosine in exercise adaptation. *Br. J. Sports Med.* **1992**, *26*, 54–58. [CrossRef] [PubMed]
129. Marcos-Contreras, O.; Martinez de Lizarrondo, S.; Bardou, I.; Orset, C.; Pruvost, M.; Anfray, A.; Frigout, Y.; Hommet, Y.; Lebouvier, L.; Montaner, J.; et al. Hyperfibrinolysis increases BBB permeability by a plasmin- and bradykinin-dependent mechanism. *Blood* **2016**, *128*, 2423–2434. [CrossRef] [PubMed]
130. Xie, Z.; Shen, Q.; Xie, C.; Lu, W.; Peng, C.; Wei, X.; Li, X.; Su, B.; Gao, C.; Liu, M. Retro-inverso bradykinin opens the door of blood-brain tumor barrier for nanocarriers in glioma treatment. *Cancer Lett.* **2015**, *369*, 144–151. [CrossRef]
131. Rodríguez-Masso', S.; Erickson, M.; Banks, W.; Ulrich, H.; Martins, A. The bradykinin B2 receptor agonist (NG291) causes rapid onset of transient BBB disruption without evidence of early brain injury. *Front. Neurosci.* **2021**, *15*, 791709. [CrossRef]
132. Domer, F.; Boertje, S.; Bing, E.; Reddix, I. Histamine- and acetylcholine-induced changes in the permeability of the BBB of normotensive and spontaneously hypertensive rats. *Neuropharmacology* **1983**, *22*, 615–619. [CrossRef]
133. Schilling, L.; Wahl, M. Opening of the BBB during cortical superfusion with histamine. *Brain Res.* **1994**, *653*, 289–296. [CrossRef]
134. Zhang, H.; Chen, Y.; Wang, Z.; Xie, G.; Liu, M.; Yuan, B.; Chai, H.; Wang, W.; Cheng, P. Implications of Gut Microbiota in Neurodegenerative Diseases. *Front. Immunol.* **2022**, *13*, 785644. [CrossRef]
135. Sherwin, E.; Bordenstein, S.R.; Quinn, J.L.; Dinan, T.G.; Cryan, J.F. Microbiota and the Social Brain. *Science* **2019**, *366*, 6465. [CrossRef]
136. Needham, B.D.; Kaddurah-Daouk, R.; Mazmanian, S.K. Gut Microbial Molecules in Behavioural and Neurodegenerative Conditions. *Nat. Rev. Neurosci.* **2020**, *21*, 717–731. [CrossRef]
137. Banks, W.A. The Blood–Brain Barrier as an Endocrine Tissue. *Nat. Rev. Endocrinol.* **2019**, *15*, 444–455. [CrossRef] [PubMed]
138. Sellge, G.; Kufer, T.A. PRR-Signaling Pathways: Learning from Microbial Tactics. *Semin. Immunol.* **2015**, *27*, 75–84. [CrossRef] [PubMed]
139. Harrington, M. For Lack of Gut Microbes, the Blood-Brain Barrier 'Leaks'. *Lab. Anim.* **2015**, *44*, 6–7. [CrossRef] [PubMed]
140. Braniste, V.; Al-Asmakh, M.; Kowal, C.; Anuar, F.; Abbaspour, A.; Tóth, M.; Korecka, A.; Bakocevic, N.; Ng, L.G.; Kundu, P.; et al. The gut microbiota influences blood-brain barrier permeability in mice. *Sci. Transl. Med.* **2014**, *6*, 263ra158, Erratum in *Sci. Transl. Med.* **2014**, *6*, 266er7.
141. Aho, V.T.E.; Houser, M.C.; Pereira, P.A.B.; Chang, J.; Rudi, K.; Paulin, L.; Hertzberg, V.; Auvinen, P.; Tansey, M.G.; Scheperjans, F. Relationships of gut microbiota, short-chain fatty acids, inflammation, and the gut barrier in Parkinson's disease. *Mol. Neurodegener.* **2021**, *16*, 6. [CrossRef] [PubMed]
142. Smith, P.M.; Howitt, M.R.; Panikov, N.; Michaud, M.; Gallini, C.A.; Bohlooly-Y, M.; Glickman, J.N.; Garrett, W.S. The microbial metabolites, short-chain fatty acids, regulate colonic Treg cell homeostasis. *Science* **2013**, *341*, 569–573. [CrossRef]
143. Honda, K.; Littman, D.R. The Microbiota in Adaptive Immune Homeostasis and Disease. *Nature* **2016**, *535*, 75–84. [CrossRef]
144. Sun, M.; He, C.; Cong, Y.; Liu, Z. Regulatory Immune Cells in Regulation of Intestinal Inflammatory Response to Microbiota. *Mucosal Immunol.* **2015**, *8*, 969–978. [CrossRef]
145. Huang, F.; Wu, X. Brain Neurotransmitter Modulation by Gut Microbiota in Anxiety and Depression. *Front. Cell Dev. Biol.* **2021**, *9*, 649103. [CrossRef]
146. Terstappen, G.; Meyer, A.; Bell, R.; Zhang, W. Strategies for delivering therapeutics across the blood-brain barrier. *Nat. Rev. Drug Discov.* **2021**, *20*, 362–383. [CrossRef]
147. Gao, X.; Xu, J.; Yao, T.; Liu, X.; Zhang, H.; Zhan, C. Peptide-decorated nanocarriers penetrating the BBB for imaging and therapy of brain diseases. *Adv. Drug Deliv. Rev.* **2022**, *187*, 114362. [CrossRef] [PubMed]
148. Zhu, Z.; Zhai, Y.; Hao, Y.; Wang, Q.; Han, F.; Zheng, W.; Hong, J.; Cui, L.; Jin, W.; Ma, S.; et al. Specific anti-glioma targeted-delivery strategy of engineered small extracellular vesicles dual-functionalised by Angiopep-2 and TAT peptides. *J. Extracell. Vesicles* **2022**, *11*, e12255. [CrossRef] [PubMed]
149. Reynolds, J.; Mahajan, S. Transmigration of tetraspanin 2 (Tspan2) siRNA via microglia derived exosomes across the blood brain barrier modifies the production of immune mediators by microglia cells. *J. NeuroImmune Pharmacol. Off. J. Soc. NeuroImmune Pharmacol.* **2020**, *15*, 554–563. [CrossRef]
150. Ma, F.; Yang, L.; Sun, Z.; Chen, J.; Rui, X.; Glass, Z.; Xu, Q. Neurotransmitter-derived lipidoids (NT-lipidoids) for enhanced brain delivery through intravenous injection. *Sci. Adv.* **2020**, *6*, eabb4429. [CrossRef] [PubMed]
151. Fenno, L.; Yizhar, O.; Deisseroth, K. The development and application of optogenetics. *Annu. Rev. Neurosci.* **2011**, *34*, 389–412. [CrossRef] [PubMed]

152. Gradinaru, V.; Mogri, M.; Thompson, K.R.; Henderson, J.M.; Deisseroth, K. Optical deconstruction of parkinsonian neural circuitry. *Science* **2009**, *324*, 354–359. [CrossRef]
153. McDannold, N.; Maier, S.E. Magnetic resonance acoustic radiation force imaging. *Med. Phys.* **2015**, *42*, 4838–4846. [CrossRef]
154. Zhu, L.; Wang, L.V. Photoacoustic tomography: Applications and advances. *Photons Plus Ultrasound Imaging Sens.* **2013**, *8581*, 85810V.
155. Zlokovic, B.V. The blood-brain barrier in health and chronic neurodegenerative disorders. *Neuron* **2008**, *57*, 178–201. [CrossRef]
156. Pardridge, W.M. Receptor mediated peptide transport through the blood-brain barrier. *Endocr. Metab. Immune Disord.-Drug Targets* **2016**, *16*, 182–187.
157. Spencer, B.J.; Verma, I.M. Targeted delivery of proteins across the blood-brain barrier. *Proc. Natl. Acad. Sci. USA* **2007**, *104*, 7594–7599. [CrossRef] [PubMed]
158. Zhang, B.; Sun, X.; Mei, H.; Wang, Y.; Liao, Z.; Chen, J.; Zhang, Q. LDLR-mediated peptide-22-conjugated nanoparticles for dual-targeting therapy of brain glioma. *Biomaterials* **2019**, *217*, 119264. [CrossRef] [PubMed]
159. Yu, Y.J.; Zhang, Y.; Kenrick, M.; Hoyte, K.; Luk, W.; Lu, Y.; Atwal, J.; Elliott, J.M.; Prabhu, S.; Watts, R.J.; et al. Boosting brain uptake of a therapeutic antibody by reducing its affinity for a transcytosis target. *Sci. Transl. Med.* **2011**, *3*, 84ra44. [CrossRef]
160. Niewoehner, J.; Bohrmann, B.; Collin, L.; Urich, E.; Sade, H.; Maier, P.; Neumann, U. Increased brain penetration and potency of a therapeutic antibody using a monovalent molecular shuttle. *Neuron* **2014**, *81*, 49–60. [CrossRef] [PubMed]
161. Couch, J.A.; Yu, Y.J.; Zhang, Y. The blood-brain barrier and beyond: Strategies for advancing brain drug delivery. *Drug Discov. Today Technol.* **2017**, *25*, 63–71.
162. Haney, M.; Klyachko, N.; Zhao, Y.; Gupta, R.; Plotnikova, E.; He, Z.; Patel, T.; Piroyan, A.; Sokolsky, M.; Kabanov, A.; et al. Exosomes as drug delivery vehicles for Parkinson's disease therapy. *J. Control. Release Off. J. Control. Release Soc.* **2015**, *207*, 18–30. [CrossRef]
163. Wang, J.; Shi, Y.; Yu, S.; Wang, Y.; Meng, Q.; Liang, G.; Eckenhoff, M.; Wei, H. Intranasal administration of dantrolene increased brain concentration and duration. *PLoS ONE* **2020**, *15*, e0229156. [CrossRef]
164. Qweider, M.; Gilsbach, J.; Rohde, V. Inadvertent intrathecal vincristine administration: A neurosurgical emergency. *Case Rep. J. Neurosurg. Spine* **2007**, *6*, 280–283. [CrossRef]
165. Nassan, M.; Videnovic, A. Circadian rhythms in neurodegenerative disorders. *Nat. Rev. Neurol.* **2022**, *18*, 7–24. [CrossRef]
166. Zhang, S.; Yue, Z.; Arnold, D.; Artiushin, G.; Sehgal, A. A circadian clock in the BBB regulates xenobiotic efflux. *Cell* **2018**, *173*, 130–139. [CrossRef]
167. Deisseroth, K. Optogenetics. *Nat. Methods* **2011**, *8*, 26–29. [CrossRef] [PubMed]
168. Moriyama, Y.; Nguyen, J. Rapid initiation of guided focused ultrasound-induced BBB disruption using radiofrequency. *Ultrasonics* **2009**, *49*, 566–573.
169. Dromi, S.; Frenkel, V.; Luk, A.; Traughber, B.; Angstadt, M.; Bur, M.; Wood, B.J. Pulsed-high intensity focused ultrasound and low temperature–sensitive liposomes for enhanced targeted drug delivery and antitumor effect. *Clin. Cancer Res.* **2007**, *13*, 2722–2727. [CrossRef] [PubMed]
170. Poon, C.; McMahon, D.; Hynynen, K. Noninvasive and targeted drug delivery to the brain using focused ultrasound. *ACS Chem. Neurosci.* **2017**, *8*, 16–26.
171. Cui, B.; Cho, S. Blood-brain barrier-on-a-chip for brain disease modeling and drug testing. *BMB Rep.* **2022**, *55*, 213–219. [CrossRef]
172. Hajal, C.; Le Roi, B.; Kamm, R.; Maoz, B. Biology and Models of the Blood-Brain Barrier. *Annu. Rev. Biomed. Eng.* **2021**, *23*, 359–384. [CrossRef]
173. Peng, B.; Hao, S.; Tong, Z.; Bai, H.; Pan, S.; Lim, K.; Li, L.; Voelcker, N.; Huang, W. Blood-brain barrier (BBB)-on-a-chip: A promising breakthrough in brain disease research. *Lab. Chip* **2022**, *22*, 3579–3602. [CrossRef]
174. Hynynen, K.; McDannold, N. MRI-guided focused ultrasound for brain therapy. *Handb. Clin. Neurol.* **2019**, *161*, 323–335.
175. O'Reilly, M.A.; Hynynen, K. Blood-brain barrier: Real-time feedback-controlled focused ultrasound disruption by using an acoustic emissions-based controller. *Radiology* **2012**, *263*, 96–106. [CrossRef]
176. Dammann, P.; Krafft, A.J.; Robertson, V. Overcoming the blood-brain barrier: An overview of intranasal, magnetic, and ultrasound-mediated drug delivery. *J. Control. Release* **2020**, *329*, 471–482.
177. Jordão, J.F.; Thévenot, E.; Hynynen, K. Focused ultrasound-mediated BBB disruption as a strategy for the treatment of Alzheimer's disease. *J. Alzheimer's Dis.* **2013**, *34*, 289–294.
178. Mesiwala, A.H.; Farrell, L.; Wenzel, H.J. High-intensity focused ultrasound selectively disrupts the BBB in vivo. *Appl. Phys. Lett.* **2002**, *80*, 4201–4203.
179. Ting, C.Y.; Fan, C.H.; Liu, H.L. Combining microbubbles and ultrasound for drug delivery to brain tumors: Current progress and overview. *Theranostics* **2018**, *8*, 1054.
180. Yang, F.Y.; Liu, S.H. Enhancing of BBB permeability using ultrasound. *World J. Radiol.* **2012**, *4*, 345.
181. Cho, E.E.; Drazic, J.; Hynynen, K. Biophysical mechanisms of BBB opening using focused ultrasound and microbubbles. *APL Bioeng.* **2018**, *2*, 031701.
182. Frenkel, V. Ultrasound mediated delivery of drugs and genes to solid tumors. *Adv. Drug Deliv. Rev.* **2008**, *60*, 1193–1208. [CrossRef]
183. Price, R.J.; Fisher, D.G.; Suk, J.S. Targeted drug delivery with focused ultrasound-induced BBB opening using acoustically-activated nanodroplets. *J. Control. Release* **2020**, *293*, 210–220.

184. Staahl, B.T.; Doudna, J.A. CRISPR-Cas9: A tool for qualitative and quantitative genetic assessment. *ACS Chem. Biol.* **2016**, *11*, 532–534.
185. Yang, F.; Li, X. Using artificial intelligence to improve the precision of focused ultrasound therapy. *Ultrasound Med. Biol.* **2019**, *45*, 12–25.
186. Chaplin, V.; Lafon, C. Machine learning-based prediction of therapeutic outcomes in focused ultrasound. *Ultrasound Med. Biol.* **2020**, *46*, 427–437.

*pharmaceutics*

MDPI

*Review*

# Cell-Penetrating and Targeted Peptides Delivery Systems as Potential Pharmaceutical Carriers for Enhanced Delivery across the Blood–Brain Barrier (BBB)

**Soma Mondal Ghorai [1], Auroni Deep [1], Devanshi Magoo [2], Chetna Gupta [3] and Nikesh Gupta [4,*]**

1 Department of Zoology, Hindu College, University of Delhi, Delhi 110007, India
2 Department of Chemistry, Hindu College, University of Delhi, Delhi 110007, India
3 Department of Chemistry, Hansraj College, University of Delhi, Delhi 110007, India
4 Pharmaceutical Sciences Division, School of Pharmacy, University of Wisconsin-Madison, WI 53705, USA
* Correspondence: nikesh.gupta@wisc.edu or nikeshgupta@yahoo.com

**Citation:** Ghorai, S.M.; Deep, A.; Magoo, D.; Gupta, C.; Gupta, N. Cell-Penetrating and Targeted Peptides Delivery Systems as Potential Pharmaceutical Carriers for Enhanced Delivery across the Blood–Brain Barrier (BBB). *Pharmaceutics* **2023**, *15*, 1999. https://doi.org/10.3390/pharmaceutics15071999

Academic Editors: Nicolas Tournier and Toshihiko Tashima

Received: 16 March 2023
Revised: 25 June 2023
Accepted: 11 July 2023
Published: 21 July 2023



**Abstract:** Among the challenges to the 21st-century health care industry, one that demands special mention is the transport of drugs/active pharmaceutical agents across the blood–brain barrier (BBB). The epithelial-like tight junctions within the brain capillary endothelium hinder the uptake of most pharmaceutical agents. With an aim to understand more deeply the intricacies of cell-penetrating and targeted peptides as a powerful tool for desirable biological activity, we provide a critical review of both CPP and homing/targeted peptides as intracellular drug delivery agents, especially across the blood–brain barrier (BBB). Two main peptides have been discussed to understand intracellular drug delivery; first is the cell-penetrating peptides (CPPs) for the targeted delivery of compounds of interest (primarily peptides and nucleic acids) and second is the family of homing peptides, which specifically targets cells/tissues based on their overexpression of tumour-specific markers and are thus at the heart of cancer research. These small, amphipathic molecules demonstrate specific physical and chemical modifications aimed at increased ease of cellular internalisation. Because only a limited number of drug molecules can bypass the blood–brain barrier by free diffusion, it is essential to explore all aspects of CPPs that can be exploited for crossing this barrier. Considering siRNAs that can be designed against any target RNA, marking such molecules with high therapeutic potential, we present a synopsis of the studies on synthetic siRNA-based therapeutics using CPPs and homing peptides drugs that can emerge as potential drug-delivery systems as an upcoming requirement in the world of pharma- and nutraceuticals.

**Keywords:** cell-penetrating peptides (CPPs); endosomal entrapment; homing peptides; blood–brain barrier (BBB); tumour-specific markers; siRNA-CPP delivery

## 1. Introduction

There are considerable breakthrough discoveries on the structure and development of synthetic and natural drugs that have gained importance in science and clinical studies. Often, scientists from around the globe create compounds that possess the potential to revolutionise health sciences. However, not all of them produce significant results when administered. Brain tumours and associated cancers are often fatal to patients because treatment such as chemotherapy is complicated due to extensive intratumoral heterogeneity that renders poor penetration of the drugs through the blood–brain barrier (BBB), causing less bioavailability of drugs and a lack of selective tumour targeting [1]. Thus, the success of any drug requires a comprehensive analysis of its mode of action as well as a study of the system targeted by the compound of interest.

A very superficial drug classification involves two terms in daily use: (i) extracellular and (ii) intracellular drug delivery. The latter has captured the attention of medicine because the introduction of various biomolecules into the cytosol (or a targeted intracellular compartment) is a powerful tool for the manifestation of desired biological activities. For a long time, transport across the lipid bilayer remained the major challenge. Micelles provided a solution to this long-encountered transportation hurdle as they could transport a series of different molecules ranging from hydrophobic drugs and proteins to genes [2]. Transport systems soon became increasingly sophisticated, and today we are the proud possessors of multiple techniques that make targeted drug delivery feasible (Figure 1). Such techniques can be conveniently identified as macro, micro, or nano techniques based on their impact resolution [3]. The passage of compounds across the plasma membrane can be obtained by membrane fusion, endocytic pathways, trans-membrane transporter proteins, and membrane-disruption-facilitated techniques such as direct cell penetration or increased permeability [4]. The last decade has witnessed a plethora of the latest techniques enabling small cell-penetrating peptides (CPPs), peptide shuttles, and brain-permeable peptide–drug conjugates (PDCs) to cross the formidable barrier of the brain parenchyma and endothelial cells. In order to achieve a delayed-release pattern, it is essential that our drugs of interest be encapsulated within biocompatible carriers that increase their plasma life and stability. As a result, peptide-based drug delivery systems have an advantage over current medications [5]. One such mechanism of intracellular drug delivery brings CPPs into the picture. Furthermore, most circulating physiological ligands are either proteins/peptides or peptide-conjugated complexes; thus, peptides are also considered the better choice for specific or targeted drug delivery.

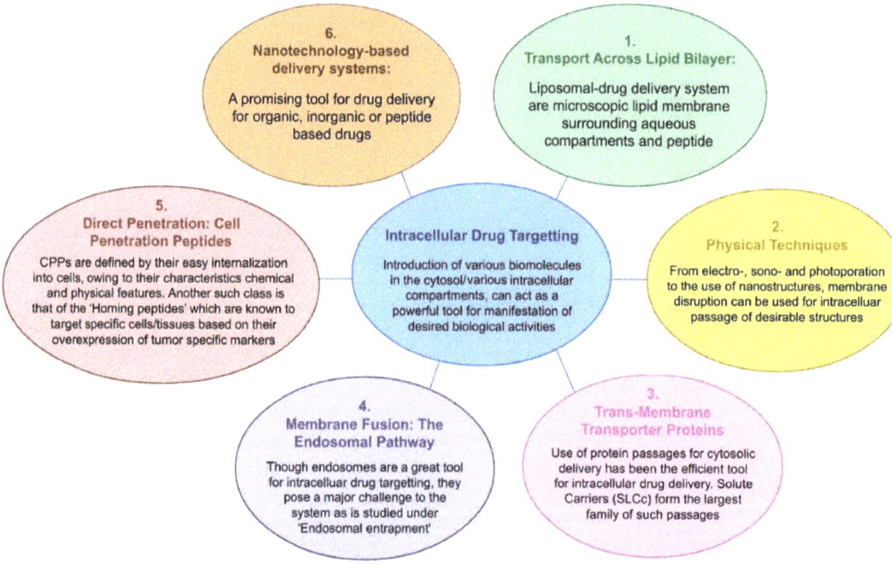


**Figure 1.** Intracellular drug targeting and the various drug-delivery pathways (the figure has been prepared using Adobe Animate CC software, https://www.adobe.com/in/products/animate.html (accessed on 24 June 2023)).

Despite the number of advantages that this system possesses, one cannot completely rule out the advantages of the lipid-mediated mechanism, which practically started the science of intracellular molecular delivery [2]. Hence, lipid–peptide conjugates have arisen as the new mediators of nutraceuticals, with increased biological stability and mechanical strength, controlled release, greater circulation time, targeted delivery, and decreased cytotoxicity [4,6]. Moreover, passage through the lipid bilayer demands optimal hydrophobicity. These distinct structural features have rendered CPPs as potential molecules in the science of drug (both biomolecule and nanoparticle) delivery. TAT-peptides conjugated to iron oxide nanoparticles were the first to be used for CPP-mediated nanoparticle delivery across the BBB [7]. Similarly, solid-lipid nanoparticles (SLNs) conjugated to TAT-peptides have been delivered to CNS without compromising the integrity of the BBB [8]. CPP-modified quantum dot-loaded polymeric micelles were prepared from a copolymer polyethylene glycol phosphatidyl ethanolamine (PEG–PE) bearing the TAT–PEG–PE linker and have been the most used CPPs for therapeutic delivery across the BBB [9].

Additional classes of targeting peptides are the 'homing peptides'. These classes of peptides have become helpful in cancer research, especially for brain tumours, as they are known to target specific cells/tissues based on their overexpression of tumour-antigens or specific markers [10]. This article focuses on peptide-based delivery systems and the implications of various ways of reaching tissues by penetrating the blood–brain barrier.

## 2. Cell-Penetrating Peptides (CPPs)

Two decades ago, the concept of peptide-transduction domains (PTDs) emerged with the observation of transcription factors that could move to and from the cell membrane as well as from one cell to another [11]. The 1988 discovery is credited to Frankel and Pabo, who demonstrated that the HIV-1 Tat (transcription-transactivating) protein not only enters the cells but also relocates to the nucleus [12]. A series of such observations, studies, and discoveries finally led to the era wherein the PTDs of CPPs can deliver drugs/medication(s) into cells of interest. Simply, CPPs can be considered the hitchhiker's ride to a predetermined destination. The transport can take place either by covalent bonding, leading to the formation of a drug–CPP conjugate [13], or by the formation of non-covalent conjugates [11]. CPPs are essentially a 15–25 long amino-acid sequence of amphipathic molecules rich in positively charged amino acids, primarily arginine. Arginine is preferred over lysine owing to the extra H-bond of the guanidium group. Naturally, all characteristic features of CPPs are primarily aimed at improving internalisation into the cells.

The Pep- and MPG families of small peptides are instances of such amphipathic cell-penetrating molecules that can form conjugates with proteins and nucleic acids, respectively, and can aid in obtaining the desired results [14]. CPPs can form peptide nucleic acid (PNA) conjugates, which can increase the uptake of therapeutic nucleic acids by cells of interest. This increase in PNA uptake by hepatocytes was studied by Ndeboko et al. to inhibit replication in duck hepatitis-B virus following a low-dose administration [15].

### *2.1. Various Strategies of CPP-Mediated Drug Delivery*

CPPs are designed to successfully deliver macromolecules into the cytosol; thus, they are used as delivery systems rather than therapeutic agents [16]. CPPs may be transported directly across the cellular membrane or by entrapment as peptides/cargo within the endosomes. Endocytic pathways usually involve one of the energy-dependent mechanisms such as phagocytosis, caveolae-mediated endocytosis (CvME), clathrin-mediated endocytosis (CME), or cholesterol-dependent endocytosis. In the uptake of peptides like TAT, polyarginine, and NickFect families of peptides (NF51/NF1), it was observed that macropinosomes are formed by rearrangement of actinic cytoskeletal elements and invagination of the cellular membrane, thus entrapping extracellular fluid [17,18]. Similarly, reordering the actinic cytoskeletal elements by clustering the caveolin-1 proteins was used for the uptake of CPPs with cargoes such as p18, p28 azurin fragment, CVP1 (chicken anaemia-derived CPP), PepFect14/DNA conjugate, and TAT via the CvME pathway [19,20]. In clathrin-mediated endocytosis (CME), the interaction of peptides with specific cell surface receptors leads to the formation of vesicles in phosphatidylinositol 4,5-biphosphate-rich regions of the plasma membrane. Thereafter, an adaptor protein binds to phosphatidylinositol 4,5-biphosphate forming coated pits where dynamin, the energy-rich GTPase, cleaves and releases the clathrin-coated vesicles with their delivery to early endosomes [21,22]. Anionic CPPs, oligo-arginine, and TAT are known to involve CME in peptide delivery to the cells [23].

At physiologically low temperatures, when a positively charged CPP interacts with the negatively charged phospholipid bilayer of a membrane, it may skip adherence to the lipid bilayer and be translocated without the aid of energy [24]. This direct translocation involves four different internalisation methods, namely, the inverted micelle model, barrel stave model, carpet-like model, and toroidal pore model [25]. In the inverted micelle model, conjugated hydrophilic CPPs interact with hydrophobic inner lipid membranes, forming hexagonal micelles that release the cargo after interaction with the inner membrane, thereby destabilising the micelle [19]. At a high concentration of CPPs and high pH, perpendicular pores are formed on the cell surfaces lined by hydrophilic residues of the CPP encircling the internal milieu of the pores; this is known as the barrel stave model [24]. Böhmová et al. proposed the toroidal pore model and carpet-like model for direct translocation [22]. In the toroidal model, the hydrophilic residues of CPPs are associated with the polar lipid heads, forming a wall that houses both the inserted peptides within the hydrophilic phospholipid cell membrane and, in the carpet model, this interaction leads to remodelling of the cellular membrane as internalisation occurs without the hydrophobic core, forming a hole in the membrane (Figure 2).

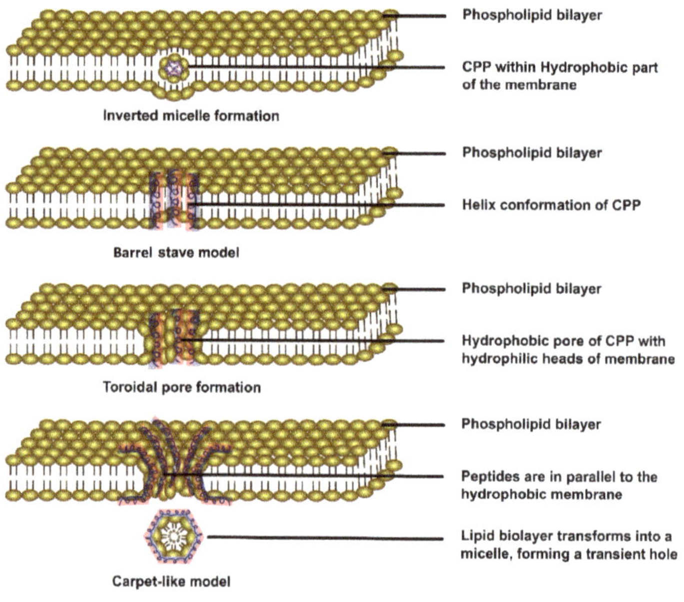


**Figure 2.** Graphical representation of the direct internalisation of CPPs via cell membranes. The blue and red colours represent the hydrophilic and hydrophilic parts of the peptide, respectively [25] (the figure has been created using Adobe Animate CC software, https://www.adobe.com/in/products/animate.html (accessed on 25 June 2023)).

### 2.2. *Escape of CPPs from Endosomal Entrapment and Protease Degradation*

CPPs at low levels are classically internalised via endocytic pathways, and the macromolecules used as therapeutic peptides often enter cells and become entrapped inside endosomes. Endosomal escape represents a major hurdle for the usage of CPPs as delivery systems and/or therapeutics [26,27]. The endosome escape route for CPPs is difficult to envisage and still not fully understood [28,29]. However, the endosomal escape of CPPs can be achieved if they are translocated in the cytosol where the therapeutic targets are situated without disturbing the endosomal membranes or causing toxicity. In this section of the manuscript, we present the many strategies mentioned in the literature as well as some future directions that indicate the mechanisms by which CPPs can escape endosomal entrapment.

Cell toxicity caused by strong peptide–lipid interactions may be harmful to the cell but may help the CPP to escape the endosomal membrane. Thus, key properties may be harnessed for the selective benefit of CPPs. Endosomes undergo the high synthesis of bis(monoacylglycerol)phosphate (BMP) in the late phase, which makes them more acidic on maturation. This shift in pH driven by a proton pump facilitates some CPPs to undergo alterations in their three-dimensional structure and helps them to cross endosomal membranes [30–32].

In some studies, it has been shown that a six-polyethylene glycol unit (PEG-P6-GFWFG) TAT used as a CPP, in combination with hydrophobic endosomal escape domains (EEDs), significantly downregulated cellular toxicity while sustaining cell-penetrating capabilities [33]. Histidine residues with the imidazole group changed to positively charged motifs at a pH below 6; hence, poly-histidine sequences contribute to endosomal escape [34]. This was successfully demonstrated in delivering plasmid DNA with the reporter protein luciferase to human glioma cells in the brain using TAT, covalently attached to 10 His residues (TAT10H) [35].

In 2014, Qian et al. proposed that the cyclic peptide cFΦR4, commonly used for stability, could be strategically internalised through endocytosis, and thereafter escape from endosomes [36]. Along similar lines, oligomerisation of CPPs is also considered a resourceful approach to counter endosomal entrapment. A CPP TAT (dfTAT) was designed to form dimers between two Cys residues, which enhanced cytosolic release by 90-fold, whereas its earlier efficiency was only 1% [37]. This suggested that these peptides reach the cytosol via endocytosis and escape because of pH acidification [38]. Moreover, chirality improved the stability and penetration ability of D-dfTAT. This peptide also showed better resistance to protease digestion and enhanced the lytic ability of the endosome membrane.

The CPPs that can successfully overcome endosomal entrapment usually employ the following mechanisms to escape endosomes: (a) Budding: This proposal has recently gained prominence as it is very likely that high concentrations of CPPs can lead to the formation of smaller vesicles by cutting off from the original endosome that readily degrades and releases their content [39]. (b) Membrane disruption: CPPs are known to possess positively charged surfaces that tend to react with negatively charged acyl chains of phospholipid headgroups of the lipid bilayer. This causes transient disruption of the endosomal membrane and the release of cargoes [40,41]. (c) Proton sponge effect: The sustained influx of protons into the luminal space of endosomes causes the internalisation of chloride ions, which leads to the osmotic imbalance and mechanical disintegration of endosomes [42,43]. Of late, studies have claimed the proton sponge hypothesis to be non-feasible and unrealistic [44,45]. (d) Pore formation: Considering CPPs as bacterial endotoxins, they behave similarly by inserting and oligomerising into the lipid bilayer. The hydrophobic cores of CPPs form defined pores that make the endosomal membrane permeable to release the inside content [46,47]. This theory has also been challenged as few macromolecules are delivered into the cytosol that are larger than the pore diameter created by peptide oligomerisation [48]. Mechanisms to escape endosomal entrapment is illustrated in Figure 3A–D.

Clearly, there is no 'rule of thumb' to overcome this challenge of endosomal entrapment. It is an uphill task to achieve a win–win situation of not breaking the cell membrane while breaking free from the endosomal membrane. To achieve endosomal selectivity, several factors that affect cellular uptake and translocation across the plasma membrane should be employed. The uptake of cargo depends first on the composition of the lipid and protein content of the plasma membrane and second on the concentration and physiochemical properties of the peptide and its cargo. CPPs with a high positive charge, e.g., more arginine domain with the guanidinium group as well as amphipathic peptides, are better suited for direct cellular uptake than endocytosis. Generally, at high concentrations, direct transportation occurs by temporarily destabilising the plasma membrane and, at low concentrations, endocytosis is observed. Transportan, a primary amphipathic CPP, and arginine-rich CPPs at low concentrations are mainly endocytosed, while rapid cytoplasm entry occurs at higher concentrations. Similarly, at higher concentrations, CPPs like R8, R9, and TAT are taken up via vesicular structures like clathrin or endosomes and, at low concentrations, uptake mainly occurs via nonendocytic nucleation zones or direct transportation across the plasma membrane. But there are many alterations to these observations. Penetratin at low concentrations leads to direct translocation, while at high quantities, endocytosis prevails [19]. Thus, CPP uptake, depending on concentration, can be more complex than envisaged.

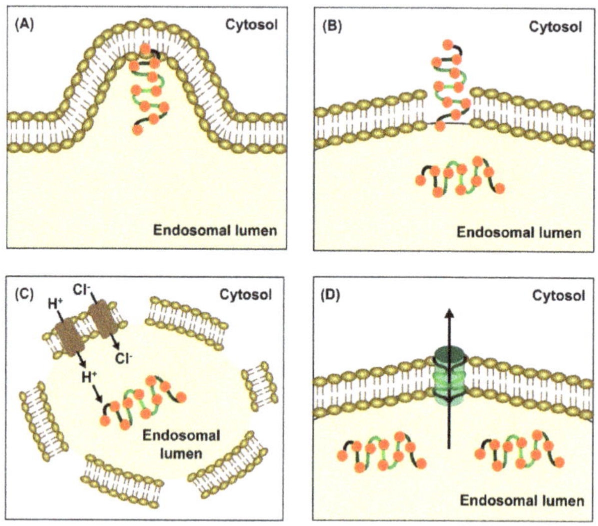


**Figure 3.** Various mechanisms to escape endosomal entrapment include (**A**) budding, (**B**) membrane disruption, (**C**) proton sponge effect, and (**D**) pore formation (the figure has been created using Adobe Animate CC software, https://www.adobe.com/in/products/animate.html (accessed on 24 June 2023)).

A recent paper by Nadal-Bufí et al. presented the strategies that form the basis of future directions towards disabling the endosomal entrapment of CPPs and releasing therapeutic peptides to their targeted site [49]. First, CPPs should be designed to deliver therapeutic peptides by the optimisation of EEDs or the identification of new EED sequences. EEDs characteristically have cationic and hydrophobic residues that can selectively bind and disrupt cell membranes and reduce toxicity. Among the natural sources, virus and antimicrobial peptides possess high lytic activity and active membrane properties; thus, they can be employed to design EEDs. Also, at an acidic pH, the overall positive charge of CPPs is enhanced, which improves cellular uptake and endosomal escape. Incorporating Arg-residues within the sequence of CPPs can be an approach to increase the positive charge against endosome membranes with a high proportion of negatively charged lipids. Thus, cyclisation of stereochemical changes in CPPs can increase their uptake as well as improve endosomal escape [50]. However, there is no certainty in some CPPs that have the capacity to permeabilise and escape from endosomal membranes to reach the cytosol [51]. Moreover, sometimes the cargo itself can change the properties of CPPs; thus, a sound understanding is required to judiciously strategise therapeutic CPPs that can target intracellular proteins as well as escape endosomal entrapment.

Targeting peptides face another problem of proteolytic degradation within the cellular compartments. Nanomaterial-based drug delivery systems have been proven to cross the BBB either by carrier-mediated transcytosis (CMT), adsorptive-mediated transcytosis (AMT), or receptor-mediated transcytosis (RMT) and have often offered protection to proteolysis. Lipid-based nanoparticles (NPs) with surface modifications via transferrin, lactoferrin, glucose, and glutathione polyethylene (PEG) are more effective in BBB permeability. PEGylation of gold and silica NPs have also been shown to increase biocompatibility. Polymeric-based NPs such as chitosan, hydroxyl polyamidoamine (PAMAM), and poly (D,L-lactide-co-glycolide) (PLGA) have better physical and chemical properties and are highly resistant to degradation [52].

The modification of peptide sequences including amino acid incorporation within the backbone or the non-canonical side chains, enantio/retro-enantio isomerisation, and the cyclisation of N and C-termini further enhances protease resistance. Peptides modified with such changes are termed 'peptidomimetics'. N and C termini modifications prevent exoprotease-mediated hydrolysis. Backbone changes like isosteric replacement of amide bonds, carbon skeleton extension or amide alkylation, N-methylation and α-methylation, or the addition of β or γ amino acid residues impart protection from endoproteases. These changes increase lipophilicity by reducing hydrogen bond formation, thereby enabling peptides to cross biological barriers. The D-enantiomeric amino acid is usually a 'retro-enantio isomer' that displays side chain topology like that of its native L-form with inverted amide bonds. Such retro-enantio isomers have reduced immunogenicity and are resistant to proteolytic degradation. Cyclical peptides have better biological activity than linear peptides as the cyclical configuration is mostly favoured for high peptide affinity due to better binding of the target protein [53].

## 3. Homing Peptides for Targeted Drug Delivery

One class of tumour-homing peptides (THPs) includes 3–15 residues and long, receptor-specific peptide molecules wherein the target receptors can vary from intracellular to cell-surface bound receptor molecules [10]. THPs can be characterised and identified based on specific sequences that can recognise and bind to receptors widely expressed in tumour cells. Integrins are among such commonly recognised cell-surface receptors. These receptors play a primary role in anchorage by binding cells to the extra-cellular matrix. These integrins can identify short peptide sequences or tripeptides like Arg-Gly-Asp (RGD) [54]. This RGD peptide was the first to be documented against endothelial cell integrins [55]. Such peptides are known to form many drug conjugates, thus easing the process of drug delivery owing to their strikingly small sizes and low molecular weights. Another similar tripeptide, NGR (Asn-Gly-Arg), is known to target the endothelial cells of neoangiogenic vessels [56]. To bring our drugs from paper to practice, these small peptides can conveniently act as vehicles for targeted drug delivery. Hence, these peptides are now at the heart of advanced cancer medicine and associated research.

Unlike the CPPs that can be internalised by diverse cell lineages, THPs show receptor-mediated, endocytic cellular internalisation and are hence increasingly relevant for lineage- or tumour-specific drug targeting [57]. Evidently, in addition to chemical composition, specificity, mode of action, and physiological impacts, another essential criterion for drug selection is the time of action. Certain conditions might demand delayed or sustained drug release while others might call for an immediate or burst release. Most SOS or over-the-counter medications should ideally belong to the latter class. Both CPPs and THPs can be manipulated for temporally monitored administration of drugs. This conclusion can be easily drawn because the collective process of THP binding and incorporation into a target cell requires less than 120 min [57]. A series of studies on colon-cancer-homing peptides (CPP2) and myeloid-leukaemia-homing peptides (CPP44) brought us to believe that these homing peptides are taken up in an ATP-dependent manner and that their internalisation is not influenced by serum components. In addition, certain CPPs such as CPP44 show selective and preferential entry in tumour cell lines only [58]. This selectivity can be a tool in minimising or altogether negating the adverse physiological impacts of cancer medications and therapies.

## 4. Peptide-Mediated Drug Delivery Systems across the Blood–Brain Barrier

### *4.1. Introduction to the Blood–Brain Barrier (BBB)*

The brain, like all other vital organs of the body, needs nutrients and gases to function properly. It is substantially protected by three coatings of meninges protecting the

BBB from overexposure to potassium, glutamate, and glycine, which, at increased concentrations, can be neurotoxic [59]. Armed with a widespread blood capillary network, the BBB is considered an important barrier that regulates drug molecule access to the brain parenchyma. Tight junctions (TJs) and adherens junctions (AJs) are the two main junctional complexes of the BBB that regulate the influx and efflux of substances through the paracellular pathway connecting the endothelial cells of brain capillaries. Apart from the BBB, the blood–cerebrospinal fluid barrier (BCSFB), circumventricular organ barrier (CVOB), and arachnoid barrier (AB) filter out small and large drug molecules and 98% of pharmaceuticals [60]. In most cases, it has been noted that most drugs remain inaccessible to the brain as they are flushed out by the BBB via the return journey of the CSF to the blood or through the transporters present in the brain parenchymal cells [61]. The extracellular base membrane, a layer of endothelial cells (ECs) connected to astrocytes (ACs) and pericytes (PCs), and microglia form the neurovascular units (NVUs) of the BBB, which stops the penetration of drugs into the CNS [62,63]. Drugs administered via intravenous routes are unable to cross NVUs, which has remained a challenge to date [64].

Several ways of transport are known that enable drug molecules, lipid-soluble small molecules, weak bases, and electrically neutral solutes to diffuse passively across the BBB, as shown in (Figure 4) [65,66]. Any drug molecules that can passively diffuse across the BBB should have a molecular weight of less than 400 Da, good lipophilicity, a log of the octanol–water partition coefficient (logPo/w) between five and six, and fewer than eight hydrogen bonding groups [67,68]. This passive diffusion may transfer nutrients/drugs by passing through the intracellular space (paracellular) or moving solutes through a cell (transcellular). Regrettably, it has been determined that more than 98% of drugs targeted to CNS cannot cross the BBB at the minimum therapeutic concentration [18]. Thus, CPPs and homing peptides are new strategies anticipated to escape the BBB, thereby improving drug delivery to the CNS [59].

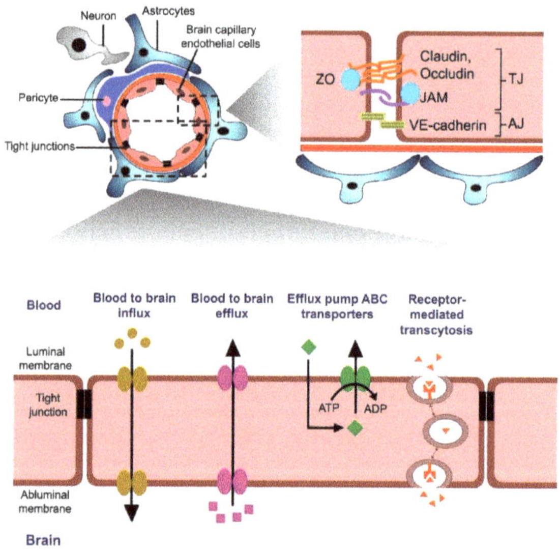


**Figure 4.** Various cellular interactions and the transport across the blood–brain barrier (the figure has been created using Adobe Animate CC software, https://www.adobe.com/in/products/animate.html (accessed on 24 June 2023)) [66,69].

### 4.2. Cell-Penetrating Peptides as Delivery Systems across the Blood–Brain Barrier

CPPs are the peptide-based drug delivery system that holds promising and attainable prospects to deliver drugs to the brain. These small synthetic peptide shuttles (containing natural amino acids) enable the influx of a varied range of small molecules across the BBB. These natural peptides are derived from various sources, namely, HIV proteins (TAT, RI-OR2-TAT), the rabies virus (RVG-29), phage receptors (Pep-22, TGN, G23, T7, THR), venom neurotoxins (Apanin, MinApa4), and neurotropic endogenous peptides (regulon polypeptides, RAP, angiopep-2). Incidentally, although these compounds are highly pathogenic or toxic, they are reported to be non-toxic to neuronal cells [70].

Despite the well-studied ability of CPPs to enter mammalian cells, it is only a few fragmentary studies that mention their transcellular aspects [71]. A study conducted on Caco-2, the human colon cancer cell line, investigated the differential penetration of three different CPPs across the plasma membrane, namely, transportan, penetratin, and TP-10, and it was concluded that Transportan and transportan analogue TP-10 traverse the membrane primarily by a transcellular mechanism [72]. Similar studies conducted for Tat proteins showed a plasma–membrane permeation barrier in well-differentiated epithelial cell lines, i.e., Caco-2 and MDCK, which was absent in HeLa [73]. A BBB transport study conducted for such peptides demonstrated wavering levels of cell penetration wherein the Tat basic proteins showed a greater degree of cellular entry compared to the transportan peptides. Also, it was deciphered that the mere cell-penetrating ability of CPPs is not indicative of their ability to traverse the BBB [71]. The blood–brain barrier is a tool for homeostasis and is selective to an extent wherein it is rendered almost impermeable [74]. As a result, certain small molecules/drugs and almost all large molecules cannot cross the BBB and hence cannot be used for therapeutic approaches. The first instance of the transport of a biologically active compound in the brain was shown by fusing the beta-galactosidase protein to the protein transduction domain (PTD) of the Tat-protein (Figure 5) [75]. Hence, experiments were conducted using conjugated drugs and the data obtained for CPP and nanomaterials showed that these conjugates could pave a path for treating CNS-associated disorders [76]. However, every advancement that has been introduced in drug delivery across the BBB has met multiple limitations and challenges owing to the complex design and the physiological impact of any disruptions that occur at the membrane. Notwithstanding these challenges, CPPs are coming up as potential tools for accomplishing such complicated drug deliveries.

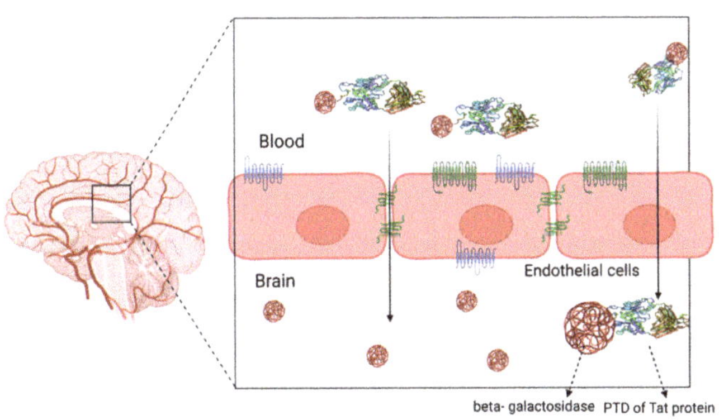


**Figure 5.** Drugs conjugated to Tat-protein can be targeted across the blood–brain barrier. CPPs can show transcellular movements either by traversing across junctions or through endocytic pathways (the figure has been created with the help of BioRender).

Most of the earlier known CPPs are either covalent or non-covalent peptide-based delivery systems. Carrier peptides have many limitations: (i) lack of biocompatibility and bioavailability; (ii) may be toxic and antigenic; (iii) lack chemical fixation; (iv) may lose specificity to the target site; and (v) may get degraded by endosomes or proteasomes. In this context, MPG and Pep families of cell-penetrating small peptides have been successfully applied to the delivery of different cargoes (siRNA and peptides) both in vitro and in vivo, especially delivering therapeutics across the BBB. Listed are those CPPs that can act as a substitute for a covalent and non-covalent strategy for the delivery of drugs across the BBB.

#### 4.2.1. Lipoprotein-Enabled Novel Shuttle Peptides

Numerous novel shuttle peptides have been explored but efficient transport to the brain must be improvised, and researchers are still seeking the perfect approach to allow drugs to pass through the BBB. Lipoproteins seem to possess a significant ability as delivery systems to cross the BBB; for example, apolipoprotein B (ApoB), and apolipoprotein E (ApoE) equivalents were found to infiltrate the BBB [77,78]. Analogues of high-affinity lipid-associated peptides, namely, Ac-mE18A-NH2, Ac-hE18A-NH2, and Ac-hE(R)18A-NH2, tagged with hApoE, showed high internalisation compared to the control (Ac-R1018A-NH2), in which the receptor-binding domain contained only the positively charged arginine (R) [79]. Brain necrosis was significantly reduced in a mouse model with a therapeutic peptide (HAYED) that was an analogue of apolipoprotein E (K16APoE) tagged to 16 lysine (K16) residue linked to a low-density lipoprotein receptor-related protein (LDLR) [80].

#### 4.2.2. Naturally Derived CPPs

Amid the naturally occurring CPPs, virus-derived peptides have revolutionised targeted drug delivery across the BBB. A rabies virus glycoprotein (RVG-29) readily docks to the nicotinic acetylcholine (nAChR) receptor located on the endothelial cell lining and neuronal cells, thus facilitating its penetration across the BBB [81]. Overexpression of the α-synuclein (α-Syn) gene is the hallmark in Parkinson's disease (PD) and the therapeutics pertain to the delivery of a shorter RVG linked to the negatively charged siRNA to suppress α-Syn. This version of RVG has a spacer of four additional glycine followed by positively charged arginine (R) at the end of the C-terminus (C2-9r (H2N-CDIFTNSRGKRAGGGGrrrrrrrrr, where r is D-arginine [82])). HIV-1-TAT peptidecan spontaneously internalise semiconductor nanowire (Si NW). TAT linked to surface SiNWs facilitates the internalisation of NW into mouse hippocampal neurons as well as into primary dorsal root ganglion (DRG) neurons [83]. Dengue virus type 2 capsid protein (*DEN2C*) can be used as a trans-BBB peptide vector as its translocation was shown to be receptor-independent while being steady with absorptive-mediated transport (AMT). One such peptide is PepH3, which shows tremendous potential for high brain penetration by crossing the BBB. This peptide is easily cleared from the brain via excretion; thus, it is a good candidate as a peptide shuttle to cargo in and out of the brain [84].

Other natural peptide-based shuttles are the venom-derived CPPs that have been demonstrated to traverse across the BBB and deliver drugs to the desired site. The monocyclic lactam-bridged peptidomimetic (MiniAp-4) analogue, derived from apamin (a neurological toxin from bee venom), was devised by minimising its intricacy, toxicity, immunogenicity, and protease resistance, while efficiently transporting drugs across the BBB into the brain parenchyma [85].

Nanoligand carrier (NLC), a brain-specific phage-derived peptide, is known to target cerebral endothelial cells via a transferrin receptor. Some phage peptides can recognise and bind their target, transit through the BBB, and reach neurons and microglial cells. NLC-β-secretase 1 (*BACE1*), another of the phage-displaying, self-assembled peptide siRNA complexes, displays effective *BACE1* suppression in the brain, without inflammation and/or toxicity. Therefore, to overcome limitations in specificity and efficacy, NLCs act as safe multifunctional CPPs or phage-display peptide nanocarriers [86]. A brain glioma cascade delivery system (AsTNP) was established by utilising an AS1411 aptamer and phage-displayed TGN peptide. The docetaxel-loaded AsTNP easily crossed the BBB and exhibited an anti-glioma effect with improved glioma survival [87]. Furthermore, two selected phage-display peptides, GLHTSATNLYLH and VAARTGEIYVPW, when co-cultured with primary rat endothelial cells and primary rat glial cells (astrocytes and microglia), crossed the BBB via active transport mechanisms [88].

#### 4.2.3. CPP-Mediated Nanocarriers

Peptidomimetic antibodies/ligands can be tailor-made by conjugating with nanocarriers that can identify transcytotic receptors on the membranous surface of the BBB for efficient delivery [89]. Nanoparticles (NPs) conjugated to drugs or diagnostics can encapsulate, adsorb, and get released at specific target sites/organs, including the brain. Biologically active polymeric NPs tagged with a TAT peptide (Tat-PEG-b-chol) can successfully deliver drugs across the BBB [90]. The polyamine (putrescine)-modified F(ab') portion of an anti-amyloid antibody formulated with chitosan nanoparticles was also delivered to the brain [91]. Polymeric NPs (PMNPs) comprised of polysaccharides, proteins, amino acids, and polyesters are most extensively studied for brain drug delivery. PMNPs allow for transit across the BBB by either disrupting the tight junctions (TJs) and mucoadhesion in the brain capillaries or via transcytosis through brain endothelial cells [92]. Poly-ethylene glycol (PEG) liposomes are extensively used to conjugate with transferrin (Tf) and poly-L-arginine (cell-penetrating peptides) for delivering brain imaging drugs and DNA [93]. TfR-specific peptide B6 and endothelial growth factor receptor (EGFR) GE11 peptide can transport siRNA across the BBB [94]. 7-amino acid glycopeptide (g7) was used to deliver responsive angiopep-2-decorated poly(lactic-co-glycolic acid) (PLGA) hybrid NPs, while methoxypolyethylene glycol (MPEG) and methoxypoly (ethylene glycol)-b-polycaprolactone (PCL) NPs conjugated with angiopep-2 accumulated in the brain [95]. K16ApoE-decorated PLGA-NPs have shown a higher uptake into the brain and provided better MRI contrast for diagnostic purposes [96].

#### 4.2.4. CPP-Enabled Metallic Nanopeptides (NPs)

Metallic NPs are another form of nanocarriers that are extensively used to improve imaging as they can effectively cross the BBB. Also, glutathione (GSH)-conjugated iron NPs (GSHIONPs) forming IONPs@Asp-PTX-PEG-GSH are steady, non-toxic, and show improved MRI contrast for brain imaging [97]. In comparison to normal NPs, maleic anhydride-coated superparamagnetic iron oxide nanoparticles (Mal-SPIONs) showed improved dissemination to the thalamus, temporal lobe, and frontal cortex, [98]. Gold NPs conjugated to TAT (AuNPs-TAT) or glioma-specific peptide chlorotoxin (CTX) (Au PENPs) and showed improved cellular uptake in the brain [99]. Silicon NPs (pSiNPs) delivered siRNA across the BBB to treat brain gliomas with rabies virus-mimetic silica-coated gold nanorods [100].

#### 4.2.5. CPP-Enabled Exosomes

Exosomes are naturally produced by dendritic cells, monocytes, and macrophages with characteristic layers of lipids containing many adhesive proteins that help them interact well with the cellular membranes without getting entrapped within mononuclear phagocytes [101]. Thus, these have been explored to enhance the delivery of incorporated drugs to target cells, including the brain [102]. Exosomes derived from dendritic cells were used for combining neuron-specific RVG peptide tagged with lysosome-associated membrane protein 2b (*Lamp2b*) to carry siRNA into mouse brains. It was observed that serum levels for interleukin (IL)-6, tumour necrosis factor (TNF)-$\alpha$, interferon gamma-induced protein (IP)-10, and interferon (IFN)-$\alpha$ serum substantially increased compared to those of siRNA-RVG-9R [103]. Dendritic cell-derived exosomes with interferon-$\gamma$ were used to deliver miR-219, which increased myelination in rats' brains [104]. The bioavailability of curcumin was increased by loading it onto exosomes, using it as a drug to treat brain lesions with cyclo-peptide (c(RGDyK)) [79,80], or as imaging material by conjugating it with a neuroleptin-1-targeted peptide [105]. Exosomes derived from bone marrow loaded with siRNA and RVG (targeting ligand) successfully decreased the $\alpha$-Syn accumulation in the brain observed in patients with progressive Parkinson's disease [106].

#### 4.2.6. CPP-Enabled Liposomes

In the last two decades, liposomes have been studied extensively as effective methods for drug delivery to the brain. Liposomal NPs usually get self-assembled within the phospholipid bilayer of the plasma membrane and can integrate into other biological membranes. The cationic liposome-siRNA-peptide (RVG-9r) containing cationic lipid octadecenolyoxy[ethyl-2-heptadecenyl-3 hydroxyethyl] imidazolinium chloride bound to the peptide moiety nAChRs penetrated the BBB to deliver siRNA into FVB mouse brains [107] with liposomes containing 1,2-dioleoyl-3-trimethylammonium-propane (DOTAP) or 1,2-distearoyl-sn-glycero-3-phosphoethanolamine (DSPE) complexed with siRNA and RVG peptides and target prions [108]. Cationic liposome-siRNA-peptide (RVG-9r) penetrated the BBB and reduced the effect of prion protein expression in the brain [109]. Analgesic peptides (kyotorphin or leu-enkephalin) self-assembled and encapsulated in a quaternary methyl ester derivative of methyl vernolate vesicles were successfully delivered to mouse brains [110]. Stable nucleic acid lipid particles (SNALPs) decorated with RVG-9r peptide liposomes crossed the BBB and delivered siRNA that eliminated mutant ataxin-3 (SCA3) in the brain of Machado–Joseph disease mouse models [111]. In certain tumour growths, liposomal receptor-related protein 1 (*LRP1*) was conjugated with GRN1005, a peptide drug that limited malignant growth [112].

#### 4.2.7. Angiopep-Conjugated Polyethyleneglycol-Adapted Polyamidoamine Dendrimer (PAMAM–PEG–Angiopep)

PAMAM–PEG–angiopep/DNA NPs are dendrimer nanoparticles that were combined with apolipoprotein A-I (ApoA-I) and NL4-peptide, shown to be efficient carriers across the BBB. PAMAM is a surface primary amino group and has shown clathrin- and caveolae-mediated endocytosis of the nanocarriers comprising angiopep peptides. Intravenous injection of dendrimer nanoparticles of PAMAM–PEG–angiopep loaded with pEGFP plasmid was given to mice. Compared to the control groups of PAMAM/DNA NPs, gene expression was observed in all four regions of the mouse brains for the PAMAM–PEG–angiopep/DNA NPs, although cationic dendrimers showed haemolytic activity and cell cytotoxicity [113]. A combination of short interfering RNA (siRNA) with polyamidoamine (PAMAM) dendrimers (D) was observed to achieve silencing activity. The silencing capacity of the complex depended on D generation (G4, G5, G6, and G7), ionic strength, and N/P ratio (nitrogen amines in D/phosphate in siRNA). This assay revealed that structurally stable complexes could be formed independent of the ionic strength with N/P ratios of 5 (for G4, G5) and 10 (for G6, G7) that could penetrate the brain with minimal cytotoxicity [114]. However, even low-generation lysine dendrons (G0 and G1) conjugated with ApoE-derived peptide traversed through the BBB without any significant cytotoxicity (as noticed in up to 400 μM concentrations) [115].

Peptide-based drug delivery systems across the BBB have pros and cons such as low alteration in the BBB integrity, specific targeting and reduced toxicity, and some concerns associated with serum stability. NPs, shuttle peptides, liposomes, exosomes, and dendrimers conjugated with CPPs have shown much-enhanced permeability across the BBB. Although advances have been achieved with CPPs to cross the BBB, it has been shown that in many cases, CPPs selectively cross the BBB, which does not qualify the peptides as having effective BBB-penetrating ability. The differential influx property exhibited by CPPs can be attributed to their cationic nature (presence or absence of arginine residues), physicochemical properties (secondary structure at the membrane interface), and biological properties (cellular uptake ability) [71]. The arena of targeting and crossing the BBB is a challenging yet promising field. In-depth understanding of drug properties (pharmacokinetics and pharmacodynamics) and BBB at the molecular level is paramount to design and develop a CNS drug. Notwithstanding the many advances in drug delivery systems, there is still an indispensable need for research into improved delivery systems with fewer limitations. Peptide-based delivery systems need further optimisation and high specificity for brain targeting.

## *4.3. Homing Peptides as Delivery Systems across the Blood–Brain Barrier (BBB)*

Brain tumours and cancers are often fatal to patients because treatments such as chemotherapy suffer from poor bioavailability and reduced permeability across the BBB coupled with extensive intratumoral heterogeneity and a lack of selective tumour targeting. Peptide–drug conjugates (PDCs) are designed to link targeted peptides via a chemical linker to a therapeutic payload that can mimic an alternate antibody–drug conjugate (ADC) and expand the therapeutic potential of various drugs (Figure 6). In the context of BBB crossing and targeting CNS diseases, PDCs are designed to hijack the endogenous BBB influx transport mechanism and smuggle drugs into the brain parenchyma. Brain-permeable peptides or BBB shuttle peptides popularly known as brain-homing and brain-penetrating molecular transport vectors are a promising lot of molecules that can overcome the BBB and deliver drug molecules to the brain. Natural strategies like the phage, certain viruses, or natural neurotropic proteins can engage in receptor-mediated transcytosis for crossing the BBB. Thus, brain-homing peptides, linkers, and brain-permeable peptide–drug conjugates (PDCs) were shown to trick the brain by allowing the passage of molecules via the endogenous transcytosis mechanism [116].

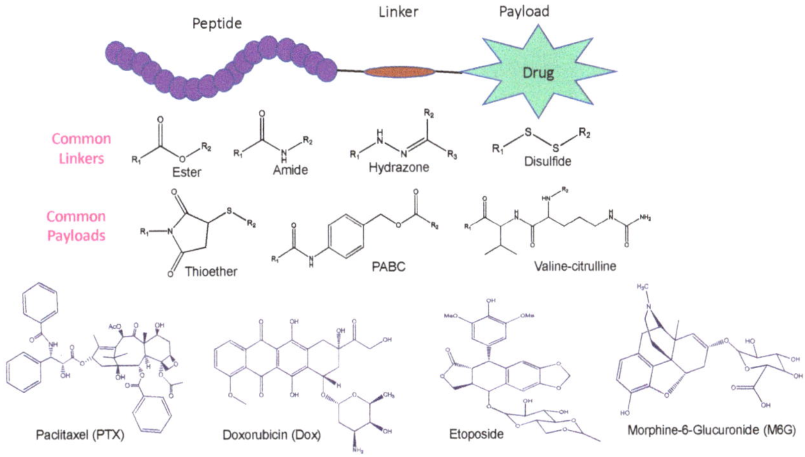


**Figure 6.** Illustration of several peptide–drug conjugates (PDCs), the chemical linkers, and the therapeutic payloads to which they are joined, and which can imitate an alternate antibody–drug conjugate (ADC).

Brain-homing peptide (BH) CNAFTPD is used to enhance the transfection efficacy of pDNA delivery across the BBB by forming biodegradable core–shell polyplexes with peptide–PEG–tris-acridine conjugates (pPAC) [117]. Similarly, a bacteria-based drug delivery system for glioblastoma (GBM) was employed as photothermal immunotherapy. Aptly called the 'Trojan bacteria', it was loaded with glucose polymer and photosensitive ICG silicon nanoparticles and shown to bypass the BBB, targeting and penetrating GBM tissues [118]. A brain-specific phage-derived peptide (nanoligand carrier, NLC) targets cerebral endothelial cells through the transferrin receptor and the receptor for advanced glycation end products. NLC-β-secretase 1 (*BACE1*) siRNA complexes are successfully delivered to neurons and microglial cells. Therefore, NLCs act as safe multifunctional nanocarriers with a wide receptor repertoire of the display peptide, which can effectively overcome the blood–brain barrier without toxicity and inflammation [119]. Recently, CNSRLHLRC, CENWWGDVC, and WRCVLREGPAGGCAWFNRHRL peptides were shown to mediate the selective localisation of phage to brain and kidney blood vessels. These peptide sequences identify selective endothelial markers to target drugs and genes in the brain and other selected tissues [120].

In glioblastoma (GBM), a debilitating brain tumour disease, a small, soluble peptide (BTP-7) covalently attaches to an insoluble anti-cancer drug, camptothecin (CPT), targeting the human GBM extracellular matrix (ECM) across the BBB [121]. Gliomas are other therapeutically problematic brain cancers with poor patient prognosis, and new drug delivery strategies are needed to achieve a more efficient chemotherapy-based approach against brain tumours. Using an in vitro phage display, fusion constructs with peptides and drugs forming Dox-SMCC-gHoPe2 have been studied where tumour-homing peptide gHo was identified as an efficient, in vivo-working vector [122]. A comprehensive summary of the cell-penetrating peptides and homing peptides used as brain drug delivery systems is provided in Table 1.

**Table 1.** List of probable CPP/homing peptides and their sequence, source, and formulations used as a target molecule against the blood–brain barrier.

| Name of the Peptide | Sequence of the Peptide | Peptide Source | Formulations/Carriers | Ref. No. |
|---|---|---|---|---|
| ApoE | LRKLRKRLL | Apolipoprotein E | Shuttle synthetic peptides | [77] |
| ApoB | SSVIDALQYKLEGTTRLTRKRGLKLA TALSLSNKFVEGS | Apolipoprotein B | Shuttle synthetic peptides | [78] |
| hApoE | LRKLRKRLLR | Human apolipoprotein E (hApoE) | Shuttle synthetic peptides | [79] |
| RVG-29 | YTIWMPENPRPGTPCDIFTNSRGKRASNG | Rabies virus glycoprotein | Shuttle natural peptide | [81] |
| TAT | GGGGYGRKKRRQRRR | Human immunodeficiency virus 1 | Shuttle natural peptide | [83] |
| PepH3 | AGILKRW | Dengue virus type 2 capsid protein (*DEN2C*) | Shuttle natural peptide | [84] |
| Apamin | H-CNCKAPETALCARRCQQH-NH2 | Venom neurotoxin | Shuttle natural peptide | [85] |
| MiniAp-4 | H-DapKAPETALD-NH2 | Venom neurotoxin | Shuttle natural peptide | [85] |
| THRre | PWVPSWMPPRHT | Phage display | Shuttle natural peptide | [86] |
| TGN | TGNYKALHPHNG | Phage display | Shuttle natural peptide | [87] |
| THR | THRPPMWSPVWP | Phage display | Shuttle natural peptide | [123] |
| THRre_2f | (PWVPSWMPPRHT)2KKGK(CF)G | Phage display | Shuttle natural peptide | [124] |
| K16APoE | HAYED | Apolipoprotein E (LDLR) | Shuttle natural peptide | [125] |
| TAT peptide | Tat-PEG-b-chol | Nanoparticles | NPs (PMNPs) | [90] |
| Polyamine (putrescine) | F(ab′) anti-amyloid antibody | Nanoparticles | Polymeric NPs (PMNPs) | [91] |
| TfR-peptide | TfR poly-L-arginine | Poly-ethylene glycol liposomes | Polymeric NPs (PMNPs) | [93] |
| GE11 peptide | TfR-endothelial factor receptor (EGFR) | siRNA/TMC–PEG-RV | Polymeric NPs (PMNPs) | [94] |
| Angiopep-2 | TFFYGGSRGKRNNFKTEEY | Neurotropic endogenous protein | Polymeric NPs (PMNPs) | [95] |
| K16APoE | HAYED | PLGA-NPs | Polymeric NPs (PMNPs) | [96] |
| g7 | GFtGPLS (O-β-d-glucose) CONH2 | Enkephalin analogues/opioid | Polymeric NPs (PMNPs) | [119,126] |
| Mal-SPIONs | $[C_2H_2(CO)_2O]Fe_2O_3$ | Superparamagnetic iron oxide nanoparticles | Metallic NPs | [88] |
| GSH-peptide | IONPs@Asp-PTX-PEG-GSH | Glutathione nanoparticles (GSHIONPs) | Metallic NPs | [97] |
| Silicon NPs | pSiNPs | Rabies virus-mimetic silica-coated gold nanorods | Metallic NPs | [100] |
| cyclo-peptide | c(RGDy)K | Macrophages/monocytes | Exosomes | [80] |
| neuron-specific RVG peptide | siRNA-RVG-9R | Dendritic cells | Exosomes | [103] |
| miR-219 | | Dendritic cells | Exosomes | [104] |
| siRNA3 RVG | | Bone marrow | Exosomes | [106] |
| siRNA-peptide | octadecenolyoxy[ethyl-2-heptadecenyl-3 hydroxyethyl] imidazolinium chloride | Bone marrow | Exosomes | [107] |
| neuroleptin-1-targeted peptide | RGERPRR | Macrophages/monocytes | Exosomes | [127] |
| siRNA-RVG peptide | 1,2-dioleoyl-3-trimethylammonium-propane (DOTAP) | Cationic liposomes | Liposomes | [108] |

**Table 1.** *Cont.*

| Name of the Peptide | Sequence of the Peptide | Peptide Source | Formulations/Carriers | Ref. No. |
|---|---|---|---|---|
| siRNA-RVG peptide | 1,2-distearoyl-sn-glycero-3-phosphoethanolamine (DSPE) | Cationic liposomes | Liposomes | [108] |
| siRNA-peptide (RVG-9r) | RVG-29-PEG-PLGA/DTX | Cationic liposomes | Liposomes | [109] |
| kyotorphin or leu-enkephalin | methyl ester-methyl vernolate | Self-assembled liposomes | Liposomes | [110] |
| siRNA-RVG peptide | Stable nucleic acid lipid particles [SNALPs] | Self-assembled liposomes | Liposomes | [111] |
| *LRP1* | ANG-PEG– poly($\varepsilon$-caprolactone) | Self-assembled liposomes | Liposomes | [102,112] |
| Angiopep peptide | TFFYGGSRGKRNNFKTEEYC | PAMAM–PEG–Angiopep/DNA | Dendrimer nanoparticles | [113] |
| ApoE derived peptide | LRKLRKRLLR | Lysine dendrons | Dendrimer nanoparticles | [115] |
| pPAC | CNAFTPD | Peptide-PEG-tris-acridine conjugates (pPAC) | Brain-homing peptide (BH) | [117] |
| phage-derived peptide | NLC-β-secretase 1 (*BACE1*) siRNA | Photosensitive ICG silicon-nanoparticles | Brain-homing peptide (BH) | [119] |
| phage-derived peptide | CNSRLHLRC, CENWWGDVC, WRCVLREGPAGGCAWFNRHRL | Nanoparticles | Brain-homing peptide (BH) | [120] |
| BTP-7 | BTP-7-Camptothecin (CPT) | Patient-derived GBM stem cells | Brain-homing peptide (BH) | [121] |
| gHoPe2 | NHQQQNPHQPPM | Phage-derived | Glioma-homing peptide (gHo) | [122] |

## 5. Cell-Penetrating Peptides and siRNA Delivery to the Central Nervous System

In the early 1990s, Napoli and Jorgensen reported posttranscriptional gene silencing in plants by RNA interference (RNAi). RNAi cleaves double-stranded or short hairpin RNA (shRNA) into functional, small interfering RNA (siRNA) with the aid of 'dicer', an endogenous mammalian protein complex that mediates RNAi. siRNAs are usually short (20–25 bp), exogenous, double-stranded RNA molecules that silence gene expression either by inhibiting transcription or by the degradation of sequence-specific target mRNA [128]. Since synthetic siRNAs can be intended against any target RNA, they have gained high therapeutic value. Indeed, siRNA-based therapeutics using small-molecule drugs can be positioned for the treatment of extensive neuronal diseases and cancers. siRNA therapeutics can also address the concerns usually posed by small-molecule drugs currently being used for targeted therapy. In vivo, targeted delivery of siRNA molecules remains a challenge due to its poor stability, reduced permeability across cellular membranes, poor endosomal escape, degradation by RNases, and rapid renal clearance. Therefore, to be effective delivery systems, siRNAs need a carrier for their protection from degradation [129]. Recently, many different approaches have been devised to deliver siRNAs into living cells by a broad variety of peptides. The simplicity of the synthesis, use, and versatility of CPPs have enabled siRNA delivery with promising strategies such as covalent conjugation, non-covalent complex formation, and CPP-decorated (functionalised) nano-complexes [130].

The first strategy is the **CPP covalently conjugated to the siRNA (CPP-siRNA)** delivery system. This method prevents separation among the CPP and its conjugate cargo both in vivo and/or in vitro. In this method, strong binding is attained between the CPP and its cargo via a cleavable linker such as the disulfide linkage, which leads to its lower molar ratio and low toxicity. This allows the components of the conjugate to be separated only in the reducing environment of the cytoplasm, e.g., by glutathione, thus avoiding its localisation in the nucleus (Figure 7) [131]. In contrast to the more cytotoxic liposome-based siRNA strategy, the penetratin-siRNA covalent approach was developed on neuron cells (in vitro) and the central nervous system (in vivo). However, there is still less clarity on the movement of siRNAs across the BBB and whether the internalisation and silencing effect is due to the covalently conjugated or the complexed species [132]. Apart from Tat and penetratin, siRNA conjugated to a low molecular weight protamine (LMWP) carrier via a cytosol-cleavable disulfide linkage using PEG as a spacer was developed, but this method was not successful [133].

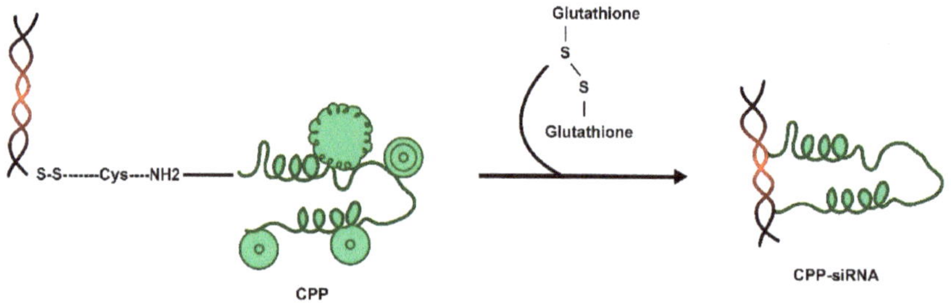


**Figure 7.** siRNA cargo covalently conjugated to the CPP is delivered via a cytosol-cleavable disulfide linkage that is separated in the reducing environment of the cytoplasm.

The second strategy is the formation of **non-covalent complexes (CPP: siRNA),** which are designed for an optimal balance between the peptide and siRNA. The stability of the complex depends upon the structure of the CPP as it must avoid charge neutralisation, thus preserving an overall positive charge [134]. In this strategy, called CLIP-RNAi, the complexes can enter the cells via an endocytic pathway and later encourage endosomal escape via photo-stimulation, letting gene silencing [135]. Specific CPPs called homing peptides can bind to the vasculature of the tumour tissues and have been used to 'aim' them at a specific tissue of the central nervous system.

A short peptide derived from rabies virus glycoprotein (RVG) and conjugated with nona-arginine peptide (RVG-9R) could bind to the acetylcholine receptor expressed by neuronal cells, resulting in specific gene silencing within the brain [136]. A widespread study of siRNA transfection by means of nona-arginine (L and D) conjugated with diverse targeting ligands was evaluated for transfection and mRNA knockdown mechanism [136]. Another peptide myristic acid-conjugated transportan (TP) conjugated to transferrin receptor-targeting peptide (myr-TP-Tf) was successfully encapsulated, and siRNA was delivered to brain endothelial cells and glioma cells [137]. Notwithstanding these heartening outcomes, the use of siRNA and the advances in novel CPPs anticipated for targeted delivery have many challenges [138].

The third strategy is using **CPP-decorated multifunctional nano-complexes,** which use amalgamations of CPPs and other carriers for siRNA delivery. These multifunctional nano-complexes possess the characteristics of multiple compounds and have a better half-life in the bloodstream. Polyethylenimine (PEI) moiety tagged with a micelle-like nanoparticle (MNP) was replaced with nona-arginine (R9), forming lipid–peptide hybrid nanoparticles (hNPs) that could readily form complexes and transfer oligonucleotides. In addition, the hNPs modified with Tat 48–60 (T-hNP) were shown to improve cellular transfection. This formulation has been reported with a better gene-silencing effect in vivo as it readily accumulates in brain tumour tissue [139]. A stearylated octaarginine multifunctional envelope-type nano device (R8-MEND) was modified using a pH-sensitive fusogenic peptide GALA that facilitated endosomal escape when fused with small unilamellar vesicles (SUVs). R8:GALA-MENDSUV allowed RNA interference and downregulated the expression of the suppressor of the cytokine-signalling 1 (SOCS1) gene in primary mouse bone marrow-derived dendritic cells (BMDCs). Later, the R8-MEND system was equipped with a PEG–peptide–lipid ternary conjugate (PEG–peptide–DOPE conjugate (PPD) that acted as a PEG shield in the tumour tissue environment [140]. It was noted that in vivo, PPD-MEND clustered in tumours and exhibited silencing activity, with negligible hepatotoxicity and immune hyperactivity [141]. Another activatable CPP (DSPE-PEG2000-ACPP) liposome-based siRNA delivery system was developed that is made of an octaarginine peptide linked to a polyanionic 'shielding domain' of glutamate and histidine by means of an acid-labile linker (hydrazone). Within the mildly acidic pH in the tumour microenvironment, the linker is cleaved, and the histidine becomes protonated. This aids the interaction of octaarginine with the plasma membrane and lets the modified liposomes pass through the BBB and deliver the siRNA cargo [142]. To facilitate selective siRNA transfection both in vitro and in vivo, a photo-pH-responsive polypeptide (PPP) decorated with poly(lactic-co-glycolic acid) (PLGA) nanoparticles was developed. At the lower pH of the tumour environment, this system was exposed to infrared (NIR) that led to the cleaving of the photo-degradable group of CPPs and the freeing of the nanoparticle to traverse through the plasma membrane and deliver the siRNA in the cytoplasm [143].

## 6. siRNA-CPP Therapeutics of the Central Nervous System

### 6.1. siRNA Delivery by Virus

Additional challenges are posed to therapeutics targeted to specific cell types of CNS such as astrocytes, neurons, or glia cells to cross the blood–brain barrier (BBB). Hence, early attempts to deliver RNAi in the CNS were performed by intracranial injections of lentiviral vectors encoding shRNA, but the method showed diminished efficacy. Lentiviral vectors crossed the BBB poorly. The inadequate neuro-invasion led to decreased and localised hRNA expression only around the injection site. This method also lacked temporal control and caused limited knockdown of protein expression. Another major concern regarding lentiviral vector technology and construction is its capacity to turn brain cells cancerous [144,145]. Another small, modified peptide that reduces siRNA off-target effects is obtained from the rabies virus glycoprotein (RVG-9r). Additionally, nicotinic acetylcholine receptors in the CNS are targeted by cationic liposomes with siRNA peptide complexes (LSPCs) and a targeting peptide (RVG-9r). Some modified siRNA-peptide complexes are encapsulated in either cationic or anionic liposomes with RVG-9r and bonded to lipid PEG either electrostatically or covalently; these are called peptide-addressed liposome-encapsulated therapeutic siRNA (PALETS) [146]. It was proven that LSPCs and PALETS reduced the surface cellular prion protein (PrPC) up to 70% in neuronal cells, while PALETS downregulated the total number of PrPC-expressing cells.

### 6.2. Non-Viral Route of siRNA Delivery

Cationic small-cell-penetrating peptides capable of crossing plasma membranes were the alternate nonviral strategy used for delivering siRNA molecules to the CNS [147,148]. The thiol linkages allow the siRNA–peptide complexes to easily dissociate in the cytoplasm by reduction of the disulfide bond. To overcome this, liposomal siRNA delivery vehicles conjugated to peptides were designed for transport to the CNS by means of the thin-film hydration method. The cationic or anionic liposomes saved the siRNAs from nucleases and proteases, whereas the combination with a peptide helped them bind to nicotinic acetylcholine receptors (nAchRs) on the brain cell surface [136]. Notwithstanding the therapeutic possibilities, this method remains plagued by important concerns regarding drug delivery to the brain such as cell specificity and transport of its cargo across the BBB. Most of these naked complexes become significantly degraded in the blood during transport as there was little or no detection of siRNA in the treated mouse brains. Moreover, there is also the problem of these complexes getting immune cleared or degraded by serum nuclease and protease.

### 6.3. Liposome–siRNA–Peptide Complexes (LSPCs)

Alternatively, more direct routes to the CNS should be explored and, in this regard, liposomes are extensively used as delivery vehicles for siRNA. Improved delivery of the liposome-encapsulated siRNA was observed with minimal siRNA degradation within the blood [149]. Cationic liposomes are the most common choice as they interact both with the anionic phosphate head groups of cell membranes and the negatively charged phosphate backbone of RNA [150,151]. Although less immunogenic, anionic liposomes are used less frequently because they repel the negative charge of the siRNA backbone and cannot penetrate the plasma membrane [152]. Liposome–siRNA complexes covalently bound to peptides have an affinity for receptors on specific cell types and thus can avoid off-target binding [153]. The mononuclear phagocyte system of the immune system has the tendency to recognise serum proteins and engulfing liposomes. Thus, PEGylated liposomes can avoid immune clearance and increase bioavailability and circulation duration in the blood [154]. However, bare liposomes are neither transported across the BBB nor provide cell-specific delivery. Surprisingly, PEGylated liposomes are known to reduce the serum degradation of siRNA to target sites in the brain, but coupling with a monoclonal antibody against glial fibrillary acidic protein (GFAP) failed to deliver itself across the astrocytes in mouse brains [155]. Thus, an effective and efficient delivery system must (1) gain access to the brain by crossing the BBB, (2) provide a molecular address for delivery to neuronal cells, and (3) protect from serum degradation.

### *6.4. Intranasal Delivery of siRNA*

Systemic transit through the vasculature of the CNS may lead therapeutic drugs to encounter immune cells, causing hypersensitivity or clearance from the system. An alternate method of administering drugs or stem cells into the nasal cavity can shorten the route across the BBB [156–158]. Neurodegenerative diseases like Alzheimer's and Parkinson's were shown to be treated by delivering mesenchymal stem cells intranasally [159,160]. Therapeutic targeting with a more direct route to the CNS combined with specific delivery to brain cells has been observed in other brain pathologies. Brain tumours and perinatal and ischaemic brain damage can also be treated using intranasally administrated mesenchymal stem cells [161–163].

### *6.5. siRNA-Loaded Exosomes*

Viral vectors or liposomes fail to deliver specifically and safely into the brain as their approaches are invasive and hindered by the immune system. Liposomes lack a long-term treatment method as they tend to elicit immune responses followed by subsequent clearance, while the use of a viral vector requires stereotaxic surgery, and the delivery is restricted to specific brain regions. These disadvantages can be overcome by the intravenous (iv) injection of modified exosomes for nucleic acid delivery into the brain. Exosomes are nanosized extracellular vesicles (30–100 nm in diameter) formed by an endocytic pathway [164]. Exosomes represent a promising drug delivery system and act as natural carriers of mRNA, microRNA, and proteins between cells [165]. Izco and co-workers developed a modified exosome that specifically targets the brain by delivering genetic material into the brain via intravenous injection. siRNAs-RVG-exosomes have been delivered for an effective knockdown of expression for both the Aβ and tau peptides of Alzheimer's disease and the alpha-synuclein of Parkinson's disease as a long-term treatment for these neurodegenerative diseases [166]. However, it was also noted that a defective endolysosomal system may interfere with the delivery of siRNAs. Thus, strategies must be devised to not only inhibit exosome secretion but also modify the content of exosomes by decreasing the exosomal cargo of pathological proteins, neuroinflammatory factors, or altered miRNAs. Increasing the cargo of trophic factors in glial-derived exosomes could also create new therapeutic strategies to halt the progression of neurodegenerative diseases [167].

Although the abovementioned siRNA delivery strategies have proven to be successful, some of the basic guidelines will become clearer after elaborating on the in vivo studies and clinical trials (Table 2). In the case of complexation-based systems, PEGylation or similar surface modification is necessary for longevity in circulation to shield the positive charge. This prevents nonspecific interaction and reduces toxicity. However, after delivering the siRNA to the target site, it must ensure endo/lysosomal escape following internalisation by the target cells. Despite the cost and regulatory hurdles associated with the targeting strategy, the siRNA-CPP delivery system is a big incentive, and the benefits are irrefutable [168].

**Table 2.** A list of various formulations and presumptive concerns for the use of siRNA–peptide conjugates.

| S. No. | siRNA-CPP Therapeutics | Route of Delivery | Formulations | Consequences/Concerns | Refs. |
|---|---|---|---|---|---|
| 1. | Virus-delivered siRNAs | | | | |
| | a. Lentivirus vector | Intracranial injections of hRNA to CNS | Vesicular stomatitis virus glycoprotein envelope (VSV-G) | Can turn brain cells cancerous | [144] |
| | b. RVG-9r | Intravascular injection targeted to neuronal PrPC | siRNA encapsulated in either cationic or anionic liposomes | Decreased levels of cellular prion protein (PrPC) | [146] |
| 2. | Non-viral delivery of siRNAs | Intravenous administration of cholesterol-conjugated siRNA lipoplexes | Cationic, anionic, or neutral, or a mixture, liposomes | 1. Significant degradation during blood transport.<br>2. Degradation by serum nuclease and protease.<br>3. Immune clearance. | [148] |
| 3. | Liposome-siRNA-peptide complexes (LSPCs) | In vitro RNA transfection with DOTMA-containing liposomes (lipofectin) | Cationic liposome | 1. Immune clearance.<br>2. Poor transport capability. | [149] |
| | | In vitro transfection with anionic lipoplexes (DOPG:DOPE) | Anionic liposome | 1. Repel the negative charge of the siRNA backbone.<br>2. Poor penetration through plasma membrane. | [152] |
| | | Intravenous injection | PEGylated liposomes | 1. Good bioavailability.<br>2. No immune clearance. | [154] |
| | | Intravenous injection | PEGylated liposomes plus monoclonal antibody | 1. Poor transport across the astrocytes in mouse brains. | [155] |
| 4. | Intranasal delivery of siRNA | Direct administration of drugs or stem cells into the nasal cavity | Human bone marrow-derived mesenchymal stem cells (MSC) | 1. Shorter route to CNS. | [159–161] |
| 5. | siRNA-loaded exosomes | Intravenous injection | Exosomes | 1. Increased cargo interferes with endosomal system. | [164] |

## 7. Conclusions and Perspectives

Diseases of the central nervous system (CNS) are the most difficult to treat, mainly because of the obstacle of the blood–brain barrier (BBB). A vast majority of drugs fail to reach the brain because of their inability to cross the BBB. Undoubtedly, the most promising studies are those that unravel strategies to deliver CNS-active drugs and peptides targeted at the BBB. Small peptides as nanoparticles or nanocarriers can be conjugated to drugs to either form a steady link or act as pro-drugs. The last decade witnessed a plethora of uses of both small molecules and proteins in diverse therapeutic areas such as diagnostics, brain cancers, and neurodegenerative disorders. Peptides can be generally classified as 'receptor-targeted' (e.g., angiopep2, CDX, and iRGD), recognising membrane proteins expressed by the BBB microvessels; 'cell-penetrating peptides' (e.g., TAT47−57, SynB1/3, and Penetratin), undergoing transcytosis through unspecific mechanisms; or 'homing peptides' (e.g., glioma-homing peptide (gHo) NHQQQNPHQPPM; brain-homing peptides CNAFTPDY, CLEVSRKNC, and CLSSRLDAC), used for DNA delivery. RNA interference (RNAi) conjugated to CPPs can become a new tool to target defective genes in the brain by inducing gene silencing and has enormous clinical potential for the treatment of various neurodegenerative disorders. Most RNAi trials use small interfering RNAs (siRNAs) but, despite the enormous potential of RNAi, only 24 clinical trials have applied siRNA-CPP-mediated therapy to date. Notwithstanding their great therapeutic potential, the successful implementation of siRNAs in vivo is hampered by the low bioavailability of these hydrophilic compounds and their inability to cross the BBB [169]. We hope that future directions of peptide therapy will offer a completely different approach to treating these progressive neurodegenerative illnesses and change the lives of those with these debilitating conditions.

In theory, both CPPs and homing peptides can be exploited to transform a large range of pharmaceuticals from paper to practice, but there exists a hindrance when it comes to replicating the in vitro results within physiological systems. Undeniably, despite having a generally good safety profile, some peptide conjugates may display toxicological features, causing antigenicity, cardiovascular alterations, or hemolysis. Furthermore, the life span of these peptides largely depends on their dodging capability in the presence of peptidases, endosomal/lysosomal degradation, and endosomal entrapment, making them unavailable to the target site [69].

Despite numerous data pertaining to the basics and applications of CPPs, the efficacy of such conjugations is still debatable, primarily when it comes to the blood–brain barrier. Endogenous analysis of CPP-mediated drug targeting in cell cultures does not necessarily indicate their behaviour at the organismal level. As discussed in the text, mere penetration inside cells does not mean that a given CPP can traverse the blood–brain barrier. Such limitations necessitate further in-vivo analysis of multiple CPPs as well as additional penetrating peptides and expand the existing database. The study of CPPs should also consider the differential expression of transporter proteins, primarily solute carriers on cell surfaces since the expression levels of these transmembrane proteins are strongly associated with various normal and anomalous conditions. Certain biologically active chemical compounds might also be studied for their cell-penetration and transcellular traversing activities so that the additional conjugation step can be eliminated.

Even though modern-day medicine has tapped the potential of many physiological loopholes to the advantage of humankind, a broad area remains unexplored. A significant proportion of our physiology and metabolism is influenced by the dark matter in our system. Despite null results, unknown interactions can also lead to negative results, which are commonly referred to as side effects. For most pharmaceuticals, these side effects exceed what has been documented or studied. One way to minimise these undocumented results is to take the dark matter into consideration. This is possible owing to the CPP/homing peptide specificity. However, despite this specificity, drugs can frequently target more than one macromolecule in an organism. Additionally, drug-bound CPPs can exhibit altered behaviours that further interfere with their normal roles in biological systems, specifically, brain activity. This can be negated by using pre-conjugated drug–CPP or drug–homing peptide combinations to minimise unwanted interactions within physiological systems. The careful optimisation of this and additional techniques can aid in moving many potential pharmaceuticals from texts to tables. An underestimated yet large number of efficient drugs fail to reach the counters owing to the lack of a delivery mechanism. Potent drugs (biomolecules and nanoparticles) that can be used to cure fatal disorders of the CNS, such as Parkinson's and Alzheimer's disease, or treat various brain tumours, do not exhibit any significant results if not coupled with an adequate transport and translocation system. Thus, a detailed analysis of both the available and the potential drug delivery systems that can effectively cross the blood–brain barrier has emerged as a critical requirement in the world of pharma- and nutraceuticals.

**Funding:** This research received no external funding.

**Institutional Review Board Statement:** Not applicable.

**Informed Consent Statement:** Not applicable.

**Data Availability Statement:** Not applicable.

**Acknowledgments:** The authors are thankful to the Hindu and Hansraj College, University of Delhi, India, and the University of Wisconsin–Madison, USA, for providing access to scientific articles and research journals.

**Conflicts of Interest:** The authors declare no conflict of interest.

## References

1. Bhowmik, A.; Khan, R.; Ghosh, M.K. Blood brain barrier: A challenge for effectual therapy of brain tumours. *BioMed. Res. Int.* **2015**, *2015*, 320941. [CrossRef] [PubMed]
2. Lu, Y.; Zhang, E.; Yang, J.; Cao, Z. Strategies to improve micelle stability for drug delivery. *Nano. Res.* **2018**, *11*, 4985–4998. [CrossRef]
3. Morshedi Rad, D.; Alsadat Rad, M.; Razavi Bazaz, S.; Kashaninejad, N.; Jin, D.; Ebrahimi Warkiani, M. A comprehensive review on intracellular delivery. *Adv. Mater.* **2021**, *33*, 2005363. [CrossRef]
4. Stewart, M.P.; Sharei, A.; Ding, X.; Sahay, G.; Langer, R.; Jensen, K.F. In vitro and ex vivo strategies for intracellular delivery. *Nature* **2016**, *538*, 183–192. [CrossRef]
5. Berillo, D.; Yeskendir, A.; Zharkinbekov, Z.; Raziyeva, K.; Saparov, A. Peptide-based drug delivery systems. *Medicina* **2021**, *57*, 1209. [CrossRef]
6. Gayraud, F.; Klugman, M.; Neundorf, I. Recent Advances and Trends in Chemical CPP–Drug Conjugation Techniques. *Molecules* **2021**, *26*, 1591. [CrossRef]
7. Josephson, L.; Tung, C.H.; Moore, A.; Weissleder, R. High-efficiency intracellular magnetic labeling with novel superparamagnetic-Tat peptide conjugates. *Bioconjug. Chem.* **1999**, *10*, 186–191. [CrossRef]
8. Blasi, P.; Giovagnoli, S.; Schoubben, A.; Ricci, M.; Rossi, C. Solid lipid nanoparticles for targeted brain drug delivery. *Adv. Drug Deliv. Rev.* **2007**, *59*, 454–477. [CrossRef]
9. Malhotra, M.; Prakash, S. Targeted drug delivery across blood-brain-barrier using cell penetrating peptides tagged nanoparticles. *Curr. Nanosci.* **2011**, *7*, 81–93. [CrossRef]
10. Goyal, R. Peptide-Based Molecular Constructs for Cellular Targeting and Small Molecule Delivery. Ph.D. Thesis, Indian Institute of Technology, Guwahati, India, 2020.
11. Heitz, F.; Morris, M.C.; Divita, G. Twenty years of cell-penetrating peptides: From molecular mechanisms to therapeutics. *Br. J. Pharmacol.* **2009**, *157*, 195–206. [CrossRef] [PubMed]
12. Frankel, A.D.; Pabo, C.O. Cellular uptake of the TAT protein from human Immunodeficiency virus. *Cell* **1988**, *55*, 1189–1193. [CrossRef]
13. Nagahara, H.; Vocero-Akbani, A.M.; Snyder, E.L.; Ho, A.; Latham, D.G.; Lissy, N.A.; Becker-Hapak, M.; Ezhevsky, S.A.; Dowdy, S.F. Transduction of full-length TAT fusion proteins into mammalian cells: TAT-p27Kip1 induces cell migration. *Nat. Med.* **1998**, *4*, 1449–1452. [CrossRef] [PubMed]
14. Morris, M.C.; Deshayes, S.; Heitz, F.; Divita, G. Cell-penetrating peptides: From molecular mechanisms to therapeutics. *Biol. Cell* **2008**, *100*, 201–217. [CrossRef] [PubMed]
15. Ndeboko, B.; Ramamurthy, N.; Lemamy, G.J.; Jamard, C.; Nielsen, P.E.; Cova, L. Role of cell-penetrating peptides in intracellular delivery of peptide nucleic acids targeting hepadnaviral replication. *Mol. Ther.-Nucleic Acids* **2017**, *9*, 162–169. [CrossRef] [PubMed]
16. Zhang, D.; Wang, J.; Xu, D. Cell-penetrating peptides as noninvasive transmembrane vectors for the development of novel multifunctional drug-delivery systems. *J. Control. Release* **2016**, *229*, 130–139. [CrossRef] [PubMed]
17. Komin, A.; Russell, L.; Hristova, K.; Searson, P. Peptide-based strategies for enhanced cell uptake, transcellular transport, and circulation: Mechanisms and challenges. *Adv. Drug Deliv. Rev.* **2017**, *110*, 52–64. [CrossRef]
18. Arukuusk, P.; Pärnaste, L.; Margus, H.; Eriksson, N.J.; Vasconcelos, L.; Padari, K.R.; Pooga, M.; Langel, U.L. Differential endosomal pathways for radically modified peptide vectors. *Bioconjugate Chem.* **2013**, *24*, 1721–1732. [CrossRef]

19. Ruseska, I.; Zimmer, A. Internalization mechanisms of cell-penetrating peptides. *Beilstein J. Nanotechnol.* **2020**, *11*, 101–123. [CrossRef]
20. Hu, G.; Zheng, W.; Li, A.; Mu, Y.; Shi, M.; Li, T.; Zou, H.; Shao, H.; Qin, A.; Ye, J. A novel CAV derived cell-penetrating peptide efficiently delivers exogenous molecules through caveolae-mediated endocytosis. *Vet. Res.* **2018**, *49*, 16. [CrossRef]
21. Haucke, V.; Kozlov, M.M. Membrane remodeling in clathrin-mediated endocytosis. *J. Cell Sci.* **2018**, *131*, jcs216812. [CrossRef]
22. Kaksonen, M.; Roux, A. Mechanisms of clathrin-mediated endocytosis. *Nat. Rev. Mol. Cell Biol.* **2018**, *19*, 313–326. [CrossRef]
23. Futaki, S.; Nakase, I. Cell-surface interactions on arginine-rich cell-penetrating peptides allow for multiplex modes of internalization. *Acc. Chem. Res.* **2017**, *50*, 2449–2456. [CrossRef]
24. Guidotti, G.; Brambilla, L.; Rossi, D. Cell-penetrating peptides: From basic research to clinics. *Trends Pharmacol. Sci.* **2017**, *38*, 406–424. [CrossRef]
25. Böhmová, E.; Machová, D.; Pechar, M.; Pola, R.; Venclíková, K.; Janoušková, O.; Etrych, T. Cell-penetrating peptides: A useful tool for the delivery of various cargoes into cells. *Physiol. Res.* **2018**, *67*, S267–S279. [CrossRef] [PubMed]
26. Erazo-Oliveras, A.; Muthukrishnan, N.; Baker, R.; Wang, T.-Y.; Pellois, J.-P. Improving the endosomal escape of cell-penetrating peptides and their cargos: Strategies and challenges. *Pharmaceuticals* **2012**, *5*, 1177–1209. [CrossRef] [PubMed]
27. Smith, S.A.; Selby, L.I.; Johnston, A.P.R.; Such, G.K. The Endosomal Escape of Nanoparticles: Toward More Efficient Cellular Delivery. *Bioconjugate Chem.* **2019**, *30*, 263–272. [CrossRef]
28. Varkouhi, A.K.; Scholte, M.; Storm, G.; Haisma, H.J. Endosomal escape pathways for delivery of biologicals. *J. Control. Release* **2011**, *151*, 220–228. [CrossRef]
29. Martens, T.F.; Remaut, K.; Demeester, J.; De Smedt, S.C.; Braeckmans, K. Intracellular delivery of nanomaterials: How to catch endosomal escape in the act. *Nano Today* **2014**, *9*, 344–364. [CrossRef]
30. Meyer, M.; Philipp, A.; Oskuee, R.; Schmidt, C.; Wagner, E. Breathing life into polycations: Functionalization with pH-responsive endosomolytic peptides and polyethylene glycol enables siRNA delivery. *J. Am. Chem. Soc.* **2008**, *130*, 3272–3273. [CrossRef] [PubMed]
31. Kobayashi, S.; Nakase, I.; Kawabata, N.; Yu, H.-H.; Pujals, S.; Imanishi, M.; Giralt, E.; Futaki, S. Cytosolic targeting of macromolecules using a pH-dependent fusogenic peptide in combination with cationic liposomes. *Bioconjugate Chem.* **2009**, *20*, 953–959. [CrossRef]
32. Chen, R.; Khormaee, S.; Eccleston, M.E.; Slater, N.K. The role of hydrophobic amino acid grafts in the enhancement of membrane-disruptive activity of pH-responsive pseudo-peptides. *Biomaterials* **2009**, *30*, 1954–1961. [CrossRef]
33. Lonn, P.; Kacsinta, A.; Cui, X.; Hamil, A.; Kaulich, M.; Gogoi, K.; Dowdy, S. Enhancing endosomal escape for intracellular delivery of macromolecular biologic therapeutics. *Sci. Rep.* **2016**, *6*, 32301. [CrossRef] [PubMed]
34. Han, K.; Chen, S.; Chen, W.-H.; Lei, Q.; Liu, Y.; Zhuo, R.-X.; Zhang, X.-Z. Synergistic gene and drug tumour therapy using a chimeric peptide. *Biomaterials* **2013**, *34*, 4680–4689. [CrossRef] [PubMed]
35. Lo, S.L.; Wang, S. An endosomolytic Tat peptide produced by incorporation of histidine and cysteine residues as a nonviral vector for DNA transfection. *Biomaterials* **2008**, *29*, 2408–2414. [CrossRef] [PubMed]
36. Qian, Z.; LaRochelle, J.R.; Jiang, B.; Lian, W.; Hard, R.L.; Selner, N.G.; Luechapanichkul, R.; Barrios, A.M.; Pei, D. Early endosomal escape of a cyclic cell-penetrating peptide allows effective cytosolic cargo delivery. *Biochemistry* **2014**, *53*, 4034–4046. [CrossRef]
37. Erazo-Oliveras, A.; Najjar, K.; Truong, D.; Wang, T.Y.; Brock, D.J.; Prater, A.R.; Pellois, J.P. The Late Endosome and Its Lipid BMP Act as Gateways for Efficient Cytosolic Access of the Delivery Agent dfTAT and Its Macromolecular Cargos. *Cell Chem. Biol.* **2016**, *23*, 598–607. [CrossRef]
38. Erazo-Oliveras, A.; Najjar, K.; Dayani, L.; Wang, T.Y.; Johnson, G.A.; Pellois, J.P. Protein delivery into live cells by incubation with an endosomolytic agent. *Nat. Methods* **2014**, *11*, 861–867. [CrossRef]
39. Qian, Z.; Martyna, A.; Hard, R.L.; Wang, J.; Appiah-Kubi, G.; Coss, C.; Phelps, M.A.; Rossman, J.S.; Pei, D. Discovery and Mechanism of Highly Efficient Cyclic Cell-Penetrating Peptides. *Biochemistry* **2016**, *55*, 2601–2612. [CrossRef]
40. Appelbaum, J.S.; LaRochelle, J.R.; Smith, B.A.; Balkin, D.M.; Holub, J.M.; Schepartz, A. Arginine topology controls escape of minimally cationic proteins from early endosomes to the cytoplasm. *Chem. Biol.* **2012**, *19*, 819–830. [CrossRef]
41. Bus, T.; Traeger, A.; Schubert, U.S. The great escape: How cationic polyplexes overcome the endosomal barrier. *J. Mater. Chem. B* **2018**, *6*, 6904–6918. [CrossRef]
42. Pack, D.W.; Putnam, D.; Langer, R. Design of imidazole-containing endosomolytic biopolymers for gene delivery. *Biotechnol. Bioeng.* **2000**, *67*, 217–223. [CrossRef]
43. Sonawane, N.D.; Szoka, F.C., Jr.; Verkman, A.S. Chloride accumulation and swelling in endosomes enhances DNA transfer by polyamine-DNA polyplexes. *J. Biol. Chem.* **2003**, *278*, 44826–44831. [CrossRef]
44. Benjaminsen, R.V.; Mattebjerg, M.A.; Henriksen, J.R.; Moghimi, S.M.; Andresen, T.L. The possible "proton sponge" effect of polyethylenimine (PEI) does not include change in lysosomal pH. *Mol. Ther.* **2013**, *21*, 149–157. [CrossRef]
45. Vermeulen, L.M.P.; De Smedt, S.C.; Remaut, K.; Braeckmans, K. The proton sponge hypothesis: Fable or fact? *Eur. J. Pharm. Biopharm.* **2018**, *129*, 184–190. [CrossRef]
46. Tweten, R.K. Cholesterol-dependent cytolysins, a family of versatile pore-forming toxins. *Infect. Immun.* **2005**, *73*, 6199–6209. [CrossRef]
47. Gruenberg, J.; van der Goot, F.G. Mechanisms of pathogen entry through the endosomal compartments. *Nat. Rev. Mol. Cell Biol.* **2006**, *7*, 495–504. [CrossRef]

48. Herce, H.D.; Garcia, A.E.; Litt, J.; Kane, R.S.; Martin, P.; Enrique, N.; Rebolledo, A.; Milesi, V. Arginine-rich peptides destabilize the plasma membrane, consistent with a pore formation translocation mechanism of cell-penetrating peptides. *Biophys. J.* **2009**, *97*, 1917–1925. [CrossRef]
49. Nadal-Bufí, F.; Henriques, S.T. How to overcome endosomal entrapment of cell-penetrating peptides to release the therapeutic potential of peptides? *Pept. Sci.* **2020**, *112*, e24168. [CrossRef]
50. Mandal, D.; Nasrolahi Shirazi, A.; Parang, K. Cell-penetrating homochiral cyclic peptides as nuclear-targeting molecular transporters. *Angew. Chem. Int. Ed. Engl.* **2011**, *50*, 9633–9637. [CrossRef]
51. Lee, Y.J.; Johnson, G.; Peltier, G.C.; Pellois, J.P. A HA2-Fusion tag limits the endosomal release of its protein cargo despite causing endosomal lysis. *Biochim. Biophys. Acta* **2011**, *1810*, 752–758. [CrossRef]
52. Song, J.; Lu, C.; Leszek, J.; Zhang, J. Design and Development of Nanomaterial-Based Drug Carriers to Overcome the Blood–Brain Barrier by Using Different Transport Mechanisms. *Int. J. Mol. Sci.* **2021**, *22*, 10118. [CrossRef] [PubMed]
53. Lucana, M.C.; Arruga, Y.; Petrachi, E.; Roig, A.; Lucchi, R.; Oller-Salvia, B. Protease-Resistant Peptides for Targeting and Intracellular Delivery of Therapeutics. *Pharmaceutics* **2021**, *13*, 2065. [CrossRef] [PubMed]
54. Varner, J.A.; Cheresh, D.A. Integrins and cancer. *Curr. Opin. Cell Biol.* **1996**, *8*, 724–730. [CrossRef]
55. Koivunen, E.; Wang, B.; Ruoslahti, E. Phage libraries displaying cyclic peptides with different ring sizes: Ligand specificities of the RGD-directed integrins. *Biotechnology* **1995**, *13*, 265–270. [CrossRef]
56. Corti, A.; Curnis, F. Tumour vasculature targeting through NGR peptide-based drug delivery systems. *Curr. Pharm. Biotechnol.* **2011**, *12*, 1128–1134. [CrossRef]
57. Kondo, E.; Iioka, H.; Saito, K. Tumour-homing peptide and its utility for advanced cancer medicine. *Cancer Sci.* **2021**, *112*, 2118–2125. [CrossRef]
58. Kondo, E.; Saito, K.; Tashiro, Y.; Kamide, K.; Uno, S.; Furuya, T.; Mashita, M.; Nakajima, K.; Tsumuraya, T.; Kobayashi, N.; et al. Tumour lineage-homing cell-penetrating peptides as anticancer molecular delivery systems. *Nat. Commun.* **2012**, *3*, 951. [CrossRef]
59. Pardridge, W.M. The blood-brain barrier: Bottleneck in brain drug development. *NeuroRx* **2005**, *2*, 3–14. [CrossRef]
60. Treat, L.H.; McDannold, N.; Zhang, Y.; Vykhodtseva, N.; Hynynen, K. Improved anti-tumour effect of liposomal doxorubicin after targeted blood-brain barrier disruption by MRI-guided focused ultrasound in rat glioma. *Ultrasound. Med. Biol.* **2012**, *38*, 1716–1725. [CrossRef]
61. Rip, J.; Schenk, G.J.; de Boer, A.G. Differential receptor-mediated drug targeting to the diseased brain. *Expert. Opin. Drug. Deliv.* **2009**, *6*, 227–237. [CrossRef]
62. Gururangan, S.; Friedman, H.S. Innovations in design and delivery of chemotherapy for brain tumours. *Neuroimaging Clin. N. Am.* **2002**, *12*, 583–597. [CrossRef] [PubMed]
63. Saraiva, C.; Praça, C.; Ferreira, R.; Santos, T.; Ferreira, L.; Bernardino, L. Nanoparticle-mediated brain drug delivery: Overcoming blood-brain barrier to treat neurodegenerative diseases. *J. Control. Release* **2016**, *235*, 34–47. [CrossRef] [PubMed]
64. Sweeney, M.D.; Ayyadurai, S.; Zlokovic, B.V. Pericytes of the neurovascular unit: Key functions and signaling pathways. *Nat. Neurosci.* **2016**, *19*, 771–783. [CrossRef] [PubMed]
65. Abbott, N.J.; Romero, I.A. Transporting therapeutics across the blood-brain barrier. *Mol. Med. Today* **1996**, *2*, 106–113. [CrossRef] [PubMed]
66. Abbott, N.J.; Rönnbäck, L.; Hansson, E. Astrocyte-endothelial interactions at the blood-brain barrier. *Nat. Rev. Neurosci.* **2006**, *7*, 41–53. [CrossRef]
67. Pajouhesh, H.; Lenz, G.R. Medicinal chemical properties of successful central nervous system drugs. *NeuroRx* **2005**, *2*, 541–553. [CrossRef]
68. Lipinski, C.A.; Lombardo, F.; Dominy, B.W.; Feeney, P.J. Experimental and computational approaches to estimate solubility and permeability in drug discovery and development settings. *Adv. Drug Deliv. Rev.* **2001**, *46*, 3–26. [CrossRef]
69. Parrasia, S.; Szabò, I.; Zoratti, M.; Biasutto, L. Peptides as Pharmacological Carriers to the Brain: Promises, Shortcomings and Challenges. *Mol. Pharm.* **2022**, *19*, 3700–3729. [CrossRef]
70. Reissmann, S. State of art: Cell penetration and cell-penetrating peptides and proteins. *Health Educ. Public Health* **2021**, *4*, 393–410.
71. Stalmans, S.; Bracke, N.; Wynendaele, E.; Gevaert, B.; Peremans, K.; Burvenich, C.; Polis, I.; De Spiegeleer, B. Cell-Penetrating Peptides Selectively Cross the Blood-Brain Barrier In Vivo. *PLoS ONE* **2015**, *10*, e0139652. [CrossRef]
72. Lindgren, M.E.; Hällbrink, M.M.; Elmquist, A.M.; Langel, U. Passage of cell-penetrating peptides across a human epithelial cell layer in vitro. *Biochem. J.* **2004**, *377*, 69–76. [CrossRef] [PubMed]
73. Violini, S.; Sharma, V.; Prior, J.L.; Dyszlewski, M.; Piwnica-Worms, D. Evidence for a plasma membrane-mediated permeability barrier to Tat basic domain in well-differentiated epithelial cells: Lack of correlation with heparan sulfate. *Biochemistry* **2002**, *41*, 12652–12661. [CrossRef] [PubMed]
74. Chen, Y.; Liu, L. Modern methods for delivery of drugs across the blood-brain barrier. *Adv. Drug Deliv. Rev.* **2012**, *64*, 640–665. [CrossRef] [PubMed]
75. Schwarze, S.R.; Ho, A.; Vocero-Akbani, A.; Dowdy, S.F. In vivo protein transduction: Delivery of a biologically active protein into the mouse. *Science* **1999**, *285*, 1569–1572. [CrossRef]
76. Zhang, Y.; Guo, P.; Ma, Z.; Lu, P.; Kebebe, D.; Liu, Z. Combination of cell-penetrating peptides with nanomaterials for the potential therapeutics of central nervous system disorders: A review. *J. Nanobiotechnol.* **2021**, *19*, 255. [CrossRef]

77. Datta, G.; Chaddha, M.; Garber, D.W.; Chung, B.H.; Tytler, E.M.; Dashti, N.; Bradley, W.A.; Gianturco, S.H.; Anantharamaiah, G.M. The receptor binding domain of apolipoprotein E, linked to a model class A amphipathic helix, enhances internalization and degradation of LDL by fibroblasts. *Biochemistry* **2000**, *39*, 213–220. [CrossRef] [PubMed]
78. Spencer, B.J.; Verma, I.M. Targeted delivery of proteins across the blood-brain barrier. *Proc. Natl. Acad. Sci. USA* **2007**, *104*, 7594–7599. [CrossRef]
79. Wang, D.; El-Amouri, S.S.; Dai, M.; Kuan, C.Y.; Hui, D.Y.; Brady, R.O.; Pan, D. Engineering a lysosomal enzyme with a derivative of receptor-binding domain of apoE enables delivery across the blood-brain barrier. *Proc. Natl. Acad. Sci. USA* **2013**, *110*, 2999–3004. [CrossRef]
80. Tian, T.; Zhang, H.X.; He, C.P.; Fan, S.; Zhu, Y.L.; Qi, C.; Huang, N.P.; Xiao, Z.D.; Lu, Z.H.; Tannous, B.A.; et al. Surface functionalized exosomes as targeted drug delivery vehicles for cerebral ischemia therapy. *Biomaterials* **2018**, *150*, 137–149. [CrossRef]
81. Kumar, P.; Wu, H.; McBride, J.L.; Jung, K.E.; Kim, M.H.; Davidson, B.L.; Lee, S.K.; Shankar, P.; Manjunath, N. Transvascular delivery of small interfering RNA to the central nervous system. *Nature* **2007**, *448*, 39–43. [CrossRef]
82. Javed, H.; Menon, S.A.; Al-Mansoori, K.M.; Al-Wandi, A.; Majbour, N.K.; Ardah, M.T.; Varghese, S.; Vaikath, N.N.; Haque, M.E.; Azzouz, M.; et al. Development of Nonviral Vectors Targeting the Brain as a Therapeutic Approach for Parkinson's Disease and Other Brain Disorders. *Mol. Ther.* **2016**, *24*, 746–758. [CrossRef]
83. Lee, J.H.; Zhang, A.; You, S.S.; Lieber, C.M. Spontaneous Internalization of Cell Penetrating Peptide-Modified Nanowires into Primary Neurons. *Nano Lett.* **2016**, *16*, 1509–1513. [CrossRef]
84. Neves, V.; Aires-da-Silva, F.; Morais, M.; Gano, L.; Ribeiro, E.; Pinto, A.; Aguiar, S.; Gaspar, D.; Fernandes, C.; Correia, J.D.G.; et al. Novel Peptides Derived from Dengue Virus Capsid Protein Translocate Reversibly the Blood-Brain Barrier through a Receptor-Free Mechanism. *ACS Chem. Biol.* **2017**, *12*, 1257–1268. [CrossRef]
85. Oller-Salvia, B.; Sánchez-Navarro, M.; Ciudad, S.; Guiu, M.; Arranz-Gibert, P.; Garcia, C.; Gomis, R.R.; Cecchelli, R.; García, J.; Giralt, E.; et al. MiniAp-4: A Venom-Inspired Peptidomimetic for Brain Delivery. *Angew. Chem. Int. Ed. Engl.* **2016**, *55*, 572–575. [CrossRef]
86. Wu, C.H.; Liu, I.J.; Lu, R.M.; Wu, H.C. Advancement and applications of peptide phage display technology in biomedical science. *J. Biomed. Sci.* **2016**, *23*, 8. [CrossRef] [PubMed]
87. Gao, H.; Qian, J.; Cao, S.; Yang, Z.; Pang, Z.; Pan, S.; Fan, L.; Xi, Z.; Jiang, X.; Zhang, Q. Precise glioma targeting of and penetration by aptamer and peptide dual-functioned nanoparticles. *Biomaterials* **2012**, *33*, 5115–5123. [CrossRef] [PubMed]
88. Majerova, P.; Hanes, J.; Olesova, D.; Sinsky, J.; Pilipcinec, E.; Kovac, A. Novel blood–brain barrier shuttle peptides discovered through the phage display method. *Molecules* **2020**, *25*, 874. [CrossRef] [PubMed]
89. Torchilin, V.P. Recent approaches to intracellular delivery of drugs and DNA and organelle targeting. *Annu. Rev. Biomed. Eng.* **2006**, *8*, 343–375. [CrossRef] [PubMed]
90. Liu, L.; Guo, K.; Lu, J.; Venkatraman, S.S.; Luo, D.; Ng, K.C.; Ling, E.A.; Moochhala, S.; Yang, Y.Y. Biologically active core/shell nanoparticles self-assembled from cholesterol-terminated PEG-TAT for drug delivery across the blood-brain barrier. *Biomaterials* **2008**, *29*, 1509–1517. [CrossRef]
91. Agyare, E.K.; Curran, G.L.; Ramakrishnan, M.; Yu, C.C.; Poduslo, J.F.; Kandimalla, K.K. Development of a smart nano-vehicle to target cerebrovascular amyloid deposits and brain parenchymal plaques observed in Alzheimer's disease and cerebral amyloid angiopathy. *Pharm. Res.* **2008**, *25*, 2674–2684. [CrossRef]
92. Dong, X. Current Strategies for Brain Drug Delivery. *Theranostics* **2018**, *8*, 1481–1493. [CrossRef] [PubMed]
93. Sharma, G.; Modgil, A.; Layek, B.; Arora, K.; Sun, C.; Law, B.; Singh, J. Cell penetrating peptide tethered bi-ligand liposomes for delivery to brain in vivo: Biodistribution and transfection. *J. Control. Release* **2013**, *167*, 1–10. [CrossRef] [PubMed]
94. Urbiola, K.; Blanco-Fernández, L.; Ogris, M.; Rödl, W.; Wagner, E.; Tros de Ilarduya, C. Novel PAMAM-PEG-Peptide Conjugates for siRNA Delivery Targeted to the Transferrin and Epidermal Growth Factor Receptors. *Pers. Med.* **2018**, *8*, 4. [CrossRef] [PubMed]
95. Lu, F.; Pang, Z.; Zhao, J.; Jin, K.; Li, H.; Pang, Q.; Zhang, L.; Pang, Z. Angiopep-2-conjugated poly(ethylene glycol)-co- poly(ε-caprolactone) polymersomes for dual-targeting drug delivery to glioma in rats. *Int. J. Nanomed.* **2017**, *12*, 2117–2127. [CrossRef] [PubMed]
96. Ahlschwede, K.M.; Curran, G.L.; Rosenberg, J.T.; Grant, S.C.; Sarkar, G.; Jenkins, R.B.; Ramakrishnan, S.; Poduslo, J.F.; Kandimalla, K.K. Cationic carrier peptide enhances cerebrovascular targeting of nanoparticles in Alzheimer's disease brain. *Nanomedicine* **2019**, *16*, 258–266. [CrossRef]
97. Nosrati, H.; Tarantash, M.; Bochani, S.; Charmi, J.; Bagheri, Z.; Fridoni, M.; Abdollahifar, M.A.; Davaran, S.; Danafar, H.; Kheiri Manjili, H. Glutathione (GSH) peptide conjugated magnetic nanoparticles as blood–brain barrier shuttle for MRI-monitored brain delivery of paclitaxel. *ACS Biomater. Sci. Eng.* **2019**, *5*, 1677–1685. [CrossRef]
98. Wang, S.; Zhang, B.; Su, L.; Nie, W.; Han, D.; Han, G.; Zhang, H.; Chong, C.; Tan, J. Subcellular distributions of iron oxide nanoparticles in rat brains affected by different surface modifications. *Biomed. Mater. Res. A* **2019**, *107*, 1988–1998. [CrossRef]
99. Yang, L.; Qian, W.; Scott, P.; Shao, X. Towards the development of brain-penetrating gold nanoparticle-transactivator of transcription (TAT) peptide conjugates. *J. Nucl. Med.* **2018**, *59*, 1034.

100. Kang, J.; Joo, J.; Kwon, E.J.; Skalak, M.; Hussain, S.; She, Z.G.; Ruoslahti, E.; Bhatia, S.N.; Sailor, M.J. Self-Sealing Porous Silicon-Calcium Silicate Core-Shell Nanoparticles for Targeted siRNA Delivery to the Injured Brain. *Adv. Mater.* **2016**, *28*, 7962–7969. [CrossRef]
101. Haney, M.J.; Klyachko, N.L.; Zhao, Y.; Gupta, R.; Plotnikova, E.G.; He, Z.; Patel, T.; Piroyan, A.; Sokolsky, M.; Kabanov, A.V.; et al. Exosomes as drug delivery vehicles for Parkinson's disease therapy. *J. Control. Release* **2015**, *207*, 18–30. [CrossRef]
102. Luan, X.; Sansanaphongpricha, K.; Myers, I.; Chen, H.; Yuan, H.; Sun, D. Engineering exosomes as refined biological nanoplatforms for drug delivery. *Acta Pharmacol. Sin.* **2017**, *38*, 754–763. [CrossRef]
103. Alvarez-Erviti, L.; Seow, Y.; Yin, H.; Betts, C.; Lakhal, S.; Wood, M.J. Delivery of siRNA to the mouse brain by systemic injection of targeted exosomes. *Nat. Biotechnol.* **2011**, *29*, 341–345. [CrossRef]
104. Pusic, A.D.; Pusic, K.M.; Clayton, B.L.; Kraig, R.P. IFNγ-stimulated dendritic cell exosomes as a potential therapeutic for remyelination. *J. Neuroimmunol.* **2014**, *266*, 12–23. [CrossRef] [PubMed]
105. Islam, Y.; Leach, A.G.; Smith, J.; Pluchino, S.; Coxonl, C.R.; Sivakumaran, M.; Downing, J.; Fatokun, A.A.; Teixidò, M.; Ehtezazi, T. Peptide based drug delivery systems to the brain. *Nano. Express* **2020**, *1*, 012002. [CrossRef]
106. Cooper, J.M.; Wiklander, P.B.; Nordin, J.Z.; Al-Shawi, R.; Wood, M.J.; Vithlani, M.; Schapira, A.H.; Simons, J.P.; El-Andaloussi, S.; Alvarez-Erviti, L. Systemic exosomal siRNA delivery reduced alpha-synuclein aggregates in brains of transgenic mice. *Mov. Disord.* **2014**, *29*, 1476–1485. [CrossRef]
107. Pulford, B.; Reim, N.; Bell, A.; Veatch, J.; Forster, G.; Bender, H.; Meyerett, C.; Hafeman, S.; Michel, B.; Johnson, T.; et al. Liposome-siRNA-peptide complexes cross the blood-brain barrier and significantly decrease PrP on neuronal cells and PrP in infected cell cultures. *PLoS ONE* **2010**, *5*, e11085. [CrossRef] [PubMed]
108. Bender, H.R.; Kane, S.; Zabel, M.D. Delivery of Therapeutic siRNA to the CNS Using Cationic and Anionic Liposomes. *J. Vis. Exp.* **2016**, *113*, e54106.
109. Grinberg, S.; Linder, C.; Kolot, V.; Waner, T.; Wiesman, Z.; Shaubi, E.; Heldman, E. Novel cationic amphiphilic derivatives from vernonia oil: Synthesis and self-aggregation into bilayer vesicles, nanoparticles, and DNA complexants. *Langmuir* **2005**, *21*, 7638–7645. [CrossRef] [PubMed]
110. Popov, M.; Abu Hammad, I.; Bachar, T.; Grinberg, S.; Linder, C.; Stepensky, D.; Heldman, E. Delivery of analgesic peptides to the brain by nano-sized bolaamphiphilic vesicles made of monolayer membranes. *Eur. J. Pharm. Biopharm.* **2013**, *85*, 381–389. [CrossRef]
111. Conceição, M.; Mendonça, L.; Nóbrega, C.; Gomes, C.; Costa, P.; Hirai, H.; Moreira, J.N.; Lima, M.C.; Manjunath, N.; Pereira de Almeida, L. Intravenous administration of brain-targeted stable nucleic acid lipid particles alleviates Machado-Joseph disease neurological phenotype. *Biomaterials* **2016**, *82*, 124–137. [CrossRef]
112. Lu, M.; Xing, H.; Xun, Z.; Yang, T.; Zhao, X.; Cai, C.; Wang, D.; Ding, P. Functionalized extracellular vesicles as advanced therapeutic nanodelivery systems. *Eur. J. Pharm. Sci.* **2018**, *121*, 34–46. [CrossRef] [PubMed]
113. Ke, W.; Shao, K.; Huang, R.; Han, L.; Liu, Y.; Li, J.; Kuang, Y.; Ye, L.; Lou, J.; Jiang, C. Gene delivery targeted to the brain using an Angiopep-conjugated polyethyleneglycol-modified polyamidoamine dendrimer. *Biomaterials* **2009**, *30*, 6976–6985. [CrossRef]
114. Perez, A.P.; Romero, E.L.; Morilla, M.J. Ethylendiamine core PAMAM dendrimers/siRNA complexes as in vitro silencing agents. *Int. J. Pharm.* **2009**, *380*, 189–200. [CrossRef] [PubMed]
115. Al-Azzawi, S.; Masheta, D.; Guildford, A.; Phillips, G.; Santin, M. Designing and Characterization of a Novel Delivery System for Improved Cellular Uptake by Brain Using Dendronised Apo-E-Derived Peptide. *Front. Bioeng. Biotechnol.* **2019**, *7*, 49. [CrossRef] [PubMed]
116. Zhou, X.; Smith, Q.R.; Liu, X. Brain penetrating peptides and peptide-drug conjugates to overcome the blood-brain barrier and target CNS diseases. *Wiley Interdiscip. Rev. Nanomed. Nanobiotechnol.* **2021**, *13*, e1695. [CrossRef] [PubMed]
117. Zhang, H.; Gerson, T.; Varney, M.L.; Singh, R.K.; Vinogradov, S.V. Multifunctional peptide-PEG intercalating conjugates: Programmatic of gene delivery to the blood-brain barrier. *Pharm. Res.* **2010**, *27*, 2528–2543. [CrossRef]
118. Sun, R.; Liu, M.; Lu, J.; Chu, B.; Yang, Y.; Song, B.; Wang, H.; He, Y. Bacteria loaded with glucose polymer and photosensitive ICG silicon-nanoparticles for glioblastoma photothermal immunotherapy. *Nat. Commun.* **2022**, *13*, 5127. [CrossRef]
119. Wu, L.P.; Ahmadvand, D.; Su, J.; Hall, A.; Tan, X.; Farhangrazi, Z.S.; Moghimi, S.M. Crossing the blood-brain-barrier with nanoligand drug carriers self-assembled from a phage display peptide. *Nat. Commun.* **2019**, *10*, 4635. [CrossRef]
120. Smith, T.L.; Sidman, R.L.; Arap, W.; Pasqualini, R. Targeting vascular zip codes: From combinatorial selection to drug prototypes. In *The Vasculome*; Elsevier: Amsterdam, The Netherlands, 2022; pp. 393–401.
121. Cho, C.F.; Farquhar, C.E.; Fadzen, C.M.; Scott, B.; Zhuang, P.; von Spreckelsen, N.; Loas, A.; Hartrampf, N.; Pentelute, B.L.; Lawler, S.E. A Tumour-Homing Peptide Platform Enhances Drug Solubility, Improves Blood-Brain Barrier Permeability and Targets Glioblastoma. *Cancers* **2022**, *14*, 2207. [CrossRef]
122. Eriste, E.; Kurrikoff, K.; Suhorutšenko, J.; Oskolkov, N.; Copolovici, D.M.; Jones, S.; Laakkonen, P.; Howl, J.; Langel, Ü. Peptide-based glioma-targeted drug delivery vector gHoPe2. *Bioconjug. Chem.* **2013**, *24*, 305–313. [CrossRef]
123. Prades, R.; Oller-Salvia, B.; Schwarzmaier, S.M.; Selva, J.; Moros, M.; Balbi, M.; Grazú, V.; de La Fuente, J.M.; Egea, G.; Plesnila, N.; et al. Applying the retro-enantio approach to obtain a peptide capable of overcoming the blood-brain barrier. *Angew. Chem. Int. Ed. Engl.* **2015**, *54*, 3967–3972. [CrossRef] [PubMed]

124. Prades, R.; Guerrero, S.; Araya, E.; Molina, C.; Salas, E.; Zurita, E.; Selva, J.; Egea, G.; López-Iglesias, C.; Teixidó, M. Delivery of gold nanoparticles to the brain by conjugation with a peptide that recognizes the transferrin receptor. *Biomaterials* **2012**, *33*, 7194–7205. [CrossRef] [PubMed]
125. Zou, Z.; Shen, Q.; Pang, Y.; Li, X.; Chen, Y.; Wang, X.; Luo, X.; Wu, Z.; Bao, Z.; Zhang, J. The synthesized transporter K16APoE enabled the therapeutic HAYED peptide to cross the blood-brain barrier and remove excess iron and radicals in the brain, thus easing Alzheimer's disease. *Drug Deliv. Transl. Res.* **2019**, *9*, 394–403. [CrossRef] [PubMed]
126. Tosi, G.; Badiali, L.; Ruozi, B.; Vergoni, A.V.; Bondioli, L.; Ferrari, A.; Rivasi, F.; Forni, F.; Vandelli, M.A. Can leptin-derived sequence-modified nanoparticles be suitable tools for brain delivery? *Nanomedicine* **2012**, *7*, 365–382. [CrossRef] [PubMed]
127. Zhuang, X.; Xiang, X.; Grizzle, W.; Sun, D.; Zhang, S.; Axtell, R.C.; Ju, S.; Mu, J.; Zhang, L.; Steinman, L.; et al. Treatment of brain inflammatory diseases by delivering exosome encapsulated anti-inflammatory drugs from the nasal region to the brain. *Mol. Ther.* **2011**, *19*, 1769–1779. [CrossRef] [PubMed]
128. Napoli, C.; Lemieux, C.; Jorgensen, R. Introduction of a chimeric chalcone synthase gene into petunia results in reversible co-suppression of homologous genes in trans. *Plant Cell* **1990**, *2*, 279–289. [CrossRef] [PubMed]
129. Tatiparti, K.; Sau, S.; Kashaw, S.K.; Iyer, A.K. siRNA delivery strategies: A comprehensive review of recent developments. *Nanomaterials* **2017**, *7*, 77. [CrossRef]
130. Xie, X.; Lin, W.; Li, M.; Yang, Y.; Deng, J.; Liu, H.; Chen, Y.; Fu, X.; Liu, H.; Yang, Y. Efficient siRNA delivery using novel cell-penetrating peptide-siRNA conjugate-loaded nanobubbles and ultrasound. *Ultrasound. Med. Biol.* **2016**, *42*, 1362–1374. [CrossRef]
131. Pratt, A.J.; MacRae, I.J. The RNA-induced silencing complex: A versatile gene-silencing machine. *J. Biol. Chem.* **2009**, *284*, 17897–17901. [CrossRef]
132. Mathupala, S.P. Delivery of small-interfering RNA (siRNA) to the brain. *Expert. Opin. Ther. Pat.* **2009**, *19*, 137–140. [CrossRef]
133. Yu, Z.; Ye, J.; Pei, X.; Sun, L.; Liu, E.; Wang, J.; Huang, Y.; Lee, S.J.; He, H. Improved method for synthesis of low molecular weight protamine–siRNA conjugate. *Acta Pharm. Sin. B* **2018**, *8*, 116–126. [CrossRef] [PubMed]
134. Pärnaste, L.; Arukuusk, P.; Langel, K.; Tenson, T.; Langel, Ü. The Formation of Nanoparticles between Small Interfering RNA and Amphipathic Cell-Penetrating Peptides. *Mol. Ther. Nucleic Acids* **2017**, *7*, 1–10. [CrossRef]
135. Matsushita-Ishiodori, Y.; Ohtsuki, T. Photoinduced RNA interference. *Acc. Chem. Res.* **2012**, *45*, 1039–1047. [CrossRef] [PubMed]
136. Zeller, S.; Choi, C.S.; Uchil, P.D.; Ban, H.-S.; Siefert, A.; Fahmy, T.M.; Mothes, W.; Lee, S.-K.; Kumar, P. Attachment of cell-binding ligands to arginine-rich cell-penetrating peptides enables cytosolic translocation of complexed siRNA. *Chem. Biol.* **2015**, *22*, 50–62. [CrossRef] [PubMed]
137. Youn, P.; Chen, Y.; Furgeson, D.Y. A myristoylated cell-penetrating peptide bearing a transferrin receptor-targeting sequence for neuro-targeted siRNA delivery. *Mol. Pharm.* **2014**, *11*, 486–495. [CrossRef] [PubMed]
138. Xu, Y.Y.; Cao, X.W.; Fu, L.Y.; Zhang, T.Z.; Wang, F.J.; Zhao, J. Screening and characterization of a novel high-efficiency tumour-homing cell-penetrating peptide from the buffalo cathelicidin family. *J. Pept. Sci.* **2019**, *25*, e3201. [CrossRef]
139. Kang, J.H.; Battogtokh, G.; Ko, Y.T. Self-assembling lipid–peptide hybrid nanoparticles of phospholipid–nonaarginine conjugates for enhanced delivery of nucleic acid therapeutics. *Biomacromolecules* **2017**, *18*, 3733–3741. [CrossRef]
140. Hatakeyama, H.; Akita, H.; Kogure, K.; Oishi, M.; Nagasaki, Y.; Kihira, Y.; Ueno, M.; Kobayashi, H.; Kikuchi, H.; Harashima, H. Development of a novel systemic gene delivery system for cancer therapy with a tumour-specific cleavable PEG-lipid. *Gene Ther.* **2007**, *14*, 68–77. [CrossRef]
141. Xiang, B.; Jia, X.-L.; Qi, J.-L.; Yang, L.-P.; Sun, W.-H.; Yan, X.; Yang, S.-K.; Cao, D.-Y.; Du, Q.; Qi, X.-R. Enhancing siRNA-based cancer therapy using a new pH-responsive activatable cell-penetrating peptide-modified liposomal system. *Int. J. Nanomed.* **2017**, *12*, 2385. [CrossRef]
142. Yang, Y.; Xie, X.; Yang, Y.; Li, Z.; Yu, F.; Gong, W.; Li, Y.; Zhang, H.; Wang, Z.; Mei, X. Polymer nanoparticles modified with photo-and pH-dual-responsive polypeptides for enhanced and targeted cancer therapy. *Mol. Pharm.* **2016**, *13*, 1508–1519. [CrossRef]
143. Richard, C.M. The basic science of gene therapy. *Science* **1993**, *260*, 926–932.
144. Quinonez, R.; Sutton, R.E. Lentiviral vectors for gene delivery into cells. *DNA Cell Biol.* **2002**, *21*, 937–951. [CrossRef] [PubMed]
145. Zabel, M.D.; Mollnow, L.; Bender, H. siRNA Therapeutics for Protein Misfolding Diseases of the Central Nervous System. *Des. Deliv. SiRNA Ther.* **2021**, *2282*, 377–394.
146. Chiu, Y.L.; Ali, A.; Chu, C.Y.; Cao, H.; Rana, T.M. Visualizing a correlation between siRNA localization, cellular uptake, and RNAi in living cells. *Chem. Biol.* **2004**, *11*, 1165–1175. [CrossRef] [PubMed]
147. Meade, B.R.; Dowdy, S.F. Enhancing the cellular uptake of siRNA duplexes following noncovalent packaging with protein transduction domain peptides. *Adv. Drug. Deliv. Rev.* **2008**, *60*, 530–536. [CrossRef]
148. Barichello, J.M.; Ishida, T.; Kiwada, H. Complexation of siRNA and pDNA with cationic liposomes: The important aspects in lipoplex preparation. *Liposomes Methods Protoc. Pharm. Nanocarriers* **2010**, *605*, 461–472.
149. Malone, R.W.; Felgner, P.L.; Verma, I.M. Cationic liposome-mediated RNA transfection. *Proc. Natl. Acad. Sci. USA* **1989**, *86*, 6077–6081. [CrossRef]
150. Balazs, D.A.; Godbey, W. Liposomes for use in gene delivery. *J. Drug Deliv.* **2011**, *2011*, 326497. [CrossRef]
151. Patil, S.D.; Burgess, D.J. DNA-based Biopharmaceuticals: Therapeutics for the 21st Century. *AAPS Newsmag.* **2003**, *6*, 27.

152. Georgieva, J.V.; Hoekstra, D.; Zuhorn, I.S. Smuggling drugs into the brain: An overview of ligands targeting transcytosis for drug delivery across the blood–brain barrier. *Pharmaceutics* **2014**, *6*, 557–583. [CrossRef]
153. Uno, Y.; Piao, W.; Miyata, K.; Nishina, K.; Mizusawa, H.; Yokota, T. High-density lipoprotein facilitates in vivo delivery of α-tocopherol–conjugated short-interfering RNA to the brain. *Hum. Gene Ther.* **2011**, *22*, 711–719. [CrossRef]
154. Papahadjopoulos, D.; Allen, T.; Gabizon, A.; Mayhew, E.; Matthay, K.; Huang, S.; Lee, K.; Woodle, M.; Lasic, D.; Redemann, C. Sterically stabilized liposomes: Improvements in pharmacokinetics and antitumour therapeutic efficacy. *Proc. Natl. Acad. Sci. USA* **1991**, *88*, 11460–11464. [CrossRef]
155. Zamboni, W.C.; Ramalingam, S.; Friedland, D.M.; Edwards, R.P.; Stoller, R.G.; Strychor, S.; Maruca, L.; Zamboni, B.A.; Belani, C.P.; Ramanathan, R.K. Phase I and pharmacokinetic study of pegylated liposomal CKD-602 in patients with advanced malignancies. *Clin. Cancer Res.* **2009**, *15*, 1466–1472. [CrossRef] [PubMed]
156. Battaglia, L.; Panciani, P.P.; Muntoni, E.; Capucchio, M.T.; Biasibetti, E.; De Bonis, P.; Mioletti, S.; Fontanella, M.; Swaminathan, S. Lipid nanoparticles for intranasal administration: Application to nose-to-brain delivery. *Expert Opin. Drug Deliv.* **2018**, *15*, 369–378. [CrossRef] [PubMed]
157. Erdő, F.; Bors, L.A.; Farkas, D.; Bajza, Á.; Gizurarson, S. Evaluation of intranasal delivery route of drug administration for brain targeting. *Brain Res. Bull.* **2018**, *143*, 155–170. [CrossRef] [PubMed]
158. Danielyan, L.; Schäfer, R.; von Ameln-Mayerhofer, A.; Buadze, M.; Geisler, J.; Klopfer, T.; Burkhardt, U.; Proksch, B.; Verleysdonk, S.; Ayturan, M.; et al. Intranasal delivery of cells to the brain. *Eur. J. Cell Biol.* **2009**, *88*, 315–324. [CrossRef] [PubMed]
159. Danielyan, L.; Schäfer, R.; von Ameln-Mayerhofer, A.; Bernhard, F.; Verleysdonk, S.; Buadze, M.; Lourhmati, A.; Klopfer, T.; Schaumann, F.; Schmid, B. Therapeutic efficacy of intranasally delivered mesenchymal stem cells in a rat model of Parkinson disease. *Rejuvenation Res.* **2011**, *14*, 3–16. [CrossRef]
160. Danielyan, L.; Beer-Hammer, S.; Stolzing, A.; Schäfer, R.; Siegel, G.; Fabian, C.; Kahle, P.; Biedermann, T.; Lourhmati, A.; Buadze, M. Intranasal delivery of bone marrow-derived mesenchymal stem cells, macrophages, and microglia to the brain in mouse models of Alzheimer's and Parkinson's disease. *Cell Transplant.* **2014**, *23*, 123–139. [CrossRef]
161. Donega, V.; Nijboer, C.H.; van Tilborg, G.; Dijkhuizen, R.M.; Kavelaars, A.; Heijnen, C.J. Intranasally administered mesenchymal stem cells promote a regenerative niche for repair of neonatal ischemic brain injury. *Exp. Neurol.* **2014**, *261*, 53–64. [CrossRef]
162. Oppliger, B.; Joerger-Messerli, M.; Mueller, M.; Reinhart, U.; Schneider, P.; Surbek, D.V.; Schoeberlein, A. Intranasal delivery of umbilical cord-derived mesenchymal stem cells preserves myelination in perinatal brain damage. *Stem Cells Dev.* **2016**, *25*, 1234–1242. [CrossRef]
163. Balyasnikova, I.V.; Prasol, M.S.; Ferguson, S.D.; Han, Y.; Ahmed, A.U.; Gutova, M.; Tobias, A.L.; Mustafi, D.; Rincón, E.; Zhang, L. Intranasal delivery of mesenchymal stem cells significantly extends survival of irradiated mice with experimental brain tumours. *Mol. Ther.* **2014**, *22*, 140–148. [CrossRef]
164. Raposo, G.; Stoorvogel, W. Extracellular vesicles: Exosomes, microvesicles, and friends. *J. Cell Biol.* **2013**, *200*, 373–383. [CrossRef] [PubMed]
165. Valadi, H.; Ekström, K.; Bossios, A.; Sjöstrand, M.; Lee, J.J.; Lötvall, J.O. Exosome-mediated transfer of mRNAs and microRNAs is a novel mechanism of genetic exchange between cells. *Nat. Cell Biol.* **2007**, *9*, 654–659. [CrossRef] [PubMed]
166. Izco, M.; Carlos, E.; Alvarez-Erviti, L. The two faces of Exosomes in Parkinson's disease: From pathology to therapy. *Neuroscientist* **2022**, *28*, 180–193. [CrossRef] [PubMed]
167. Cheng, Z.; Al Zaki, A.; Hui, J.Z.; Muzykantov, V.R.; Tsourkas, A. Multifunctional nanoparticles: Cost versus benefit of adding targeting and imaging capabilities. *Science* **2012**, *338*, 903–910. [CrossRef]
168. Torchilin, V.P. Multifunctional, stimuli-sensitive nanoparticulate systems for drug delivery. *Nat. Rev. Drug Discov.* **2014**, *13*, 813–827. [CrossRef]
169. Castanotto, D.; Rossi, J.J. The promises and pitfalls of RNA-interference-based therapeutics. *Nature* **2009**, *457*, 426–433. [CrossRef]

*pharmaceutics*

MDPI

*Communication*

# Novel Human/Non-Human Primate Cross-Reactive Anti-Transferrin Receptor Nanobodies for Brain Delivery of Biologics

**Laura Rué [1,2,3,†], Tom Jaspers [1,†], Isabelle M. S. Degors [2,3], Sam Noppen [4], Dominique Schols [4], Bart De Strooper [2,3,5,*] and Maarten Dewilde [1,*]**

1 Laboratory for Therapeutic and Diagnostic Antibodies, Department of Pharmaceutical and Pharmacological Sciences, KU Leuven, 3000 Leuven, Belgium
2 VIB-KU Leuven Center for Brain & Disease Research, 3000 Leuven, Belgium
3 Laboratory for the Research of Neurodegenerative Diseases, Department of Neurosciences, Leuven Brain Institute (LBI), KU Leuven, 3000 Leuven, Belgium
4 Laboratory of Virology and Chemotherapy, Department of Microbiology, Immunology and Transplantation, Rega Institute, KU Leuven, 3000 Leuven, Belgium
5 UK Dementia Research Institute, University College London, London WC1E 6BT, UK
* Correspondence: bart.destrooper@kuleuven.be (B.D.S.); maarten.dewilde@kuleuven.be (M.D.)
† These authors contributed equally to this work.

**Abstract:** The blood-brain barrier (BBB), while being the gatekeeper of the central nervous system (CNS), is a bottleneck for the treatment of neurological diseases. Unfortunately, most of the biologicals do not reach their brain targets in sufficient quantities. The antibody targeting of receptor-mediated transcytosis (RMT) receptors is an exploited mechanism that increases brain permeability. We previously discovered an anti-human transferrin receptor (TfR) nanobody that could efficiently deliver a therapeutic moiety across the BBB. Despite the high homology between human and cynomolgus TfR, the nanobody was unable to bind the non-human primate receptor. Here we report the discovery of two nanobodies that were able to bind human and cynomolgus TfR, making these nanobodies more clinically relevant. Whereas nanobody BBB00515 bound cynomolgus TfR with 18 times more affinity than it did human TfR, nanobody BBB00533 bound human and cynomolgus TfR with similar affinities. When fused with an anti-beta-site amyloid precursor protein cleaving enzyme (BACE1) antibody (1A11AM), each of the nanobodies was able to increase its brain permeability after peripheral injection. A 40% reduction of brain $A\beta_{1\text{-}40}$ levels could be observed in mice injected with anti-TfR/BACE1 bispecific antibodies when compared to vehicle-injected mice. In summary, we found two nanobodies that could bind both human and cynomolgus TfR with the potential to be used clinically to increase the brain permeability of therapeutic biologicals.

**Keywords:** nanobody; VHH; transferrin receptor; blood-brain barrier; receptor-mediated transcytosis

**Citation:** Rué, L.; Jaspers, T.; Degors, I.M.S.; Noppen, S.; Schols, D.; De Strooper, B.; Dewilde, M. Novel Human/Non-Human Primate Cross-Reactive Anti-Transferrin Receptor Nanobodies for Brain Delivery of Biologics. *Pharmaceutics* **2023**, *15*, 1748. https://doi.org/10.3390/pharmaceutics15061748

Academic Editors: Xavier Declèves and Inge S. Zuhorn

Received: 27 April 2023
Revised: 6 June 2023
Accepted: 8 June 2023
Published: 16 June 2023



## 1. Introduction

The blood-brain barrier (BBB) is a very specialized organ that, together with the other brain barriers such as the blood-cerebrospinal fluid barrier and blood-arachnoid barrier, contributes to the isolation of the central nervous system (CNS) from the rest of the organism. This ensures that harmful circulating substances in the peripheral blood flow do not freely reach the CNS, while still allowing a selective influx of required elements such as nutrients [1,2]. Hence the BBB represents a bottleneck for the treatment of neurological diseases, as most of the biologicals are not able to reach their brain targets or only do so in very small quantities, i.e., less than 0.1% of peripherally administered doses [3–5]. Therefore, the high doses that need to be administered result in potential side effects and high treatment costs. The BBB is composed of an endothelial layer which is surrounded by pericytes and astrocyte end-feet [1]. Tight junctions expressed by the BBB endothelium limit the paracellular diffusion of substances. Most of the required substances in the brain that come from the periphery follow an active route of entry via specific channels and transporters [6]. Receptor-mediated transcytosis (RMT) is one such physiological mechanism in which nutrients are recognized by specific receptors that are expressed on the surface of the endothelial cells, internalized in intracellular vesicles, and finally released in the brain parenchyma [7]. Targeting such RMT receptors with antibodies is a valid strategy to increase the brain permeabilities of biologicals [8]. Among these receptors, the transferrin receptor (TfR) is one of the most exploited RMT mechanisms for brain drug delivery [9–18]. Recently, an anti-TfR-idursulfase conjugate drug (Izcargo®) was approved in Japan for the treatment of Hunter syndrome [19].

Nanobodies, which are the variable domain of camelid heavy chain-only antibodies, have ideal properties that allow the engineering of multispecific constructs [20]. Several nanobodies that successfully deliver biologicals over the BBB by targeting RMT receptors such as TfR, IGF1R, or TMEM30A have been described [11,15,16,21,22]. In a previous work, we obtained a set of mouse TfR binders and a set of human TfR binders [15,16]. Unfortunately, our human TfR nanobodies did not bind cynomolgus TfR despite the high sequence homology between both proteins. Lack of binding to non-human primate (NHP) TfR represents an obstacle to determine the preclinical efficacy and safety of potential therapeutic conjugates. Regulatory guidelines indicate that two animal species should generally be used for non-clinical toxicity testing, thereby supporting the development of drugs for human use: a rodent (e.g., mouse or rat) and a non-rodent (e.g., dog or NHP) [23]. Here we describe the identification of two human/cynomolgus TfR-binding nanobodies and validate in vivo their potential to shuttle therapeutics into the brain.

## 2. Materials and Methods

### 2.1. Animals

All animal experiments were conducted in compliance with the commonly accepted '3Rs', according to protocols approved by the local Ethical Committee of Laboratory Animals at KU Leuven (governmental license LA1210579, ECD project number P213/2020), and following governmental and EU guidelines. Mice were housed under standard conditions according to the guidelines of KU Leuven, with a 12-h light-dark cycle and with access to food and water ad libitum. Humanized Tfrc mice (hAPI KI mice), which express a chimeric mouse TfR with the human apical domain under the endogenous promoter, were used for this study [16].

### 2.2. Immunization and Nanobody Library Preparation

Targeted nanobody libraries were obtained in collaboration with the VIB Nanobody Core (Brussles, Belgium). Three alpacas were subjected to four biweekly DNA immunizations using recombinant pVAX1 plasmid DNA (Thermo Fisher Scientific, Waltham, MA, USA) encoding for a chimeric alpaca TfR with the cynomolgus apical domain (synthesized at Twist Biosciences, South San Francisco, CA, USA). DNA solutions were injected intradermally at multiple sites on the front and back limbs near the draining lymph nodes, and this was followed by electroporation. On days 4 and 8, after the last immunization, blood samples were collected and pooled, and total RNA from peripheral blood lymphocytes was isolated to recover the nanobody-encoding genes. The phagemid library was prepared as previously prescribed [24]. Briefly, total RNA was used as a template for first-strand cDNA synthesis with oligodT primer. This cDNA was used to amplify the nanobody-encoding open reading frames by means of polymerase chain reaction (PCR), digested with *PstI* and *NotI*, and cloned into a phagemid vector (pBDS001, a modified pMECS vector with an insertion of 3xFlag/6xHis tag at the C-terminus of the nanobody insertion site). Electrocompetent *E. coli* TG1 cells (Biosearch Technologies, Middlesex, UK) were transformed to obtain the nanobody libraries.

### 2.3. Cell Line Generation

The Flp-In™-CHO™ system (Thermo Fisher Scientific) was used to generate stable Chinese hamster ovary (CHO) cell lines overexpressing cynomolgus or human TfR. DNA encoding for the cynomolgus TfR or the human TfR, tagged with hemagglutinin (HA) at the C-terminus and followed by green fluorescent protein (GFP) under the control of an internal ribosome entry site (IRES), was synthesized and subcloned by Twist Bioscience into the pcDNA™5/FRT mammalian expression vector (Thermo Fisher Scientific). Flp-In™-CHO™ cells were maintained with Gibco™ Ham's F-12 Nutrient Mix medium supplemented with GlutaMAX™ (Thermo Fisher Scientific), 10% fetal bovine serum (FBS), and 100 µg/mL Zeocin™ selection antibiotic (Invivogen, San Diego, CA, USA) until the day of transfection. Cells were transfected with the TransIT-PRO® Transfection kit (Mirus, Madison, WI, USA) and maintained in Gibco™ Ham's F-12 Nutrient Mix medium supplemented with GlutaMAX™ (Thermo Fisher Scientific), 10% FBS, and Hygromycin B Gold (Invivogen) to select for stable transfectants. Stable transfectants were then amplified and frozen with 10% dimethyl sulfoxide (DMSO) for further use.

### 2.4. Nanobody Selection, Expression and Purification

Nanobody-displaying M13 phage libraries were prepared according to standard protocols [24] and selected twice on TfR-overexpressing cells. Briefly, $6 \times 10^{11}$ cfu of phages were blocked with phosphate-buffered saline (PBS)/10% FBS and incubated for an hour with 5 million cells of CHO-cynomolgus TfR-overexpressing cells in the first selection round and CHO-human TfR-overexpressing cells in the second selection round. Non-binding phages were discarded with 5 consecutive washing steps with PBS/10% FBS, whereas bound phages were eluted by means of trypsinization. The output phage library of the second selection round was subcloned into an expression vector (pBDS119, a modified pHEN6 vector with an OmpA signal peptide and a C-terminal 3xFlag/6xHis tag) and transformed in *E. coli* TG1 cells. Single clones were picked, sequenced (Eurofins, Luxembourg), and clustered according to sequence homology with PipeBio (Horsens, Denmark). In addition, the small-scale expression of sequenced clones was performed and periplasmic extracts were prepared as previously described [24] and screened for direct binding to CHO-human TfR-overexpressing cells. Nanobody leads were expressed and purified according to the protocol provided by Pardon et al. [24].

### 2.5. Flow Cytometry-Based Binder Screening and Validation

Periplasmic extracts that were diluted 1:10 in PBS 2% FBS, or a dilution range of different nanobody or bispecific antibody concentrations prepared in PBS 2% FBS, were incubated with 0.1 million CHO cells overexpressing either the human, cynomolgus, or mouse TfR for 30 min at 4 °C. As control for background binding, periplasmic extracts, nanobodies, or bispecific antibodies were also incubated with 0.1 million CHO cells overexpressing GFP. The binding of nanobodies was next resolved by a 30-min incubation at 4 °C with an anti-FLAG-iFluor647 antibody (A01811, Genscript, Piscataway, NJ, USA), diluted 1:500 for screening and 1:250 for validation assays, or with anti-human IgG Fc-Alexa Fluor647 antibody (410714, BioLegend, San Diego, CA, USA) diluted 1:200. Dead cells were stained with the viability dye eFluor™780 (1:2000; 65-0865-14, Thermo Fisher Scientific) for 30 min at 4 °C. Cells were fixed with 4% paraformaldehyde before being analyzed. Flp-In™-CHO™ cells, used as unstained control and single stain controls, were used to determine the cutoff point between background fluorescence and positive populations. UltraComp eBeads™ Compensation Beads were used (Thermo Fisher Scientific) to generate single stain controls of both anti-FLAG-iFluor647 antibody and anti-human IgG Fc-Alexa Fluor647 antibody. The data was acquired by using an Attune Nxt flow cytometer (Invitrogen) and analyzed by FCS Express 7 Research Edition.

### 2.6. Surface Plasmon Resonance

Surface Plasmon Resonance (SPR) was used to measure the interactions between nanobodies and recombinant human or cynomolgus TfR receptor. Human TfR (2474-TR, R&D Systems, Minneapolis, MN, USA) and cynomolgus TfR (90253-C07H, Sino Biological, Beijing, China) were biotinylated with the EZ-Link NHS-PEG4-Biotinylation Kit (ThermoFischer Scientific) according to the manufacturer's instructions. The binding experiments were performed at 25 °C on a Biacore T200 instrument (Cytiva, Marlborough, MA, USA) in HBS-EP+ buffer (10 mM HEPES, 150 mM NaCl, 3 mM EDTA, and 0.05% *v*/*v* Surfactant P20). Biotinylated human TfR and cynomolgus TfR were captured on a streptavidin-coated SA sensor chip (Cytiva) at a density of around 250 RU. Increasing concentrations of nanobodies were sequentially injected in a single cycle at a flow rate of 30 μL/min. The dissociation was monitored for 20 min. No specific regeneration was needed. A reference flow was used as a control for non-specific binding and refractive index changes. Several buffer blanks were used for double referencing. Binding affinities ($K_D$) and kinetic rate constants ($k_a$, $k_d$) were derived after fitting the experimental data to the 1:1 binding model with the Biacore T200 Evaluation Software 3.1 using the single-cycle kinetic procedure. Each interaction was repeated at least three times.

### 2.7. Bio-Layer Interferometry (BLI)

Binding of the bispecific antibodies to beta-site amyloid precursor protein cleaving enzyme (BACE1) was assessed with an Octet RED96 (Sartorius, Göttingen, Germany). Briefly, streptavidin (SA) biosensors (18-5020, Forté Bio/Molecular Devices) were pre-wet for at least 10 min in kinetic buffer. Next, the biosensors were dipped in biotinylated BACE1 (5 μg/mL in kinetic buffer). BACE1 (Protein Service Facility, VIB) biotinylation was performed with the EZ-Link NHS-PEG4-Biotinylation Kit (ThermoFischer Scientific) according to the manufacturer's instructions. Biosensors were then sequentially submerged in baseline wells filled with PBS containing 0.02% Tween, 0.1% bovine serum albumin (BSA), and bispecific antibodies diluted in the same buffer, and finally back into baseline wells to assess dissociation. Data was recorded using the Forté Bio Octet RED data acquisition software (Forté Bio/Molecular Devices). Curve fitting and binding kinetics determination was performed with a 1:1 model interaction using the Forté Bio Octet RED analysis software (Forté Bio/Molecular Devices). Sensorgrams were generated using Graphpad.

### 2.8. Bispecific Antibodies Engineering and Expression

The anti-BACE1 affinity-matured 1A11 antibody (1A11AM) was used to generate bispecific antibodies. The engineering and expression of BBB00574 (1A11AM-BBB00515) and BBB00578 (1A11AM-BBB00533) were performed as previously described [16,25]. Briefly, the DNA sequences encoding for the heavy chain composed of BBB00515 or BBB00533 fused to an Fc with knobs-into-holes (KiH) and ablated effector function mutations (human IgG1, L234A, L235A, P329G, T350V, T366L, K392L, T394W), the 1A11AM heavy chain with KiH and ablated effector function mutations (human IgG1, L234A, L235A, P329G, T350V, L351Y, F405A, Y407V), and the 1A11AM light chain (human kappa) were synthesized by Twist Bioscience and cloned in their pTwist CMV BetaGlobin WPRE Neo vector (Twist Bioscience). Expressions were performed using the Mirus CHOgro® High Yield Expression System (Mirus Bio) according to the manufacturer instructions. Briefly, ExpiCHO-S™ cells (Mirus Bio) were transfected with the nanobody-human Fc fusions and the 1A11AM heavy chain and light chain with a transfection ratio of 2:1:3 with TransIT-PRO Transfection Reagent (Mirus Bio) [25]. After an incubation time of 14 days, the antibodies were purified, first with AmMag™ Protein A Magnetic Beads (Genscript) and then over a CaptureSelect™ CH1-XL Pre-packed Column (ThermoFischer Scientific) according to the manufacturer's instructions.

### 2.9. Sample Collection, Aβ Extraction and Enzyme-Linked Immunosorbent Assay (ELISA)

Each mouse was euthanized by the intraperitoneal injection of a Dolethal overdose (150–200 mg/kg). To harvest plasma, blood was collected with a prefilled heparin syringe via cardiac puncture. Next, blood samples were spun at 2000× *g* for 10 min and plasma was collected. Brains were harvested after transcardial perfusion with heparinized PBS. Mouse $A\beta_{1-40}$ samples from brain and plasma were prepared according to the protocols used by Serneels et al. [26]. Briefly, one brain hemisphere per mouse was homogenized in buffer containing 0.4% diethylamine (Sigma, St. Louis, MO, USA) and 50 mM NaCl supplemented with cOmplete™ protease inhibitor cocktail (Roche, Basel, Switzerland) using a FastPrep-24™ Classic bead-beating lysis system (MP Biomedicals, Santa Ana, CA, USA). Next, soluble $A\beta_{1-40}$ was extracted via 0.4% diethylamine treatment for 30 min at 4 °C, high-speed centrifugation (100,000× *g*, 1 h, 4 °C), and neutralization with 0.5 M Tris-HCl (pH 6.8). Soluble $A\beta_{1-40}$ levels extracted from brain and $A\beta_{1-40}$ levels in plasma were quantified by ELISA using Meso Scale Discovery (MSD) 96-well plates and $A\beta_{1-40}$ antibodies provided by Janssen Pharmaceutica (Beerse, Belgium). JRFcAβ40/28 antibody was used as the capture antibody whereas the rodent-specific JRF/rAβ/2, labeled with sulfo-TAG, was used as the detection antibody. Soluble $A\beta_{1-40}$ levels were interpolated from a recombinant $A\beta_{1-40}$ (A-1153-2, rPeptide) standard curve with the non-linear regression fit Log (agonist) vs. response–variable slope (4 parameters) model from the Graphpad prism 9.4.1 software.

### 2.10. Statistical Analysis

Statistics were performed using the Graphpad prism 9.4.1 software. A one-way ANOVA statistical test, followed by a Dunnett's multiple comparisons test, was performed to report statistically significant differences in the levels of $A\beta_{1-40}$ in the plasma and brain samples obtained from mice injected with PBS or bispecific antibodies. Statistical significance was considered for a $p$ value $< 0.05$.

## 3. Results

### 3.1. Identification of Human/Cynomolgus TfR Binders

The currently described TfR affinity binders that are able to cross the BBB bind the TfR apical domain. To direct immunization against this region, camelids were immunized with DNA encoding for alpaca TfR with the sequence encoding for the apical domain replaced by the cynomolgus apical domain sequence. Phage libraries, generated after 4 biweekly immunizations of two different camelids, underwent two rounds of pannings on CHO cell lines, overexpressing cynomolgus TfR in the first round and human TfR in the second round (Figure 1A). A total of 95 individual clones were then picked from the resulting selected library and sequenced (Figure 1A). These nanobody sequences were clustered together to exclude identical sequences. The periplasmic extracts of all the non-redundant sequences were then prepared and screened to find binders to both human and cynomolgus TfR-overexpressing CHO cells (Figure 1A). From the 32 clones screened, only 8 bound both human and cynomolgus TfR-overexpressing CHO cells. A cluster analysis of these 8 clones revealed the high homology (above 91%) between 7 of them. Therefore, out of these 8 hits, two leads were chosen for further expression, purification, and characterization. Purified BBB00515 and BBB00533 bound both human and cynomolgus TfR-overexpressing cells whereas they did not bind mouse TfR-overexpressing cells or a control cell line only expressing GFP (Figure 1B–E). The binding kinetics to recombinant human and cynomolgus TfR were further characterized in vitro with Surface Plasmon Resonance (SPR) (Figure 1F–H). Both BBB00515 and BBB00533 bound immobilized recombinant cynomolgus TfR with similar estimated affinity constants ($K_D = 63.00 \pm 1.20$ nM for BBB00515 and $K_D = 103.77 \pm 8.14$ nM for BBB00533; Figure 1H). Both also bound to immobilized recombinant human TfR, but with higher $K_D$ values ($K_D = 1183.67 \pm 423.81$ nM for BBB00515 and $K_D = 207.00 \pm 27.84$ nM for BBB00533; Figure 1H).

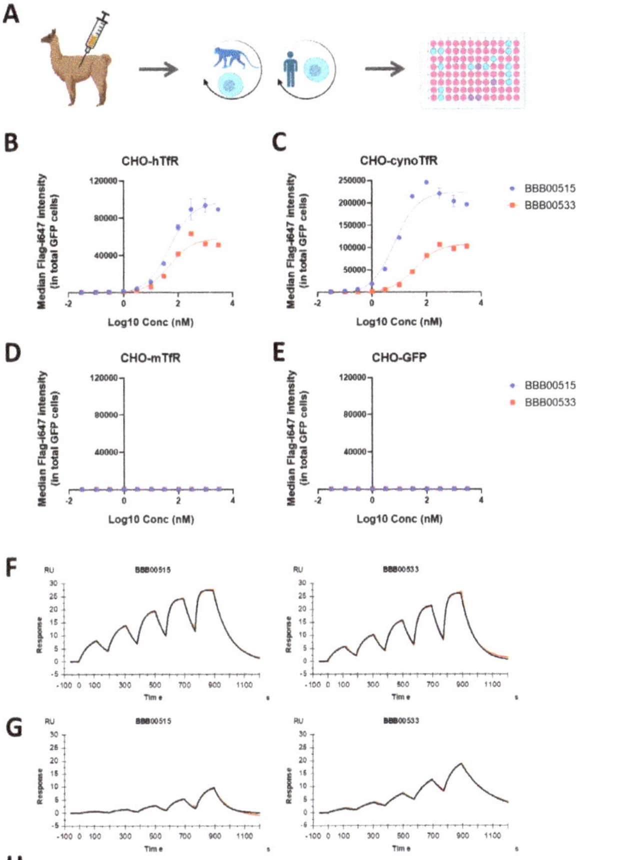


H

| Analyte | Ligand | $k_a$ (1/Ms) (x $10^5$) | $k_d$ (1/s) (x $10^{-3}$) | $K_D$ (nM) |
|---|---|---|---|---|
| BBB00515 | Cynomolgus TfR | 1.49 ± 0.05 | 9.42 ± 0.45 | 63.00 ± 1.20 |
| BBB00515 | Human TfR | 0.15 ± 0.05 | 13.68 ± 1.90 | 1183.67 ± 423.81 |
| BBB00533 | Cynomolgus TfR | 1.15 ± 0.09 | 11.83 ± 0.23 | 103.77 ± 8.14 |
| BBB00533 | Human TfR | 0.29 ± 0.01 | 5.92 ± 0.70 | 207.00 ± 27.84 |

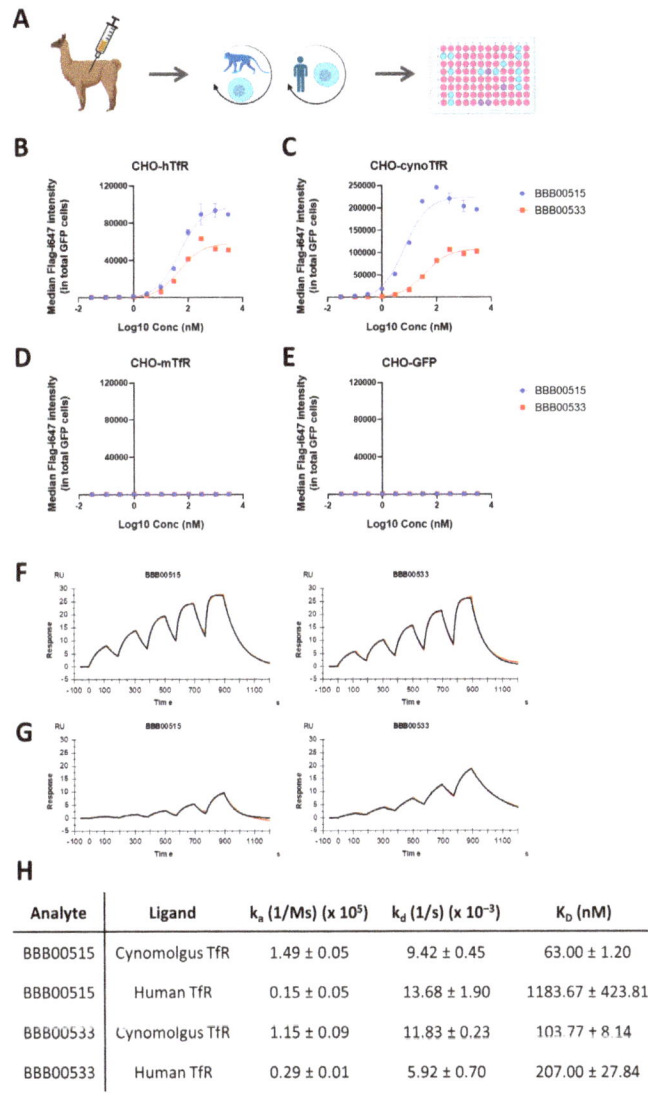

**Figure 1.** (**A**) Camelids were immunized with alpaca TfR DNA with the human apical domain sequence. Immune phage libraries were selected in the first round on CHO cells overexpressing cynomolgus TfR and on CHO cells overexpressing human TfR in the second round. The sequencing and screening of several clones was performed via flow cytometry based on the binding of periplasmic extract to CHO cells overexpressing human TfR. Graphical designs were created with BioRender.com. Different colors in 96-well plate represent different levels of binding (**B–E**) Flow cytometry analysis showing the binding of nanobodies to CHO cells overexpressing (**B**) hTfR, (**C**) cynomolgus TfR, (**D**) mouse TfR, and (**E**) GFP. The data represent means ± SEM ($n$ = 3). (**F**,**G**) SPR binding kinetics (black-colored line) and curve fitting (red-colored line) of nanobodies binding to cynomolgus TfR (**F**) and human TfR (**G**) recombinant material. (**H**) SPR kinetic analysis indicated different binding affinities of nanobodies to cynomolgus and human TfR recombinant material.

### 3.2. Anti-Human/Cynomolgus TfR Nanobodies Shuttle Anti-BACE1 mAb into the Brain

BACE1 inhibition in the brain was the paradigm used to assess the potential of the nanobodies to deliver, in vivo, biologicals in the brain [12,13,16]. BACE1 is responsible for the cleavage of APP to give rise to Aβ species [27]. BACE1-inhibiting antibody (Mab 1A11AM) is able to reduce brain $A\beta_{1-40}$ levels in vivo but does not cross the BBB in sufficient amounts when it is delivered peripherally [16,28]. Here, the abilities of BBB00515 and BBB00533 to modulate the properties of 1A11AM and improve brain accumulation after peripheral delivery were examined. Therefore, bispecific antibodies with ablated effector function were generated, with each bispecific antibody having one intact 1A11AM Fab and one nanobody, both fused to their respective Fcs (Figure 2A). BBB00574 bispecific antibody carries a BBB00515 nanobody, whereas BBB00578 carries a BBB00533 nanobody. As expected, both bispecific antibodies were still able to bind hTfR in living cells, but were not able to do so in a negative-control cell line (Figure 2B,C). Binding to BACE1 was confirmed with BLI, in which biotinylated recombinant human BACE1 protein was immobilized at the tip of streptavidin-coated biosensors (Figure 2D–F). Both bispecific antibodies bound human BACE1 with similar $K_D$ values of 0.3 nM (Figure 2F).

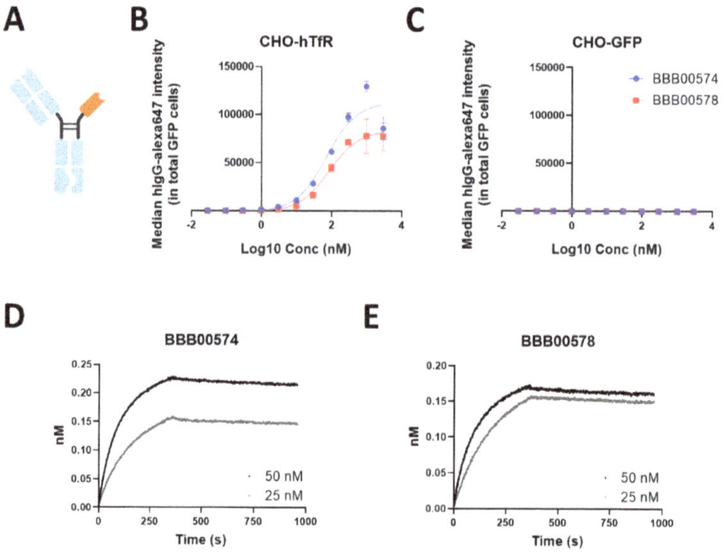


F

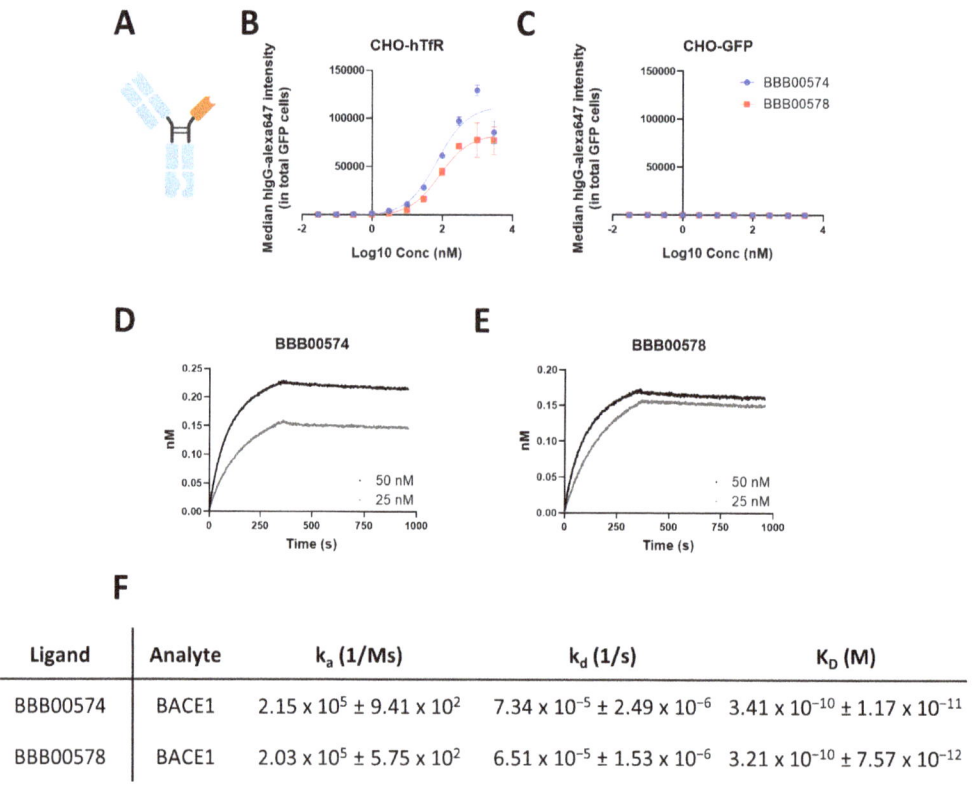

| Ligand | Analyte | $k_a$ (1/Ms) | $k_d$ (1/s) | $K_D$ (M) |
|---|---|---|---|---|
| BBB00574 | BACE1 | $2.15 \times 10^5 \pm 9.41 \times 10^2$ | $7.34 \times 10^{-5} \pm 2.49 \times 10^{-6}$ | $3.41 \times 10^{-10} \pm 1.17 \times 10^{-11}$ |
| BBB00578 | BACE1 | $2.03 \times 10^5 \pm 5.75 \times 10^2$ | $6.51 \times 10^{-5} \pm 1.53 \times 10^{-6}$ | $3.21 \times 10^{-10} \pm 7.57 \times 10^{-12}$ |

**Figure 2.** (**A**) A bispecific antibody design with one 1A11AM intact Fab and a nanobody coupled to an Fc with KiH and ablated effector function mutations. Created with BioRender.com. (**B**,**C**) Flow cytometry analysis showed bispecific antibody binding to (**B**) human TfR or (**C**) GFP-overexpressing cells. The data represent means ± SEM ($n$ = 3). (**D**,**E**) BLI binding kinetics of BBB00574 (**D**) and BBB00578 (**E**) bispecific antibodies to recombinant human BACE1. (**F**) The kinetic analysis of bispecific antibodies binding human BACE1 was performed using a 1:1 interaction model.

Next, both bispecific antibodies were administered intravenously in hAPI KI mice in which the mouse TfR apical domain had been replaced by the human sequence [16]. The chosen concentration to inject was 167 nmols/kg, which was the dose at which no central BACE1 inhibition had been observed for 1A11AM after intravenous injection [16,28]. Plasma and brains were harvested 24 h later, and $A\beta_{1-40}$ levels were quantified with ELISA. Both BBB00574 and BBB00578 bispecific antibodies could lower $A\beta_{1-40}$ levels in plasma by 60%, as compared to what had been found in samples of PBS injected mice (Figure 3A). Interestingly, $A\beta_{1-40}$ levels in the brain were reduced by 40% as compared to what had been noted in PBS injected mice (Figure 3B), suggesting the ability of both nanobodies to carry biological moieties over the BBB. 1A11AM antibody coupled to an anti-GFP nanobody and administered intravenously at the same concentration of 167 nmols/kg in hAPI KI mice did not decrease brain $A\beta_{1-40}$ levels 24 h after injection as compared to what had been noted in a PBS control group [16].

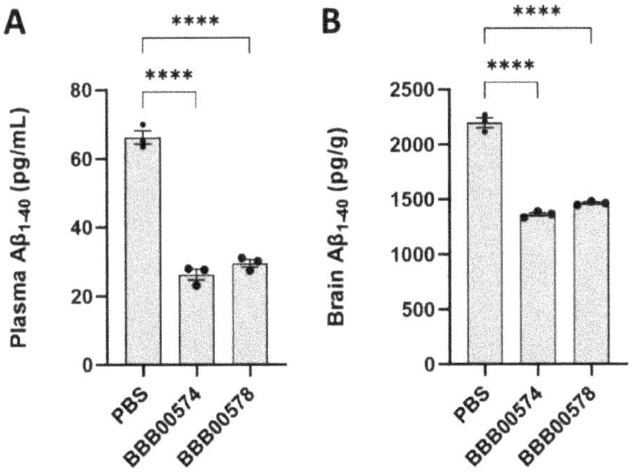


**Figure 3.** $A\beta_{1-40}$ levels were quantified in (**A**) plasma and (**B**) brain as readout of BACE1 inhibition, in mice injected intravenously with either PBS, BBB00574, or BBB00578. The data represent means ± SEM ($n$ = 3), and different conditions were compared to the PBS control group using a one-way ANOVA with Dunnett's multiple comparisons test: **** $p < 0.0001$. Each dot represents one mouse.

## 4. Discussion

In previous studies, we reported the discovery of first an anti-mouse TfR nanobody (NB62) and next an anti-human TfR nanobody (NB188) [15,16]. These could both efficiently deliver therapeutic moieties in the brain. Unfortunately, we later discovered a lack of NHP cross-reactivity for NB188, and this was a drawback for preclinical development, as safety of potential therapeutics is commonly assessed in NHPs [23]. Previous experiences from our lab and others indicate that acquiring human and cynomolgus TfR binders is challenging [12]. Currently described TfR affinity binders that are able to reach the CNS bind the TfR apical domain. Despite the fact that the apical domains of human and cynomolgus TfR have a 95% homology, there is no guarantee of cross-reactivity of antibodies [12]. We have also observed that two residues in the cynomolgus sequence that differ from those in the human sequence give rise to a glycosylation site that is absent in the human TfR, potentially hampering the binding of biologicals to TfR. To drive immunization against the cynomolgus apical domain, camelids were immunized with a chimeric DNA encoding for the alpaca TfR sequence with the apical domain sequence replaced by the cynomolgus sequence. After phage selections and screening on TfR-overexpressing cells, we found 2 nanobodies, BBB00515 and BBB00533, that were able to bind both human and cynomolgus TfR. Ideally, to be able to predict—based on the outcomes of preclinical studies—the amount of IgG that will accumulate in the brain in human patients, the binding affinities to both human and cynomolgus TfR should be similar. Although some studies have reported TfR binders with similar affinities to human and cynomolgus species [10,13], some others have reported higher affinities to human TfR than to cynomolgus TfR [12,29]. One of our two newly identified nanobodies, BBB00515, binds cynomolgus TfR with 18 times more affinity than human TfR. However, BBB00533 is only two times more affine to cynomolgus than human TfR, making it the most interesting nanobody to consider for further preclinical development.

Nanobodies were fused to a BACE1-inhibiting antibody, 1A11AM, to validate their potential to deliver biologicals into the brain. Two bispecific antibodies were engineered, and in each of them, 1A11AM Fab and one of the nanobodies (BBB00515 or BBB00533) were fused to an Fc. To provide a functional readout of BACE1 inhibition and hence BBB penetration, we chose here to quantify the $A\beta_{1-40}$ levels 24 h after injection of the bispecific antibodies. We previously demonstrated that while the 1A11AM antibody is able to reduce $A\beta_{1-40}$ levels in the periphery, it is not able to do so in the brain when injected intravenously [16,28]. Other studies showed similar findings when anti-BACE1 antibodies were injected at low concentrations and allowed to circulate for only 24 h [12,30] in each case. Interestingly, our new bispecific antibodies, BBB00574 and BBB00578—carrying either BBB00515 or BBB00533 nanobodies, respectively—were able to reduce $A\beta_{1-40}$ levels in the brain, suggesting penetration into the brain parenchyma after peripheral injection. Despite having different affinities for human TfR, both of our lead nanobodies, when fused to 1A11AM, were able to inhibit BACE1 by similar levels, resulting in a 40% reduction of $A\beta_{1-40}$ levels in the brain as compared to what had been recorded in the PBS-injected controls. This degree of BACE1 inhibition was similar to those of both Genentech's anti-human TfR/BACE1 antibodies and our previously reported anti-human TfR nanobody fused to 1A11AM antibody, all injected at equimolar concentrations [12,13,16]. Previous findings corroborate that bispecific antibodies with differing human TfR affinities can lead to similar BACE1 inhibitions 24 h after treatment [12,13]. We strongly believe that this lowering in Aβ-levels in the brain is related to an increased brain penetration of the BACE1-inhibiting antibodies and not to peripheral effects such as those suggested by the peripheral sink hypothesis in the context of Aβ clearance. This hypothesis states that Aβ clearance in blood could yield into an efflux of Aβ from the brain to blood, thereby reducing Aβ in the brain compartment [31]. However, such an effect has not been observed so far in a multitude of studies from various research groups when inhibiting peripheral BACE1 either genetically or pharmacologically, even after several months of treatment [12,16,28,30,32]. Additional experiments, such as pharmacokinetic studies of the bispecific antibodies, could potentially be performed to determine exact antibody levels in the brain over time. Finally, it would be of interest to determine the yield of BACE1 inhibition in the brain/cerebrospinal fluid (CSF) in an NHP. We expect our bispecific constructs to be efficient since their affinities to cynomolgus TfR are similar to their affinities to human TfR and in the same range as the anti-TfR1/BACE1 antibody from Genentech, which yielded a 50% BACE1 reduction in NHP CSF [13].

## 5. Conclusions

Here we have described two novel nanobodies binding to both human and non-human primate TfR and suggested that they are able to deliver biologicals into the brain in a humanized TfR mouse model. One of them, BBB00533, binds with similar affinity to human and cynomolgus TfRs. This is an important finding since cross-reactivity is a prerequisite for further clinical development. If their potentials to deliver biologicals were to be confirmed in a non-human primate, these nanobodies could be used clinically to increase the brain permeabilities of therapeutic biologicals.

**Author Contributions:** Conceptualization of the study: M.D. and B.D.S. Design, collection, analysis and interpretation of the data: L.R., T.J., I.M.S.D., S.N. and M.D. Drafting and revising the manuscript: L.R., T.J., I.M.S.D., S.N., D.S., B.D.S. and M.D. All authors have read and agreed to the published version of the manuscript.

**Funding:** Laura Rué is an Alzheimer's Association Research Fellow (AARF-22–928639). Bart De Strooper and Maarten Dewilde were supported by the Cure Alzheimer's Fund, VIB Grand Challenges and FWO (grant no. S007918N). Work in the Laboratories of Dewilde and Schols was additionally supported by Interne Fondsen KU Leuven/Internal Funds KU Leuven. Work in the De Strooper laboratory was supported by KU Leuven, VIB, and a Methusalem grant from KU Leuven and the Flemish Government, the 'Geneeskundige Stichting Koningin Elisabeth', the MRC, the Alzheimer Society, and Alzheimer Research UK. Bart De Strooper is holder of the Bax-Vanluffelen Chair for Alzheimer's Disease.

**Institutional Review Board Statement:** All animal experiments were conducted according to protocols approved by the local Ethical Committee of Laboratory Animals at KU Leuven (governmental license LA1210579, ECD project number 213/2020) and following governmental and EU guidelines.

**Informed Consent Statement:** Consent to participate was not applicable since no human subjects were involved.

**Data Availability Statement:** Data presented in this study is openly available in KU Leuven Research Data Repository (RDR) at https://doi.org/10.48804/GXJABW.

**Acknowledgments:** We thank Veronique Hendrickx for animal husbandry. We would like to thank the VIB Nanobody Core for performing the immunizations and generating the VHH-displaying phage library.

**Conflicts of Interest:** The authors declare no conflict of interest.

## References

1. Daneman, R.; Prat, A. The Blood–Brain Barrier. *Cold Spring Harb. Perspect. Biol.* **2015**, *7*, a020412. [CrossRef] [PubMed]
2. Abbott, N.J.; Patabendige, A.A.K.; Dolman, D.E.M.; Yusof, S.R.; Begley, D.J. Structure and Function of the Blood–Brain Barrier. *Neurobiol. Dis.* **2010**, *37*, 13–25. [CrossRef]
3. Freskgård, P.-O.; Urich, E. Antibody Therapies in CNS Diseases. *Neuropharmacology* **2017**, *120*, 38–55. [CrossRef] [PubMed]
4. St-Amour, I.; Paré, I.; Alata, W.; Coulombe, K.; Ringuette-Goulet, C.; Drouin-Ouellet, J.; Vandal, M.; Soulet, D.; Bazin, R.; Calon, F. Brain Bioavailability of Human Intravenous Immunoglobulin and Its Transport through the Murine Blood–Brain Barrier. *J. Cereb Blood Flow Metab.* **2013**, *33*, 1983–1992. [CrossRef]
5. Poduslo, J.F.; Curran, G.L.; Berg, C.T. Macromolecular Permeability across the Blood-Nerve and Blood-Brain Barriers. *Proc. Natl. Acad. Sci. USA* **1994**, *91*, 5705–5709. [CrossRef] [PubMed]
6. Abbott, N.J.; Rönnbäck, L.; Hansson, E. Astrocyte–Endothelial Interactions at the Blood–Brain Barrier. *Nat. Rev. Neurosci.* **2006**, *7*, 41–53. [CrossRef]
7. Pardridge, W. Targeted Delivery of Protein and Gene Medicines through the Blood-Brain Barrier. *Clin. Pharmacol. Ther.* **2015**, *97*, 347–361. [CrossRef]
8. Pardridge, W.M. Receptor-Mediated Peptide Transport through the Blood-Brain Barrier. *Endocr. Rev.* **1986**, *7*, 314–330. [CrossRef]
9. Sehlin, D.; Stocki, P.; Gustavsson, T.; Hultqvist, G.; Walsh, F.S.; Rutkowski, J.L.; Syvänen, S. Brain Delivery of Biologics Using a Cross-Species Reactive Transferrin Receptor 1 VNAR Shuttle. *FASEB J.* **2020**, *34*, 13272–13283. [CrossRef]
10. Stocki, P.; Szary, J.; Rasmussen, C.L.M.; Demydchuk, M.; Northall, L.; Logan, D.B.; Gauhar, A.; Thei, L.; Moos, T.; Walsh, F.S.; et al. Blood-Brain Barrier Transport Using a High Affinity, Brain-Selective VNAR Antibody Targeting Transferrin Receptor 1. *FASEB J.* **2021**, *35*, e21172. [CrossRef]
11. Su, S.; Esparza, T.J.; Brody, D.L. Selection of Single Domain Anti-Transferrin Receptor Antibodies for Blood-Brain Barrier Transcytosis Using a Neurotensin Based Assay and Histological Assessment of Target Engagement in a Mouse Model of Alzheimer's Related Amyloid-Beta Pathology. *PLoS ONE* **2022**, *17*, e0276107. [CrossRef] [PubMed]
12. Kariolis, M.S.; Wells, R.C.; Getz, J.A.; Kwan, W.; Mahon, C.S.; Tong, R.; Kim, D.J.; Srivastava, A.; Bedard, C.; Henne, K.R.; et al. Brain Delivery of Therapeutic Proteins Using an Fc Fragment Blood-Brain Barrier Transport Vehicle in Mice and Monkeys. *Sci Transl. Med.* **2020**, *12*, eaay1359. [CrossRef] [PubMed]
13. Yu, Y.J.; Atwal, J.K.; Zhang, Y.; Tong, R.K.; Wildsmith, K.R.; Tan, C.; Bien-Ly, N.; Hersom, M.; Maloney, J.A.; Meilandt, W.J.; et al. Therapeutic Bispecific Antibodies Cross the Blood-Brain Barrier in Nonhuman Primates. *Sci. Transl. Med.* **2014**, *6*, 261ra154. [CrossRef] [PubMed]

14. Ullman, J.C.; Arguello, A.; Getz, J.A.; Bhalla, A.; Mahon, C.S.; Wang, J.; Giese, T.; Bedard, C.; Kim, D.J.; Blumenfeld, J.R.; et al. Brain Delivery and Activity of a Lysosomal Enzyme Using a Blood-Brain Barrier Transport Vehicle in Mice. *Sci. Transl. Med.* **2020**, *12*, eaay1163. [CrossRef]
15. Wouters, Y.; Jaspers, T.; De Strooper, B.; Dewilde, M. Identification and in Vivo Characterization of a Brain-Penetrating Nanobody. *Fluids Barriers CNS* **2020**, *17*, 62. [CrossRef]
16. Wouters, Y.; Jaspers, T.; Rué, L.; Serneels, L.; De Strooper, B.; Dewilde, M. VHHs as Tools for Therapeutic Protein Delivery to the Central Nervous System. *Fluids Barriers CNS* **2022**, *19*, 79. [CrossRef] [PubMed]
17. Niewoehner, J.; Bohrmann, B.; Collin, L.; Urich, E.; Sade, H.; Maier, P.; Rueger, P.; Stracke, J.O.; Lau, W.; Tissot, A.C.; et al. Increased Brain Penetration and Potency of a Therapeutic Antibody Using a Monovalent Molecular Shuttle. *Neuron* **2014**, *81*, 49–60. [CrossRef]
18. Edavettal, S.; Cejudo-Martin, P.; Dasgupta, B.; Yang, D.; Buschman, M.D.; Domingo, D.; Van Kolen, K.; Jaiprasat, P.; Gordon, R.; Schutsky, K.; et al. Enhanced Delivery of Antibodies across the Blood-Brain Barrier via TEMs with Inherent Receptor-Mediated Phagocytosis. *Med* **2022**, *3*, 860–882.e15. [CrossRef]
19. Giugliani, R.; Martins, A.M.; So, S.; Yamamoto, T.; Yamaoka, M.; Ikeda, T.; Tanizawa, K.; Sonoda, H.; Schmidt, M.; Sato, Y. Iduronate-2-Sulfatase Fused with Anti-HTfR Antibody, Pabinafusp Alfa, for MPS-II: A Phase 2 Trial in Brazil. *Mol. Ther.* **2021**, *29*, 2378–2386. [CrossRef]
20. Muyldermans, S. Applications of Nanobodies. *Annu. Rev. Anim. Biosci.* **2021**, *9*, 401–421. [CrossRef]
21. Yogi, A.; Hussack, G.; van Faassen, H.; Haqqani, A.S.; Delaney, C.E.; Brunette, E.; Sandhu, J.K.; Hewitt, M.; Sulea, T.; Kemmerich, K.; et al. Brain Delivery of IGF1R5, a Single-Domain Antibody Targeting Insulin-like Growth Factor-1 Receptor. *Pharmaceutics* **2022**, *14*, 1452. [CrossRef]
22. Farrington, G.K.; Caram-Salas, N.; Haqqani, A.S.; Brunette, E.; Eldredge, J.; Pepinsky, B.; Antognetti, G.; Baumann, E.; Ding, W.; Garber, E.; et al. A Novel Platform for Engineering Blood-brain Barrier-crossing Bispecific Biologics. *FASEB J.* **2014**, *28*, 4764–4778. [CrossRef] [PubMed]
23. Marque, T.; Leach, M.W. Nonclinical Toxicology Testing Strategies and Applicable International Regulatory Guidelines for Using Nonhuman Primates in the Development of Biotherapeutics. In *The Nonhuman Primate in Nonclinical Drug Development and Safety Assessment*; Elsevier: Amsterdam, The Netherlands, 2015; pp. 315–336, ISBN 978-0-12-417144-2.
24. Pardon, E.; Laeremans, T.; Triest, S.; Rasmussen, S.G.F.; Wohlkönig, A.; Ruf, A.; Muyldermans, S.; Hol, W.G.J.; Kobilka, B.K.; Steyaert, J. A General Protocol for the Generation of Nanobodies for Structural Biology. *Nat. Protoc.* **2014**, *9*, 674–693. [CrossRef] [PubMed]
25. Nesspor, T.C.; Kinealy, K.; Mazzanti, N.; Diem, M.D.; Boye, K.; Hoffman, H.; Springer, C.; Sprenkle, J.; Powers, G.; Jiang, H.; et al. High-Throughput Generation of Bipod (Fab × ScFv) Bispecific Antibodies Exploits Differential Chain Expression and Affinity Capture. *Sci. Rep.* **2020**, *10*, 7557. [CrossRef] [PubMed]
26. Serneels, L.; T'Syen, D.; Perez-Benito, L.; Theys, T.; Holt, M.G.; De Strooper, B. Modeling the β-Secretase Cleavage Site and Humanizing Amyloid-Beta Precursor Protein in Rat and Mouse to Study Alzheimer's Disease. *Mol. Neurodegener.* **2020**, *15*, 60. [CrossRef] [PubMed]
27. Sinha, S.; Anderson, J.P.; Barbour, R.; Basi, G.S.; Caccavello, R.; Davis, D.; Doan, M.; Dovey, H.F.; Frigon, N.; Hong, J.; et al. Purification and Cloning of Amyloid Precursor Protein β-Secretase from Human Brain. *Nature* **1999**, *402*, 537–540. [CrossRef]
28. Zhou, L.; Chávez-Gutiérrez, L.; Bockstael, K.; Sannerud, R.; Annaert, W.; May, P.C.; Karran, E.; De Strooper, B. Inhibition of Beta-Secretase in Vivo via Antibody Binding to Unique Loops (D and F) of BACE1. *J. Biol. Chem.* **2011**, *286*, 8677–8687. [CrossRef]
29. Sonoda, H.; Morimoto, H.; Yoden, E.; Koshimura, Y.; Kinoshita, M.; Golovina, G.; Takagi, H.; Yamamoto, R.; Minami, K.; Mizoguchi, A.; et al. A Blood-Brain-Barrier-Penetrating Anti-Human Transferrin Receptor Antibody Fusion Protein for Neuronopathic Mucopolysaccharidosis II. *Mol. Ther.* **2018**, *26*, 1366–1374. [CrossRef] [PubMed]
30. Atwal, J.K.; Chen, Y.; Chiu, C.; Mortensen, D.L.; Meilandt, W.J.; Liu, Y.; Heise, C.E.; Hoyte, K.; Luk, W.; Lu, Y.; et al. A Therapeutic Antibody Targeting BACE1 Inhibits Amyloid-β Production in Vivo. *Sci. Transl. Med.* **2011**, *3*, 84ra43. [CrossRef]
31. Zhang, Y.; Lee, D.H.S. Sink Hypothesis and Therapeutic Strategies for Attenuating Aβ Levels. *Neuroscientist* **2011**, *17*, 163–173. [CrossRef]
32. Georgievska, B.; Gustavsson, S.; Lundkvist, J.; Neelissen, J.; Eketjäll, S.; Ramberg, V.; Bueters, T.; Agerman, K.; Juréus, A.; Svensson, S.; et al. Revisiting the Peripheral Sink Hypothesis: Inhibiting BACE1 Activity in the Periphery Does Not Alter β-Amyloid Levels in the CNS. *J. Neurochem.* **2015**, *132*, 477–486. [CrossRef] [PubMed]

*pharmaceutics* MDPI

*Review*

# Nanoparticle Strategies to Improve the Delivery of Anticancer Drugs across the Blood–Brain Barrier to Treat Brain Tumors

**Wouter J. F. Vanbilloen [1,2], Julian S. Rechberger [1,3], Jacob B. Anderson [1,3,4], Leo F. Nonnenbroich [1,5,6], Liang Zhang [1] and David J. Daniels [1,3,*]**

1 Department of Neurologic Surgery, Mayo Clinic, Rochester, MN 55905, USA; rechberger.julian@mayo.edu (J.S.R.)
2 Department of Neurology, Elisabeth-Tweesteden Hospital, 5022 GC Tilburg, The Netherlands
3 Department of Molecular Pharmacology and Experimental Therapeutics, Mayo Clinic, Rochester, MN 55905, USA
4 Medical Scientist Training Program, Mayo Clinic College of Medicine and Science, Rochester, MN 55905, USA
5 Hopp Children's Cancer Center Heidelberg (KiTZ), 69120 Heidelberg, Germany
6 Clinical Cooperation Unit Pediatric Oncology, German Cancer Research Center (DKFZ) and German Consortium for Translational Cancer Research (DKTK), 69120 Heidelberg, Germany
* Correspondence: daniels.david@mayo.edu

**Abstract:** Primary brain and central nervous system (CNS) tumors are a diverse group of neoplasms that occur within the brain and spinal cord. Although significant advances in our understanding of the intricate biological underpinnings of CNS neoplasm tumorigenesis and progression have been made, the translation of these discoveries into effective therapies has been stymied by the unique challenges presented by these tumors' exquisitely sensitive location and the body's own defense mechanisms (e.g., the brain–CSF barrier and blood–brain barrier), which normally protect the CNS from toxic insult. These barriers effectively prevent the delivery of therapeutics to the site of disease. To overcome these obstacles, new methods for therapeutic delivery are being developed, with one such approach being the utilization of nanoparticles. Here, we will cover the current state of the field with a particular focus on the challenges posed by the BBB, the different nanoparticle classes which are under development for targeted CNS tumor therapeutics delivery, and strategies which have been developed to bypass the BBB and enable effective therapeutics delivery to the site of disease.

**Keywords:** nanoparticle; liposome; extracellular vesicle; chemotherapy; targeted therapy; drug delivery; blood–brain barrier; brain tumor; glioma

**Citation:** Vanbilloen, W.J.F.; Rechberger, J.S.; Anderson, J.B.; Nonnenbroich, L.F.; Zhang, L.; Daniels, D.J. Nanoparticle Strategies to Improve the Delivery of Anticancer Drugs across the Blood–Brain Barrier to Treat Brain Tumors. *Pharmaceutics* **2023**, *15*, 1804. https://doi.org/10.3390/pharmaceutics15071804

Academic Editors: Nicolas Tournier and Toshihiko Tashima

Received: 22 May 2023
Revised: 14 June 2023
Accepted: 20 June 2023
Published: 23 June 2023



## 1. Introduction

### 1.1. Primary Brain and Other Central Nervous System Tumors

Primary brain and other central nervous system (CNS) tumors are a diverse group of neoplasms that occur within the brain and spinal cord. These tumors can arise from various cell types, including glial cells, neurons, meningothelial cells, and embryonic cells. In adults, brain tumors account for approximately 2% of all cancer diagnoses and 3% of deaths due to cancer [1]. It is estimated that 700,000 people in the U.S. are living with a primary brain tumor, and approximately 90,000 more will be diagnosed in 2023 [2]. More than two-thirds of patients diagnosed with glioblastoma (GBM), the most aggressive type of brain cancer in adults, will succumb to their disease within 2 years of diagnosis, and an estimated 20,000 adults in the U.S. die from primary cancerous brain tumors each year [1,3]. In individuals under the age of 20, brain tumors are the second most common category of cancer and the leading cause of cancer-related death [4,5]. In children, H3 K27-altered diffuse midline glioma (DMG) is the most lethal form of brain cancer, associated with an abysmal prognosis and a 5-year survival rate of less than 2% [4,6]. Additionally, children diagnosed with a brain tumor who survive and enter adulthood will often be affected by the long-term consequences of exposing the developing brain to medical interventions [7]. Overall, brain tumors remain a significant source of morbidity and mortality for which diagnosis and treatment require extensive resource allocation and sophisticated diagnostic and therapeutic technology [8].

Treatment options for brain tumors depend on the type, location, and stage of the tumor, as well as the patient's age and overall health [9]. Most brain tumors have proved challenging to treat, due in large part to the molecular features of these tumors, which frequently work in concert to impede advancements in therapy [10]. Surgical resection, chemotherapy, and radiation therapy (RT) remain the primary treatment modalities [11,12]. Given the lack of durable therapies for most brain tumors, there is a dire unmet gap in clinical practice for improved therapeutic modalities based on the unique molecular underpinnings of individual tumors.

As our understanding of the intricate biology that mediates tumorigenesis and progression increases, the integration of molecularly targeted agents, which can target key factors on tumor cells, the tumor microenvironment, or the patient's immune system, into conventional therapeutic regimens may provide a substantial benefit for patients with otherwise incurable brain tumors [12–15]. However, a multitude of factors, such as molecular heterogeneity, invasion of tumor cells outside the bulk tumor core identified on imaging, as well as the brain–CSF barrier and blood–brain barrier (BBB), which prevent the buildup of xenobiotics within the CNS, may limit the efficacy of these promising therapeutic strategies [16].

### *1.2. Blood–Brain Barrier*

Although progress has been made in identifying potentially targetable vulnerabilities for the treatment of brain tumors, crossing the BBB and achieving therapeutic drug levels at the tumor remain significant obstacles. The BBB is an anatomical and biochemical barrier that works by tightly controlling the permeation of ions, macromolecules, and nutrients into the brain in order safeguard it from potentially harmful substances like toxins, pathogens, and drugs present in systemic circulation [17,18]. This is accomplished with cooperative work by multiple cellular components, including brain capillary endothelial cells (ECs), pericytes, and astrocytic glia cells, which orchestrate a complex intra- and intercellular barrier network [19–21]. Together, these cells not only serve a structural purpose, but they also function as a neurovascular unit that regulates BBB integrity and affects drug penetration into the brain [22,23].

Unlike the peripheral microvasculature, ECs located at the BBB are characterized by having only few fenestrations and pinocytic vesicles and are tightly linked by tight junctions (zonulae occludentes), which together act as a physical barrier, limiting the unrestricted diffusion of substances from the bloodstream into the brain [24,25]. Claudins, occludins, and junctional adhesion molecules (JAM-A, -B, and -C) are among the most abundant proteins that make up the zonula occludens complex for restricting paracellular transport [26,27]. Molecules that cannot diffuse easily across lipid bilayers, such as small hydrophilic drugs and therapeutic macromolecules, including antibodies and antibody–drug conjugates, therefore, cannot normally accumulate in meaningful amounts due to this physical barrier [28].

Polar nutrients like some amino acids, hormones, carbohydrates, and vitamins are transported across the BBB through carrier-mediated influx transporters such as the L-type amino acid transporter 1 (LAT1), glucose transporter 1 (GLUT1), and organic anion transporter polypeptides (OATPs) [29]. Similarly, large molecules like insulin, transferrin, and some vitamins can be shuttled into the brain by multiple transport mechanisms, including receptor-mediated endocytosis and different transcytosis pathways [17,30].

Efflux transporter proteins found on the luminal and abluminal side of the EC membrane effectively transport many lipophilic molecules through the luminal EC membrane back into the capillary lumen [31]. Many small molecules including drugs that can otherwise readily diffuse across plasma membranes have substrate properties for these efflux pumps [32]. ATP-binding cassette (ABC) family members, such as P-glycoprotein (P-gp), breast cancer resistance protein (BCRP) and multidrug resistance-associated protein 1 (MRP1), have been studied in detail and reported to limit brain distribution of numerous anticancer drugs [33–37]. Therefore, the physical and biochemical characteristics of the BBB greatly restrict the delivery of therapeutic agents to the brain, which may reduce the effectiveness of many systemically administered therapies [38–40].

The integrity of the BBB within the tumor area can vary depending on the particular tumor type and is referred to as the blood–tumor barrier (BTB) by many [18,40,41]. While in the majority of brain tumor patients, the BBB is disrupted to some extent, its integrity has been shown to be variable or remain intact using dynamic contrast enhanced magnetic resonance imaging (MRI), especially in the peritumoral regions [42–44]. This is particularly true for children with DMG and some medulloblastoma subtypes (e.g., sonic hedgehog (SHH) activated tumors), where little or no contrast enhancement on MRI indicates a largely intact BBB [45]. Furthermore, the structure of the BBB and the expression pattern of efflux transporters has been shown to vary in different patient populations [46,47]. Based on age, brain location, and efflux transporter type, a distinct maturation profile was reported in brain cortical and ventricular tissue of more than 50 human patients, including fetuses, newborns, children, and adults [48]. These findings imply that major advancements in the treatment of brain tumors will require the delivery of therapeutic agents across the BBB to all tumor regions regardless of individual patient and tumor characteristics.

### *1.3. Nanoparticle Strategies in Neuro-Oncology*

Nanoparticles (NP) are a diverse group of nanoscale objects characterized by their size—usually ranging from 1 to 100 nm—which have gained attention as drug delivery systems to improve the biodistribution of therapeutic agents through improved solubility and stability, ability to cross biological barriers, and organ- or cell-specific targeting in order to either increase efficacy, reduce side effects, or both [49,50]. Several NP-based drug formulations have been approved by the U.S. Food and Drug Administration (FDA) in other oncology fields, yet no successful clinical trials have been conducted in brain tumors, highlighting an important translational gap [51]. While there exists an abundance of promising preclinical studies, the clinical failure of nanoparticle formulations in brain tumors to date is likely related to an incomplete reflection of the BBB and other anatomical and physiological hurdles that must be surmounted to obtain access to this highly protected tumor environment. In this review, we will provide an update on and highlight recent developments in NP-based drug delivery systems across the BBB, with a specific focus on the therapeutic application for brain tumors, along with existing constraints and possible future paths to overcome translational limitations (Table 1) [52–57].

**Table 1.** General strengths and weaknesses of nanoparticle classes.

| Nanoparticle Class | Strengths | Weaknesses | References |
|---|---|---|---|
| Lipid-based NP | Simplicity of manufacturing process<br>Payload flexibility<br>Potential for surface modification<br>Biocompatibility | Rapid elimination from bloodstream<br>CARPA | [58–64] |
| Polymeric NP | Precise control over physicochemical properties and drug release profile<br>Payload flexibility<br>Potential for surface modification | Rapid elimination from bloodstream<br>Relatively low drug loading capacity | [65–71] |
| Inorganic NP | Variability in sizes, shapes, and constructs<br>Unique magnetic and/or photothermal properties, allowing theragnostic applications | Low solubility, aggregation<br>Toxicity concerns | [72–76] |
| Biological NP | Biocompatibility<br>Inherently functionalized membrane<br>Payload flexibility | Rapid elimination from bloodstream<br>Low production scalability<br>More complex drug loading process<br>Low drug loading capacity | [61,77–81] |

Abbreviations: NP = nanoparticle, CARPA = complement activation-related pseudoallergy.

## 2. Nanoparticle Classes under Investigation as Drug Delivery Systems for Brain Tumors

Several classes of NPs are being pursued for the development of CNS-targeted drug delivery systems. While many paradigms are applicable across different NP categories, important differences are to be observed. Synthetic (Figure 1) and biological NPs make up the two major categories of NPs. The former are characterized by a high degree of control over pertinent physicochemical properties, such as size and surface charge, and include lipid-based NPs, polymeric NPs, and inorganic NPs, among others. Biological NPs are either fully derived from living cells or at least partly constructed through a biological process, offering biocompatibility through their intrinsically functionalized membranes while foregoing some of tunability of synthetic NPs. Although the various NP classes have been thoroughly reviewed elsewhere, we will briefly discuss the main categories that have been investigated for the application in brain tumor therapy in the following section [58,64,69,72,82–87].

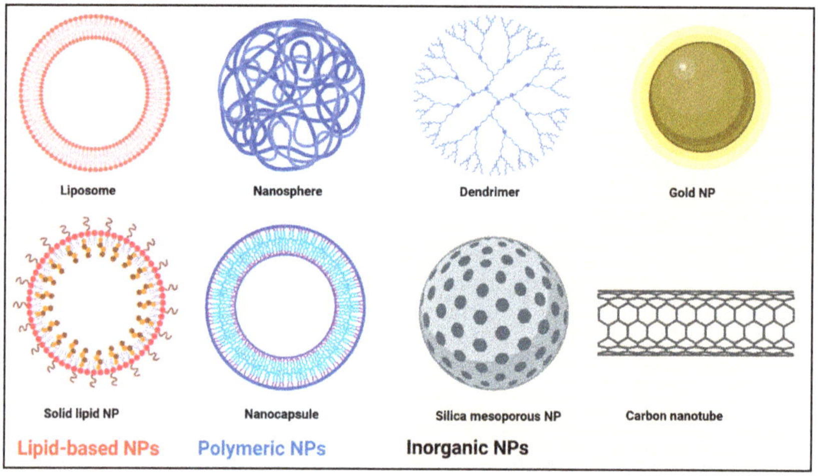


**Figure 1.** General structure of the most common synthetic nanoparticles (NPs) used for drug delivery. Created with BioRender.com.

### 2.1. Lipid-Based Nanoparticles

The two main lipid-based NPs are liposomes and solid lipid NPs (SLNs). Liposomes are spherical vesicles consisting of at least one phospholipid bilayer around an aqueous core, typically ranging from 30 to 2500 nm in size [88]. Despite the fact that several liposomal drug formulations are approved as systemic drug delivery system by the FDA, none are currently in clinical use for the treatment of brain tumors [51]. The main advantage of liposomes is the easy manufacturing process, allowing for the modulation of physicochemical properties and phospholipid composition. By introducing a double lipid bilayer or by encasing several vesicles inside a second membrane, multilaminar or multivesicular liposomes can be produced depending on the phospholipid makeup [58]. Furthermore, surface modifications using proteins, peptides or polymers are used to alter systemic circulation time and allow for targeted delivery [59,60]. A broad range of therapeutics, including both lipophilic and hydrophilic drugs, can be encapsulated in the lipid bilayer or the aqueous core, expanding the use of liposomal drug carriers [58]. An important limitation for clinical use is the low bioavailability due to efficient phagocytosis by the reticuloendothelial system (RES), resulting in preferential accumulation in the liver and spleen [61,89]. Moreover, even though liposomes are regarded as highly biocompatible, complement activation-related pseudoallergy (CARPA) is a common adverse reaction, occurring in 25–45% of patients upon first administration [62,90].

Solid lipid NPs (SLNs) are another common subset of lipid-based NPs. They differ from liposomes in that they are built from a phospholipid monolayer around a lipophilic core matrix. Within this core, micellar structures can be formed around hydrophilic cargo. SLNs have been mainly used as drug delivery systems for nucleic acids [63,91]. Ionizable phospholipids with near-neutral charge in physiologic pH form micelles around nucleic acids, while in acidic endosomes, these phospholipids become charged, promoting endosomal escape [63,91]. Combined with their simple synthesis and good biocompatibility, SLN are a promising drug delivery system for brain tumor therapy, and small molecule drugs have been successfully delivered to the brain using SLN [92–94]. However, as with liposomes, rapid accumulation in the RES is a major limiting factor [64,94].

Besides liposomes and SLNs, nanoemulsions have also been considered to improve drug delivery to CNS tumors. Nanoemulsions are colloidal suspensions, usually consisting of nanosized lipid droplets in aqueous media stabilized by surfactants [95]. They have gained attention due to their ability to cross biological barriers, increase bioavailability of hydrophobic therapeutics, ease of manufacturing, stability, and biocompatibility [95–98]. However, although some groups have been able to attach targeting ligands, the potential for modification is more restricted compared to other NPs [97]. While oral and intravenous administration have been investigated, the intranasal delivery of nanoemulsions was the most effective in the treatment of CNS tumors in animal models [99–101].

### 2.2. Polymeric Nanoparticles

Polymeric NPs are a diverse group of synthetic NPs. They are built using a natural or synthetic core polymer that either forms a solid nanosphere or a liposome-like nanocapsule, in which the core polymer forms a shell around a usually aqueous core. Most frequently used polymers in neuro-oncology research are poly (lactic-co-glycolic acid) (PLGA), poly (β-amino ester), polystyrene (PS), polyanhydride, chitosan, and polycaprolactone. Through the inclusion of various co-polymers, polymeric NPs exhibit a high potential for modifying stability and surface charge, enabling drug release timing to be altered from days to weeks [65,102–105]. As with liposomes, further surface functionalization is possible [66,67,106]. Drugs can either be attached to the surface, embedded in the nanosphere or nanocapsule shell, or can reside in the aqueous core, enabling the delivery of both lipophilic and hydrophilic cargo with different molecular weights [69].

Dendrimers are a specific type of polymeric NP that can be distinguished from other polymeric NPs by their structural differences. They are built from an initiator core that anchors a variable number of 'generations' of branched layers, terminating in an outer layer of functionalized surface groups that can harbor imaging, targeting or therapeutic moieties. Sizes typically range from 1 to 15 nm, growing 1–2 nm with each generation while doubling the amount of surface groups, allowing a high degree of control over size and surface chemistry [68]. Commonly used dendrimers to target the CNS are polamidoamine (PAMAM) and dendrigraft poly-L-lysine (DGL). Small molecule drugs and nucleic acids are the most frequent payloads, although a wide variety of therapeutics can be attached to the outer branches and encapsulated in the inner void spaces [84].

Overall, polymeric NPs are excellent candidates for drug delivery because they are biodegradable into nontoxic components, highly tunable, and several polymers have been FDA-approved for clinical use as either systemic or topical drug delivery system [51,107–113]. However, the low drug loading capacity of most polymeric NPs and rapid clearance by the RES are limiting factors [70,71]. Notwithstanding these limitations, several clinical trials of polymeric NPs for systemic drug delivery in cancer are ongoing, although none of which target CNS neoplasms [114].

### 2.3. Inorganic Nanoparticles

Inorganic NPs are synthesized from inorganic compounds, such as gold, silica, iron and carbon, and can be manufactured in a wide array of sizes and shapes. Gold NP (AuNP), for example, form nanospheres, nanorods, nanoflowers, nanoshells and nanocages [72]. Carbon forms quantum dots, fullerenes or nanotubes, and silica is usually used to make mesoporous NPs (MSN) [85,86,115]. Different inorganic NPs have unique properties, such as the photothermal properties of gold or the magnetic properties of iron NPs, giving rise to other uses such as photothermal radiosensitization therapies or imaging applications, respectively [73,74]. AuNPs, carbon nanotubes and mesoporous silica NPs in particular have been explored as drug delivery systems. AuNPs have the most diverse applications, providing a high surface-to-volume ratio and being able to conjugate a wide arrange of small molecules, proteins or nucleic acids directly to the surface [72]. MSN provide a large surface area, can be modulated to harbor different pore sizes fitting various types of drugs, and allow a high degree of control over drug release [87]. Carbon nanotubes can be loaded with hydrophobic drugs, and the surface decorated with various therapeutic and targeting moieties [116]. The main disadvantages of inorganic NPs are toxicity concerns and low solubility leading to aggregation [74,75]. While AuNPs are generally regarded as safe, MSNs are prone to causing hemolysis through interaction with the red blood cell plasma membrane, and especially prolonged exposure to carbon nanotubes induces cytotoxicity in vitro and lung and liver toxicity in rodents [76,87].

### 2.4. Biological Nanoparticles

Biological NPs (Figure 2) mainly encompass extracellular vesicles (EVs) and cell-derived nanovesicles (CDN). Extracellular vesicles (EVs) are a group of naturally occurring NPs with a phospholipid bilayer membrane that are produced by most cells studied to date [117–129]. Based on their biogenesis, EVs are classified into three main groups: exosomes, microvesicles and apoptotic bodies. Exosomes have attracted the most attention as a drug delivery mechanism, but it can be difficult to distinguish them from other EVs because of the overlap in size and biological make-up [130–133]. Therefore, in accordance with the MISEV2018 consensus paper, we will use the term EV in the rest of this review [133].

Contrary to earlier theories that EVs were primarily responsible for the removal of unwanted proteins from cells, they have been demonstrated to play a significant role in intercellular communication in both physiological and pathological processes [77,134–141]. The strict regulation of EV lipid bilayer composition, which is different from that of the parent cell, as well as the selective inclusion/exclusion of certain membrane and intravesicular proteins that are present in the parent cell, are indications of this biological function [142–146]. While some proteins are related to their biogenesis, others are important for their biological function and differ between EVs from different parent cells, e.g., combinations of α- and β-chains of integrins changing their organotropism, or the presence of MHC molecules in EVs from dendritic cells [77,147,148]. Nucleic acids relevant to their function are also regularly identified as a cargo of EVs [149]. Although the inherently functionalized membrane provides high biocompatibility and some degree of organotropism, further surface modifications have been applied in an effort to improve drug delivery [77,150–152]. Therapeutics can be introduced into EVs either before harvesting (through the overexpression of desired proteins or nucleic acids in engineered parent cells) or after harvesting (through electroporation, sonication or other loading methods) [78]. EVs have shown little to no inherent toxicity in previous in vivo studies [77,79,80,129,153]. As with other NPs, however, a large portion of EVs are captured in the RES [61,81,154]. Furthermore, harvesting and purifying EV in sufficient quantities for research or clinical purposes are time consuming and complex, limiting their application at present [78].

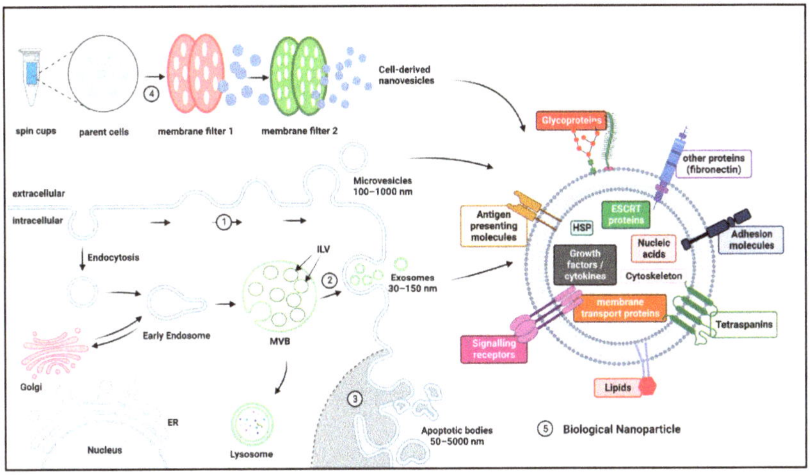


**Figure 2.** Biogenesis, production and general structure of biological NPs. (1–3) Extracellular vesicles (EVs) are differentiated into three groups based on their biogenesis (**1**) Microvesicles are small to medium sized vesicles (100–1000 nm) that originate from outward budding of the plasma membrane (PM), incorporating cytosolic proteins. (**2**) Exosomes are small, homogenous vesicles (30–150 nm), formed by inward budding of the endosomal membrane, forming intraluminal vesicles (ILVs) in an MVB and subsequently transported to either the PM, where they are released as exosomes, or to the lysosome for degradation. (**3**) Apoptotic bodies are usually large (50–5000 nm), heterogeneously shaped vesicles, shed by cells undergoing apoptosis. (**4**) Cell-derived nanovesicles (CDNs) are generated through mechanical extrusion, ultrasonication or freeze–thawing of parent cells. (**5**) EVs and CDN are both constructed from a phospholipid bilayer, inherently functionalized with various groups of membrane proteins. While some proteins are more common in certain vesicle types, there is considerable overlap. In the lumen, a diverse range of cargo proteins and nucleic acids can be identified. Abbreviations: MVB = multivesicular body, ER = endoplasmic reticulum, HSP = heat shock protein, ESCRT = endosomal sorting complexes required for transport. Created with BioRender.com.

Cell-derived nanovesicles (CDNs)—in contrast to EVs, which are created through a tightly regulated biological process—are produced through mechanical extrusion, ultrasonication, or the freeze–thawing of parent cells [155,156]. These techniques cause donor cells to release CDN in high quantities, dramatically increasing production yield compared to EVs, while preserving biological properties [155,157]. There is a substantial overlap in membrane proteins and smRNA contents between EV and CDN, although studies have demonstrated a difference in membrane lipid composition [155,156]. The in vitro and in vivo behavior of CDNs as well as the achievable drug loading capacity are also similar to EVs [155,158]. Overall, preliminary findings imply that CDNs might offer a useful EV substitute by combining the benefits of EVs with significantly improved production scalability.

## 3. Engineered Nanoparticles to Enhance Targeted Drug Delivery to CNS Tumors

Despite the abundance of available NP formulations, the majority of NPs are unable to efficiently reach the CNS, necessitating the development of advanced NP designs for brain tumor purposes that take into account the entire delivery cascade [159]. While BBB penetrance is the most widely acknowledged prerequisite, attaining adequate, persistent plasma concentrations; having the ability to migrate the extracellular matrix of the brain parenchyma; and being able to selectively deliver therapeutic payloads to tumor cells are equally important for achieving a therapeutic effect (e.g., CRITID procedure of brain-targeting drug delivery) [54]. In this section, we will review the various strategies that have been applied across NP classes to address these biological barriers in the treatment of brain tumors (Figure 3) [54,160,161].

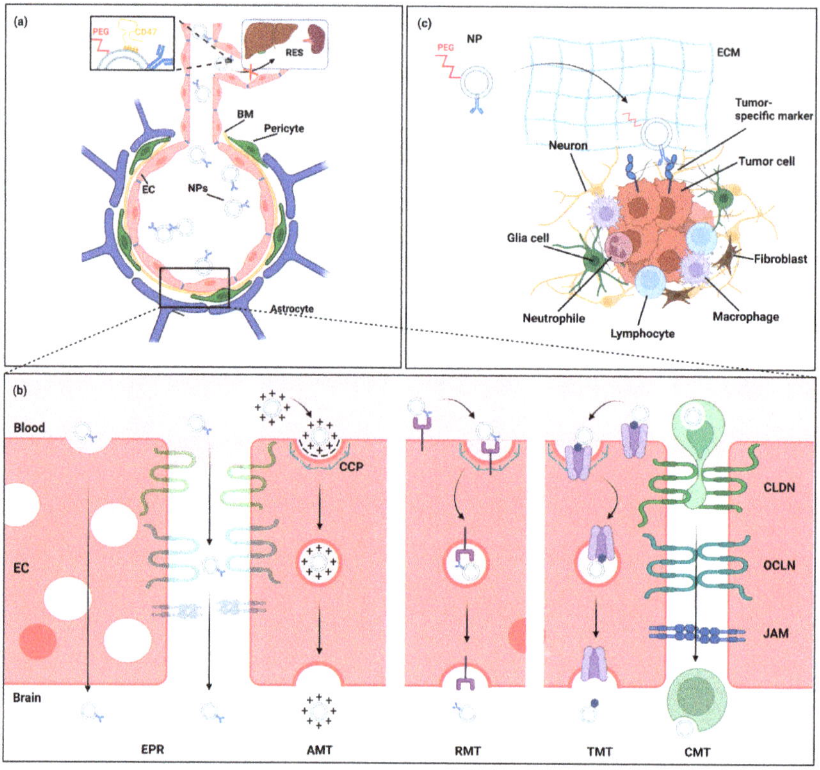


**Figure 3.** Paradigms of NP-mediated delivery to the central nervous system (CNS). (**a**) The majority of systemically administered NPs are subject to rapid clearance by the reticuloendothelial system (RES). Two important strategies to avoid recognition by macrophages and inhibit phagocytosis are PEGylation or CD47 expression, respectively. (**b**) While the blood–brain barrier (BBB) considerably impairs drug delivery to the CNS, NP-mediated drug delivery can exploit various biological transport pathways to overcome this limitation. CNS neoplasm-induced neoangiogenesis gives rise to blood vessels with an immature BBB, marked by leaky tight junctions and fenestrated endothelial cells (ECs), allowing NPs to take advantage of the enhanced permeability and retention (EPR) effect. Adsorption-mediated transcytosis (AMT), receptor-mediated transcytosis (RMT), and transporter-mediated transcytosis (TMT) are forms of endosomal transport, triggered by electrostatic interactions, ligand–receptor interactions or substrate-transporter interactions, respectively, that can be leveraged by targeted NPs. Furthermore, in cell-mediated transport (CMT), NPs have been loaded into mesenchymal stem cells (MSC) and white blood cells (WBC) that migrate over the BBB in response to tissue damage and inflammation. (**c**) PEGylation allows for improved migration through the extracellular matrix (ECM), while tumor-specific ligand conjugation increases NP targeting capabilities. Abbreviations: PEG = polyethylene glycol, BM = basal membrane, CCP = clathrin-coated pit, CLDN = claudin, OCLN = occluding, JAM = junctional adhesion molecule. Created with BioRender.com.

### *3.1. Nanoparticle Clearance and Blood Circulation Time*

Achieving adequate and persistent plasma concentrations is crucial for systemically administered drugs to achieve and maintain effective CNS concentrations in order to impart its therapeutic effect. As mentioned earlier in this review, most NPs are rapidly captured in the bloodstream by the RES. While this has been long known for liposomes and polymeric NPs, EVs show a similar clearance pattern despite their biological origin, with half lives of less than ten minutes and significant accumulation in the liver, spleen and lungs [61,71,81,89,154,162]. PEGylation is the most common modification to improve NP circulation time, but this has been shown to decrease the capacity for cellular interaction [60,71,163–165]. While the improved pharmacokinetics of PEGylated NPs have been shown to enhance CNS delivery in some scenarios, a detrimental effect on BBB crossing has been reported in others [166,167]. Furthermore, while PEG is classified by the FDA as generally regarded as safe (GRAS), production of anti-PEG antibodies has been detected after repeated dosing of PEGylated NP, resulting in accelerated blood clearance (ABC) known as the ABC effect [90,168].

A more recently explored alternative strategy is the expression of CD47, a ligand of signal-regulatory protein alpha (SIRP$\alpha$) on phagocytes, inhibiting phagocytosis, as a natural 'don't eat me' signal [169]. Kamerkar et al. showed reduced clearance of EVs and liposomes after increasing CD47 expression [152]. This strategy has been further leveraged by Belhadj et al. into a combined 'eat me/don't eat me' strategy, which consists of first administering decoy EVs to saturate the RES, followed by CD47-expressing drug-loaded EVs [170]. Using this strategy, the authors reported increased tumor accumulation of drug-loaded EVs and improved survival rates in a lung cancer mouse model. This strategy is also applicable to other NPs and has been shown to be superior to PEGylation by some studies [171,172].

Additionally, physicochemical properties such as NP size and surface charge impact systemic circulation time [173–175]. NPs smaller than 5 nm are rapidly excreted through renal glomerular filtration [176]. Zhang et al., markedly reduced renal clearance of a PAMAM dendrimer by slightly increasing the size from 4.3 nm to 6.7 nm [176]. Conversely, NPs larger than 200 nm are more likely to be captured by the RES [177]. Furthermore, in phospholipid-based NPs, lipid composition can also influence clearance rates [178–180]. More recently, the effect of different NP shapes has gained considerable interest, as it has been demonstrated that rod-shaped NPs interact with cells less frequently, leading to decreased clearance by the RES [181–183].

### 3.2. Nanoparticle Strategies to Enhance Drug Delivery Past the BBB

The inability to cross the BBB and achieve therapeutic concentrations is a significant drawback of most conventional drugs [19]. While unaltered NPs exhibit some degree of BBB penetrance, engineered NPs have been developed to improve drug delivery over the BBB. These formulations exploit biological processes such as endogenous transport pathways or the migration of mesenchymal stem cells (MSC) and white blood cells (WBC) in response to tissue damage or inflammation [128,132,184–190]. Other strategies for bypassing the BBB altogether, such as intranasal delivery, convection-enhanced delivery (CED), or temporary BBB disruption, are also being investigated in combination with NPs.

#### 3.2.1. Nanoparticle Modifications to Increase BBB Passage

Although their physicochemical properties largely prevent most NPs from crossing the BBB, they can either inherently or after surface modification take advantage of natural transcytosis pathways. Transcytosis is a form of active vesicular transport, initiated by endocytosis from the luminal side of ECs, from where endosomes are sorted to be degraded in lysosomes, returned to the bloodstream, or transported to the abluminal side of the EC. In brain capillaries, endocytosis is primarily mediated by clathrin-coated pits (CPs) [191]. Three pathways are distinguished based on the trigger for endocytosis: adsorption-mediated transcytosis (AMT), receptor-mediated transcytosis (RMT) and transporter-mediated transcytosis (TMT). Although an in-depth analysis of these pathways is beyond the scope of this review, we will provide a summary of the most common strategies. We kindly refer to reviews from Azarmi et al. and Moura et al. for a more comprehensive overview [192,193].

In AMT, endocytosis is initiated after the electrostatic adsorption of cationic particles to the anionic CPs. While cationic NPs, such as chitosan NPs and certain polyamidoamine (PAMAM) dendrimers, and NPs functionalized with cationic molecules have been shown to cross the BBB, AMT intrinsically lacks CNS specificity as negatively charged membranes are virtually universal to all living cells [185,194–196]. In contrast, RMT is a specific process, triggered by binding an EC surface receptor. Through the conjugation of either endogenous or engineered ligands for receptors predominantly expressed on brain ECs onto NPs, CNS-specific delivery of NP-encapsulated drugs can be achieved. Commonly targeted receptors include transferrin (TfR), lactoferrin (LfR), insulin, and low-density lipoprotein (LDLR) receptors as well as LDLR-related peptides (LRPs) [197–203]. Some authors further reported the expression of the nicotinic acetylcholine receptor (nAchR) on NPs to harness RMT [204]. Due to their potential as a dual target, being widely expressed in both tumor cells and brain EC, some receptors, such as the TfR, have undergone extensive research [198,205,206]. TfR ligands have been successfully conjugated to lipid-based, polymeric and inorganic NP, increasing target cell specificity in vitro while providing increased CNS uptake in vivo [206–210]. Using transferrin-coupled temozolomide-loaded PLGA NPs, Kuang et al. showed increased antitumor activity in a U87 orthotopic xenograft glioma mouse model [206]. Nonetheless, absolute NP uptake with RMT is usually low [211].

Similar to RMT, TMT is a specific process initiated by binding a transporter present on the EC surface. The most commonly investigated TMT transporters are GLUT1 and the glutathione transporter, both serving a dual role, being highly expressed on brain ECs and many tumor cells [203,212,213]. Critically, however, when targeting endogenous receptors and transporters important for brain homeostasis, the potential for serious adverse reactions should be considered, as ligand-coated NPs might competitively inhibit the transport of important nutrients to the CNS. To this end, a study using TfR-targeted oxaliplatin-loaded liposomes reported dose-dependent lethargy postinjection in mice [207]. Conversely, endogenous ligands might outcompete engineered NPs, decreasing the targeting efficiency.

Besides conjugation of targeting moieties, modulation of NP shape provides another strategy to optimize endocytosis. Anti-VCAM-1, anti-ICAM-1 and anti-TfR-coated PS nanorods showed increased brain accumulation compared to spherical PS NP in vitro and in vivo. Interestingly, spherical NPs associated significantly more with brain ECs than their rod-shaped counterparts, suggesting that spherical shapes increase nonspecific intercellular interactions [214–216]. Given that most NPs are spherical, this warrants further investigation of NPs with other shapes.

#### 3.2.2. Cell-Mediated and Cell-Mimicking Drug Delivery over the BBB

Another strategy to potentially enhance BBB passage is by loading NP into cells capable of migrating over the BBB, such as MSCs and WBCs, or coating them with cell membranes [217]. This way drug can be protected from degradation while carrier cells facilitate targeting to the tumor regions [188,189]. MSCs have been intensely investigated for cell-based therapies due to their regenerative properties and tumor-tropism, making them a prime candidate for NP-based drug delivery [190,218]. Roger et al. demonstrated the ability to load PLA NPs and SLN into MSCs without affecting their cell viability or ability to migrate towards glioma cells in vitro and in vivo in a U87MG orthotopic xenograft glioma mouse model after administration via CED [219]. Using a U251 heterotopic flank xenograft glioma mouse model, Li et al. reported prolonged retention and enhanced apoptosis after intratumoral injection of doxorubicin-loaded silica nanorattles attached to MSCs compared to both free drug and doxorubicin-loaded silica nanorattles [220]. Similarly, WBCs are capable of migrating over the BBB towards regions of tissue damage and inflammation [188]. Multiple groups demonstrated the ability of macrophages, neutrophils and T-lymphocytes to be loaded with different types of NPs [221–225]. Using monocytes as a carrier, Ibarra et al. showed enhanced accumulation of polymeric NPs in the tumor region of an GL261 orthotopic xenograft glioma mouse model [222]. Importantly, this xenograft model had a compromised BBB in the tumor region; therefore, none of these experiments were able to definitively prove NP passage over an intact BBB.

Rather than loading NPs into live cells, other groups have coated various NPs in specific cell membranes in order to attain similar benefits. For example, Zhang et al. have cloaked their NP in MSC membranes to improve BBB passage and tumor targeting, and Ji et al. packaged doxorubicin in platelet membranes as adjuvant therapy with neurosurgery, targeting the damaged vascular endothelium at the surgical margins [226,227]. Although further evaluation is needed, these 'Trojan horse'-inspired strategies hold promise to optimize NP delivery.

3.2.3. Bypassing the BBB

Rather than improving BBB penetrance, other strategies have focused on circumventing or (temporarily) disrupting the BBB entirely. Widely studied approaches include intranasal delivery, convection-enhanced delivery (CED), and focused ultrasound (FUS). While these techniques are also being investigated in combination with conventional drugs, beneficial effects of NP-encapsulation are being explored.

A systemic first pass effect and the BBB are avoided by intranasal delivery, which is envisioned by direct uptake via the olfactory and trigeminal neuroepithelia into the brain parenchyma. Upon intranasal administration of EV-encapsulated curcumin and JSI-124, a STAT3 inhibitor, Zhuang et al. demonstrated anti-inflammatory effects and reduced tumor growth in brain inflammation and orthotopic xenograft glioma mouse models, respectively [228]. Similarly, Sousa et al. reported improved antiangiogenesis, reduced tumor growth and reduced systemic drug exposure in a U87 orthotopic xenograft glioma mouse model after intranasal administration of a bevacizumab-loaded PLGA PNP compared to the free drug [229]. However, the translation relevance of intranasal delivery from animal models to humans is debated due to the relatively large size of the olfactory system in rodents, the highly variable administration efficiency, and the limited maximal doses [230].

CED is a neurosurgical technique that circumvents the BBB by directly infusing drugs into the brain parenchyma, encompassing the tumor site through the generation of a mechanical pressure gradient [231,232]. The use of convective kinetics facilitates the homogenous distribution of infused drugs at high local concentrations with minimal systemic toxicity [45,233]. Early-phase clinical trials of CED have established the safety and feasibility of this procedure in children and adults [234–238]. However, inadequate drug distribution and retention have been largely cited as the reasons for the failure of a phase III CED study performed in adult GBM [239–241]. Nanoparticle-encapsulated drugs were found to be retained in situ for longer than free drugs alone in prior in vivo experiments using CED of nanoparticles [242]. Zhang et al. further demonstrated the enhanced in vivo distribution of PEGylated liposomal doxorubicin compared to free doxorubicin in a tumor-naïve mouse model [243]. MTX110, a water-soluble nanoparticle formulation of panobinostat, distributed effectively in the brains of small and large animals following CED without clinical or neuropathological signs of toxicity up to an infused concentration of 30 μM and is currently undergoing clinical development [33,244]. Preliminary data from seven patients who received two 48 h MTX110 infusion pulses (30 or 60 μM) showed some encouraging signs of antitumor activity with repeated CED of MTX110 [237].

Lastly, a legion of options has been explored to improve brain–drug delivery via the temporary disruption of the BBB, including osmotically active agents such as mannitol and mechanical methods such as focused ultrasound (FUS). However, disruption of the BBB does not uniformly result in increased drug penetration into the brain, as it does not only increase influx but also facilitates rapid clearance out of the brain [245,246]. Notwithstanding, Nance et al. showed improved delivery of long-circulating PEGylated PS PNPs to the brain using MRI-guided FUS, suggesting that local and temporary BBB disruption in combination with longer circulating NP might improve the in vivo efficacy of administered therapeutics [247].

### 3.3. Nanoparticle Modifications to Increase Delivery to Brain Tumor Cells

After crossing or bypassing the BBB, the extracellular matrix (ECM) of the brain parenchyma forms another biological barrier NPs need to navigate to reach the target cell. While the ability to move throughout the ECM is inversely correlated with NP size, mechanical adhesion can severely limit the diffusion of NPs of any size [248]. Nance et al. demonstrated that uncoated PS PNPs of all sizes are immobilized by adhesion, and while densely PEGylated paclitaxel-loaded PLGA nanoparticles could readily move through the ECM, uncoated PLGA NPs could not [248]. The authors concluded that densely PEGylated NPs with a near-neutral charge and a size of <114 nm are most optimal for diffusion through the brain parenchyma after systemic administration. Building on these findings, Schneider et al. produced a PEGylated PS PNP decorated with a ITEM4 monoclonal antibody targeting fibroblast growth factor-inducible 14 (Fn14), which is highly expressed in high-grade glioma. The authors demonstrated specific targeting of glioma cells with retained ability to navigate the ECM in rat brain tissue and in a U87 orthotopic xenograft glioma mouse model using CED [249].

This combination of surface modifications, including targeting antibodies and peptides, is frequently used to enhance drug delivery specifically to the targeted tumor cell. While in solid tumors outside the CNS, NPs provide passive accumulation through the enhanced permeability and retention (EPR) effect (i.e., preferential tumor accumulation of nanosized particles through leaky vessels ensuing tumor-induced neoangiogenesis and accompanying inflammatory response), it is unclear whether this concept is directly translatable to brain tumors due to the unique characteristics of the BBB [250,251]. Even though passive accumulation might still occur to a certain degree through tumor-induced BBB disruption, tumor-specific targeting moieties have been used across NP classes to increase brain tumor cell delivery [185,252–254].

The most intensely investigated targets for drug delivery to high-grade gliomas are vascular endothelial growth factor (VEGF) and epidermal growth factor receptor (EGFR), including the truncated, constitutively active variant EGFRvIII [67,106,255,256]. Other commonly investigated moieties are TfR-ligands, as discussed above, and chlorotoxin, targeting a chloride ion channel and matrix metalloprotease 2, which have all been shown to be overexpressed in different neuroectodermal tumors [187,206–210,257,258]. Several of these ligands have been successfully conjugated to drug-loaded NPs and demonstrated to increase cytotoxicity and tumor cell selectivity in vitro and CNS accumulation in vivo in orthotopic xenograft glioma mouse models [67,106,229,255,256,258]. However, studies have reported the reliance on the overexpression of the target receptor in the used tumor models [67,106].

Notwithstanding the promising preclinical data, the lack of successful clinical translation highlights the inherent limitations of targeting specific receptors due to inter- and intratumoral heterogeneity, expression changes upon treatment, and the generation of alternative oncogenic mutations, which all promote the development of treatment resistance [53,259,260].

## 4. Novel Strategies and Future Directions

Notwithstanding the aforementioned strategies to specifically design CNS-targeted NPs with promising preclinical data, no successful clinical translation has been achieved. However, novel technologies are under investigation to further improve NP-based brain tumor therapy by combining several treatment modalities and defining new therapeutic targets (Figure 4).

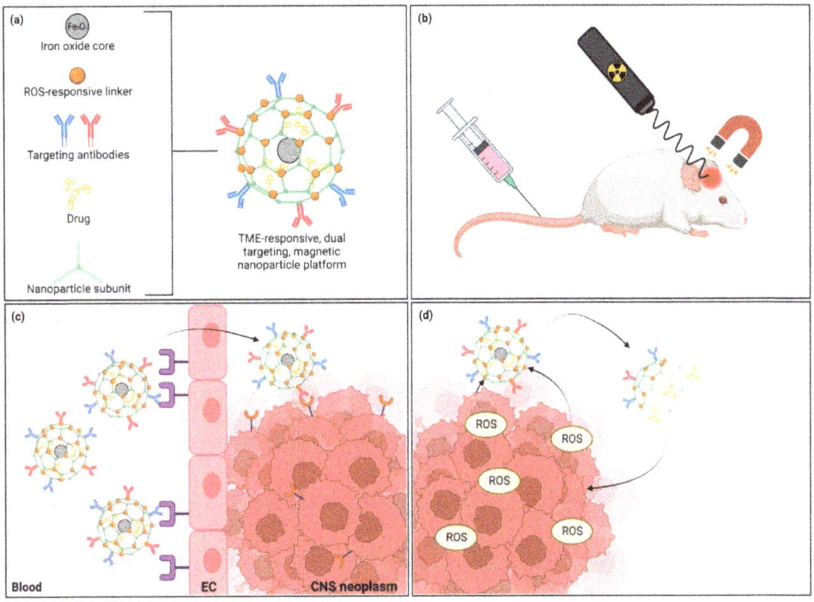


**Figure 4.** Novel strategies in NP-mediated drug delivery. (**a**) Complex NPs have been constructed, combining magnetic properties, tumor microenvironment (TME)-responsive elements, and multiple targeting strategies into one NP platform for drug delivery. (**b**) After injection, magnetic NPs can increase targeting efficiency using magnetic convection-enhanced diffusion to the region of interest. Furthermore, magnetothermal and radiosensitizing properties allow for additional therapeutic benefits. (**c**) Dual-targeting strategies for recognition of both the blood–brain barrier and brain tumor cells are commonly implemented. (**d**) TME-responsive elements can increase site-directed delivery by allowing cargo release when encountering specific molecules abundant in the TME, e.g., reactive oxygen species (ROS). Abbreviations: NP = nanoparticle, EC = endothelial cell, CNS = central nervous system. Created with BioRender.com.

While many NPs mainly focus on the efficient, targeted delivery of drugs, magnetic NPs, e.g., iron oxide (loaded) NPs, exhibit unique properties, allowing additional therapeutic benefits [261]. Using external magnetic fields, brain targeting can be improved using magnetic convection-enhanced diffusion, usually in combination with regular tumor-targeting ligands [262–265]. Furthermore, magnetic NPs induce local magnetic hyperthermia when exposed to alternating magnetic fields, providing a noninvasive method to impart local cell death, and act as a radiosensitizer, potentiating the effect of concomitant radiotherapy [266,267]. Similarly, AuNPs display a photothermal effect, providing the possibility of local hyperthermia induction using near-infrared light, while also being a potent radiosensitizer [268–270]. As such, the potential of these NPs to potentiate radiotherapy efficacy, improve chemotherapy delivery, and simultaneously allow additional local hyperthermal therapy is offering perspectives to reinforce the current treatment regimens.

The emerging appreciation of the tumor microenvironment (TME) allows ample opportunities for novel NP-based therapies, providing new therapeutic targets and creating new possibilities for TME-responsive NPs to improve site-specific delivery. For example, Hsieh et al. produced a CNS-targeted NP delivering small interfering RNA (siRNA) to silence PD-L1 expression in a GBM mouse model, increasing cytotoxic T cell infiltration and suppressing tumor progression [271]. Furthermore, several groups have created reactive oxygen species (ROS)-responsive NPs, which release their cargo when encountering high ROS concentrations as present in the GBM TME [272–274]. Seeing that novel adoptive cellular therapies are currently limited by the immunosuppressive TME and cell-mediated NP delivery has been successful preclinically, combination regimens of adoptive cellular therapies with NP-based TME modulation are under intense investigation [275,276]. Chang et al. introduced MSN loaded with the hypoxia-activated prodrug tirapazamine into anti-GBM chimeric antigen receptor (CAR) neutrophils. In a mouse model, the CAR neutrophils effectively delivered the MSN to the tumor, significantly inhibiting tumor growth and prolonging survival through the combined effect of the CAR neutrophils and the local drug delivery [277]. Furthermore, in solid tumors outside the CNS, pretreatment with TME-modulating NPs or NP-mediated photothermal therapy have also shown promising results, although this has yet to be evaluated in CNS tumors [278,279].

Increasingly, highly complex NPs are being engineered, combining multiple NP types, multiple targeting strategies and various treatment modalities in order to surmount the different biological barriers [226,265,272]. Zhang et al. produced a nanocapsule loaded with anti-VEGFR2 antibodies (inhibiting angiogenesis) crosslinked to anti-CPT1C siRNA (an essential protein for fatty acid oxidation) by a ROS-responsive disulfide crosslinker. The surface was decorated with 2-Deoxy-D-Glucose, a glycolysis inhibitor that is also a substrate for GLUT1, allowing for TMT over the BBB and targeting to the tumor cells. Upon encountering ROS in the TME, the anti-VEGFR2 antibodies, CPT1C siRNA and 2-Deoxy-D-glucose are released, inhibiting angiogenesis, fatty acid oxidation and glycolysis pathways, killing the tumor cells by effectively blocking their energy supply [272]. Another example was recently published by Li et al., combining angiopep-2-decorated EVs, targeting the LRP-1 receptor, with a magnetic NP consisting of an iron oxide core surrounded by a mesoporous silica shell, allowing for both ligand-mediated and magnetic targeting. The EVs were loaded with GPX4 siRNA and the mesoporous silica shell decorated with a dihydroorotate dehydrogenase inhibitor, targeting two important ferroptosis defense pathways, inducing cell death through their combined effect [265]. Similarly, Zhang et al. produced a CNS targeted, MSC membrane-coated, pH-responsive, cupper-based NP loaded with siRNA to induce cuproptosis, a recently uncovered form of cell death [226]. Considering the complexity of these NP platforms reflects the diversity of biological barriers that has to be surmounted, continued efforts are needed in order to achieve effective NP-based treatment strategies for CNS neoplasms.

## 5. Summary and Conclusions

To date, the therapeutic impact of advances in our knowledge of CNS tumors has been significantly hindered by the unique biology which surrounds these tumors, namely the blood–brain barrier, which not only prevents the entry of the vast majority of therapeutics, but actively removes them from the CNS space via the activity of efflux transporters. To overcome the vexing challenges posed by the BBB and increase the CNS tumor therapeutic exposure time, a variety of strategies utilizing nanoparticles have been developed, which enable greater delivery and retention of therapeutics at the site of disease. One such strategy in the CNS targeting nanoparticle space entails the modification of therapeutic-containing nanoparticles with groups which will induce nanoparticle transport into the CNS via transcytosis. To achieve this, nanoparticles are modified with ligands for receptors highly expressed on CNS endothelial cells which when bound will induce transcytosis. Alternatively, the nanoparticle can be modified with a substrate for a transporter highly expressed on CNS endothelial cells which, when bound, similarly induces transcytosis. Ideally, these receptors/transporters are both highly expressed on the CNS endothelial cells and on the tumor itself, as is the case for transferrin and GLUT1, respectively. Another approach for facilitating nanoparticle BBB circumvention involves hitching a ride with cells which are already able to enter the CNS, and which have innate tumor-tropic active homing ability. Examples of this approach have utilized MSCs and various WBCs, and although—to our knowledge—this strategy has yet to be tested in an animal model with an intact BBB, enhanced accumulation of NPs in the tumor region of orthotopic xenograft glioma mouse models has been demonstrated, indicating significant promise for the approach.

In addition to strategies which solely rely on the nanoparticle to bypass the BBB, strategies have been devised which make use of nanoparticles in combination with unique delivery methods which are designed to disrupt the BBB or bypass it entirely. These approaches include intranasal delivery, convection-enhanced delivery, and focused ultrasound. The first two delivery methods are intended to bypass the BBB, while the third attempts to temporarily disrupt the BBB, allowing therapeutics to reach the site of disease. By combining these delivery approaches with nanoparticle formulations which have an enhanced volume of distribution and extended therapeutics release profile, the hope is that the retention of therapeutics at the site of disease can be increased, and, thus, therapeutic efficacy can be achieved. These combination approaches also have the benefit of overcoming one of the major hurdles in the nanoparticle therapeutics space, namely, rapid clearance from the bloodstream by the RES. By directly delivering nanoparticles to the site of disease, this problem of rapid clearance can be ameliorated. Alternatively, the modification of nanoparticles with PEG has been shown to increase circulation time by helping the nanoparticles evade the RES. It is, however, unclear how PEGylation impacts BBB penetration ability, with some studies indicating enhanced penetrance and others indicating diminished BBB penetration. It has also been shown that CD47 expression on nanoparticles can prevent phagocytes from clearing the nanoparticles. Although in its infancy, this strategy of modifying nanoparticles with antiphagocytosis signals holds the promise of helping to defeat rapid nanoparticle clearance by the RES. Increasingly, complex nanoparticles combining several of these strategies and/or exhibiting additional magnetothermal, photothermal, or radiosensitizing effects are being evaluated and are combined with other treatment modalities. In this review, we have covered the current state of the CNS-tumor-targeting nanoparticle space, highlighting the breadth of nanoparticle types being investigated for this use, the strategies being employed to circumvent the BBB, and some of the recent advances in combining nanoparticles with unique delivery methods to overcome the myriad challenges posed by the unique biology surrounding CNS tumors. Taken together, there is significant merit in the continued investigation and development of nanoparticles as therapeutic delivery vehicles for the treatment of CNS tumors in order to translate the successful preclinical investigations into the clinic.

**Author Contributions:** Conception and design: W.J.F.V., J.S.R. and J.B.A. Drafted the article: W.J.F.V., J.S.R., J.B.A. and L.F.N. Critically revised the article: L.Z. and D.J.D. Reviewed the submitted version of the manuscript: W.J.F.V., J.S.R., J.B.A., L.F.N., L.Z. and D.J.D. Approved the final version of the manuscript on behalf of all authors: W.J.F.V., J.S.R. and J.B.A. Article supervision: D.J.D. All authors have read and agreed to the published version of the manuscript.

**Funding:** J.B.A. was supported by National Institutes of Health grants from the National Institute of General Medical Sciences (T32 GM 65841 and R25 GM 55252). The figures were created with BioRender.com.

**Institutional Review Board Statement:** Not applicable.

**Informed Consent Statement:** Not applicable.

**Data Availability Statement:** No new data were created or analyzed in this study. Data sharing is not applicable to this article.

**Conflicts of Interest:** The authors declare no conflict of interest.

## References

1. Ostrom, Q.T.; Cioffi, G.; Waite, K.; Kruchko, C.; Barnholtz-Sloan, J.S. CBTRUS Statistical Report: Primary Brain and Other Central Nervous System Tumors Diagnosed in the United States in 2014–2018. *Neuro Oncol.* **2021**, *23*, iii1–iii105. [CrossRef] [PubMed]
2. Girardi, F.; Matz, M.; Stiller, C.; You, H.; Marcos Gragera, R.; Valkov, M.Y.; Bulliard, J.-L.; De, P.; Morrison, D.; Wanner, M. Global survival trends for brain tumors, by histology: Analysis of individual records for 556,237 adults diagnosed in 59 countries during 2000–2014 (CONCORD-3). *Neuro Oncol.* **2023**, *25*, 580–592. [CrossRef] [PubMed]
3. Gittleman, H.; Boscia, A.; Ostrom, Q.T.; Truitt, G.; Fritz, Y.; Kruchko, C.; Barnholtz-Sloan, J.S. Survivorship in adults with malignant brain and other central nervous system tumor from 2000–2014. *Neuro Oncol.* **2018**, *20*, vii6–vii16. [CrossRef] [PubMed]

4. Ostrom, Q.T.; Price, M.; Ryan, K.; Edelson, J.; Neff, C.; Cioffi, G.; Waite, K.A.; Kruchko, C.; Barnholtz-Sloan, J.S. CBTRUS Statistical Report: Pediatric Brain Tumor Foundation Childhood and Adolescent Primary Brain and Other Central Nervous System Tumors Diagnosed in the United States in 2014–2018. *Neuro Oncol.* **2022**, *24*, iii1–iii38. [CrossRef]
5. Girardi, F.; Di Carlo, V.; Stiller, C.; Gatta, G.; Woods, R.R.; Visser, O.; Lacour, B.; Tucker, T.C.; Coleman, M.P.; Allemani, C. Global survival trends for brain tumors, by histology: Analysis of individual records for 67,776 children diagnosed in 61 countries during 2000–2014 (CONCORD-3). *Neuro Oncol.* **2023**, *25*, 593–606. [CrossRef]
6. Warren, K.E. Diffuse intrinsic pontine glioma: Poised for progress. *Front. Oncol.* **2012**, *2*, 205. [CrossRef]
7. Pollack, I.F.; Agnihotri, S.; Broniscer, A. Childhood brain tumors: Current management, biological insights, and future directions. *J. Neurosurg. Pediatr.* **2019**, *23*, 261–273. [CrossRef]
8. Schaff, L.R.; Mellinghoff, I.K. Glioblastoma and Other Primary Brain Malignancies in Adults: A Review. *JAMA* **2023**, *329*, 574–587. [CrossRef]
9. Louis, D.N.; Perry, A.; Wesseling, P.; Brat, D.J.; Cree, I.A.; Figarella-Branger, D.; Hawkins, C.; Ng, H.K.; Pfister, S.M.; Reifenberger, G.; et al. The 2021 WHO Classification of Tumors of the Central Nervous System: A summary. *Neuro Oncol.* **2021**, *23*, 1231–1251. [CrossRef]
10. Wen, P.Y.; Weller, M.; Lee, E.Q.; Alexander, B.M.; Barnholtz-Sloan, J.S.; Barthel, F.P.; Batchelor, T.T.; Bindra, R.S.; Chang, S.M.; Chiocca, E.A.; et al. Glioblastoma in adults: A Society for Neuro Oncol. (SNO) and European Society of Neuro-Oncology (EANO) consensus review on current management and future directions. *Neuro Oncol.* **2020**, *22*, 1073–1113. [CrossRef]
11. Stupp, R.; Mason, W.P.; van den Bent, M.J.; Weller, M.; Fisher, B.; Taphoorn, M.J.; Belanger, K.; Brandes, A.A.; Marosi, C.; Bogdahn, U.; et al. Radiotherapy plus concomitant and adjuvant temozolomide for glioblastoma. *N. Engl. J. Med.* **2005**, *352*, 987–996. [CrossRef] [PubMed]
12. Fang, F.Y.; Rosenblum, J.S.; Ho, W.S.; Heiss, J.D. New Developments in the Pathogenesis, Therapeutic Targeting, and Treatment of Pediatric Medulloblastoma. *Cancers* **2022**, *14*, 2285. [CrossRef] [PubMed]
13. Mendes, M.; Sousa, J.J.; Pais, A.; Vitorino, C. Targeted Theranostic Nanoparticles for Brain Tumor Treatment. *Pharmaceutics* **2018**, *10*, 181. [CrossRef] [PubMed]
14. Bellavance, M.A.; Blanchette, M.; Fortin, D. Recent advances in blood-brain barrier disruption as a CNS delivery strategy. *AAPS J.* **2008**, *10*, 166–177. [CrossRef]
15. Haumann, R.; Videira, J.C.; Kaspers, G.J.L.; van Vuurden, D.G.; Hulleman, E. Overview of Current Drug Delivery Methods Across the Blood-Brain Barrier for the Treatment of Primary Brain Tumors. *CNS Drugs* **2020**, *34*, 1121–1131. [CrossRef]
16. Oberoi, R.K.; Parrish, K.E.; Sio, T.T.; Mittapalli, R.K.; Elmquist, W.F.; Sarkaria, J.N. Strategies to improve delivery of anticancer drugs across the blood-brain barrier to treat glioblastoma. *Neuro Oncol.* **2016**, *18*, 27–36. [CrossRef]
17. Daneman, R.; Prat, A. The blood-brain barrier. *Cold Spring Harb. Perspect. Biol.* **2015**, *7*, a020412. [CrossRef]
18. Obermeier, B.; Daneman, R.; Ransohoff, R.M. Development, maintenance and disruption of the blood-brain barrier. *Nat. Med.* **2013**, *19*, 1584–1596. [CrossRef]
19. Pardridge, W.M. The blood-brain barrier: Bottleneck in brain drug development. *NeuroRX* **2005**, *2*, 3–14. [CrossRef]
20. Abbott, N.J.; Patabendige, A.A.; Dolman, D.E.; Yusof, S.R.; Begley, D.J. Structure and function of the blood-brain barrier. *Neurobiol. Dis.* **2010**, *37*, 13–25. [CrossRef]
21. Pardridge, W.M. The Isolated Brain Microvessel: A Versatile Experimental Model of the Blood-Brain Barrier. *Front. Physiol.* **2020**, *11*, 398. [CrossRef] [PubMed]
22. Abbott, N.J.; Rönnbäck, L.; Hansson, E. Astrocyte-endothelial interactions at the blood-brain barrier. *Nat. Rev. Neurosci.* **2006**, *7*, 41–53. [CrossRef] [PubMed]
23. Liu, L.R.; Liu, J.C.; Bao, J.S.; Bai, Q.Q.; Wang, G.Q. Interaction of Microglia and Astrocytes in the Neurovascular Unit. *Front. Immunol.* **2020**, *11*, 1024. [CrossRef] [PubMed]
24. Xu, L.; Nirwane, A.; Yao, Y. Basement membrane and blood-brain barrier. *Stroke Vasc. Neurol.* **2019**, *4*, 78–82. [CrossRef]
25. Uemura, M.T.; Maki, T.; Ihara, M.; Lee, V.M.Y.; Trojanowski, J.Q. Brain Microvascular Pericytes in Vascular Cognitive Impairment and Dementia. *Front. Aging Neurosci.* **2020**, *12*, 80. [CrossRef]
26. Ballabh, P.; Braun, A.; Nedergaard, M. The blood-brain barrier: An overview: Structure, regulation, and clinical implications. *Neurobiol. Dis.* **2004**, *16*, 1–13. [CrossRef] [PubMed]
27. Jia, W.; Lu, R.; Martin, T.A.; Jiang, W.G. The role of claudin-5 in blood-brain barrier (BBB) and brain metastases (review). *Mol. Med. Rep.* **2014**, *9*, 779–785. [CrossRef]
28. Lochhead, J.J.; Yang, J.; Ronaldson, P.T.; Davis, T.P. Structure, Function, and Regulation of the Blood-Brain Barrier Tight Junction in Central Nervous System Disorders. *Front. Physiol.* **2020**, *11*, 914. [CrossRef]
29. Tamai, I.; Tsuji, A. Transporter-mediated permeation of drugs across the blood-brain barrier. *J. Pharm. Sci.* **2000**, *89*, 1371–1388. [CrossRef]
30. Harilal, S.; Jose, J.; Parambi, D.G.T.; Kumar, R.; Unnikrishnan, M.K.; Uddin, M.S.; Mathew, G.E.; Pratap, R.; Marathakam, A.; Mathew, B. Revisiting the blood-brain barrier: A hard nut to crack in the transportation of drug molecules. *Brain Res. Bull.* **2020**, *160*, 121–140. [CrossRef]
31. Sun, H.; Dai, H.; Shaik, N.; Elmquist, W.F. Drug efflux transporters in the CNS. *Adv. Drug Deliv. Rev.* **2003**, *55*, 83–105. [CrossRef] [PubMed]

32. Löscher, W.; Potschka, H. Blood-brain barrier active efflux transporters: ATP-binding cassette gene family. *NeuroRx* **2005**, *2*, 86–98. [CrossRef] [PubMed]
33. Singleton, W.G.B.; Bienemann, A.S.; Woolley, M.; Johnson, D.; Lewis, O.; Wyatt, M.J.; Damment, S.J.P.; Boulter, L.J.; Killick-Cole, C.L.; Asby, D.J.; et al. The distribution, clearance, and brainstem toxicity of panobinostat administered by convection-enhanced delivery. *J. Neurosurg. Pediatr. PED* **2018**, *22*, 288–296. [CrossRef] [PubMed]
34. Chaves, C.; Declèves, X.; Taghi, M.; Menet, M.-C.; Lacombe, J.; Varlet, P.; Olaciregui, N.G.; Carcaboso, A.M.; Cisternino, S. Characterization of the Blood–Brain Barrier Integrity and the Brain Transport of SN-38 in an Orthotopic Xenograft Rat Model of Diffuse Intrinsic Pontine Glioma. *Pharmaceutics* **2020**, *12*, 399. [CrossRef] [PubMed]
35. Miklja, Z.; Yadav, V.N.; Cartaxo, R.T.; Siada, R.; Thomas, C.C.; Cummings, J.R.; Mullan, B.; Stallard, S.; Paul, A.; Bruzek, A.K.; et al. Everolimus improves the efficacy of dasatinib in PDGFRα-driven glioma. *J. Clin. Investig.* **2020**, *130*, 5313–5325. [CrossRef] [PubMed]
36. Oh, J.H.; Power, E.A.; Zhang, W.; Daniels, D.J.; Elmquist, W.F. Murine Central Nervous System and Bone Marrow Distribution of the Aurora A Kinase Inhibitor Alisertib: Pharmacokinetics and Exposure at the Sites of Efficacy and Toxicity. *J. Pharmacol. Exp. Ther.* **2022**, *383*, 44–55. [CrossRef]
37. Laramy, J.K.; Kim, M.; Parrish, K.E.; Sarkaria, J.N.; Elmquist, W.F. Pharmacokinetic Assessment of Cooperative Efflux of the Multitargeted Kinase Inhibitor Ponatinib Across the Blood-Brain Barrier. *J. Pharmacol. Exp. Ther.* **2018**, *365*, 249–261. [CrossRef]
38. Warren, K.E. Beyond the Blood:Brain Barrier: The Importance of Central Nervous System (CNS) Pharmacokinetics for the Treatment of CNS Tumors, Including Diffuse Intrinsic Pontine Glioma. *Front. Oncol.* **2018**, *8*, 239. [CrossRef]
39. Bhowmik, A.; Khan, R.; Ghosh, M.K. Blood brain barrier: A challenge for effectual therapy of brain tumors. *Biomed. Res. Int.* **2015**, *2015*, 320941. [CrossRef]
40. Banks, W.A. From blood–brain barrier to blood–brain interface: New opportunities for CNS drug delivery. *Nat. Rev. Drug Discov.* **2016**, *15*, 275–292. [CrossRef]
41. Rathi, S.; Griffith, J.I.; Zhang, W.; Zhang, W.; Oh, J.H.; Talele, S.; Sarkaria, J.N.; Elmquist, W.F. The influence of the blood-brain barrier in the treatment of brain tumours. *J. Intern. Med.* **2022**, *292*, 3–30. [CrossRef] [PubMed]
42. Varlet, P.; Le Teuff, G.; Le Deley, M.C.; Giangaspero, F.; Haberler, C.; Jacques, T.S.; Figarella-Branger, D.; Pietsch, T.; Andreiuolo, F.; Deroulers, C.; et al. WHO grade has no prognostic value in the pediatric high-grade glioma included in the HERBY trial. *Neuro Oncol.* **2020**, *22*, 116–127. [CrossRef] [PubMed]
43. Sarkaria, J.N.; Hu, L.S.; Parney, I.F.; Pafundi, D.H.; Brinkmann, D.H.; Laack, N.N.; Giannini, C.; Burns, T.C.; Kizilbash, S.H.; Laramy, J.K.; et al. Is the blood-brain barrier really disrupted in all glioblastomas? A critical assessment of existing clinical data. *Neuro Oncol.* **2018**, *20*, 184–191. [CrossRef] [PubMed]
44. Pafundi, D.H.; Laack, N.N.; Youland, R.S.; Parney, I.F.; Lowe, V.J.; Giannini, C.; Kemp, B.J.; Grams, M.P.; Morris, J.M.; Hoover, J.M.; et al. Biopsy validation of 18F-DOPA PET and biodistribution in gliomas for neurosurgical planning and radiotherapy target delineation: Results of a prospective pilot study. *Neuro Oncol.* **2013**, *15*, 1058–1067. [CrossRef]
45. Himes, B.T.; Zhang, L.; Daniels, D.J. Treatment Strategies in Diffuse Midline Gliomas With the H3K27M Mutation: The Role of Convection-Enhanced Delivery in Overcoming Anatomic Challenges. *Front. Oncol.* **2019**, *9*, 31. [CrossRef]
46. Ek, C.J.; Wong, A.; Liddelow, S.A.; Johansson, P.A.; Dziegielewska, K.M.; Saunders, N.R. Efflux mechanisms at the developing brain barriers: ABC-transporters in the fetal and postnatal rat. *Toxicol. Lett.* **2010**, *197*, 51–59. [CrossRef]
47. Saunders, N.R.; Liddelow, S.A.; Dziegielewska, K.M. Barrier mechanisms in the developing brain. *Front. Pharmacol.* **2012**, *3*, 46. [CrossRef]
48. Verscheijden, L.F.M.; van Hattem, A.C.; Pertijs, J.; de Jongh, C.A.; Verdijk, R.M.; Smeets, B.; Koenderink, J.B.; Russel, F.G.M.; de Wildt, S.N. Developmental patterns in human blood-brain barrier and blood-cerebrospinal fluid barrier ABC drug transporter expression. *Histochem. Cell Biol.* **2020**, *154*, 265–273. [CrossRef]
49. Mazumder, S.; Dewangan, A.K.; Pavurala, N. Enhanced dissolution of poorly soluble antiviral drugs from nanoparticles of cellulose acetate based solid dispersion matrices. *Asian J. Pharm. Sci.* **2017**, *12*, 532–541. [CrossRef]
50. Caraway, C.A.; Gaitsch, H.; Wicks, E.E.; Kalluri, A.; Kunadi, N.; Tyler, B.M. Polymeric Nanoparticles in Brain Cancer Therapy: A Review of Current Approaches. *Polymers* **2022**, *14*, 2963. [CrossRef]
51. Anselmo, A.C.; Mitragotri, S. Nanoparticles in the clinic: An update. *Bioeng. Transl. Med.* **2019**, *4*, e10143. [CrossRef] [PubMed]
52. Genovesi, L.A.; Puttick, S.; Millar, A.; Kojic, M.; Ji, P.; Lagendijk, A.K.; Brighi, C.; Bonder, C.S.; Adolphe, C.; Wainwright, B.J. Patient-derived orthotopic xenograft models of medulloblastoma lack a functional blood-brain barrier. *Neuro Oncol.* **2021**, *23*, 732–742. [CrossRef] [PubMed]
53. Becker, A.; Sells, B.; Haque, S.; Chakravarti, A. Tumor Heterogeneity in Glioblastomas: From Light Microscopy to Molecular Pathology. *Cancers* **2021**, *13*, 761. [CrossRef]
54. Ruan, S.; Zhou, Y.; Jiang, X.; Gao, H. Rethinking CRITID Procedure of Brain Targeting Drug Delivery: Circulation, Blood Brain Barrier Recognition, Intracellular Transport, Diseased Cell Targeting, Internalization, and Drug Release. *Adv. Sci.* **2021**, *8*, 2004025. [CrossRef]
55. Niu, X.; Chen, J.; Gao, J. Nanocarriers as a powerful vehicle to overcome blood-brain barrier in treating neurodegenerative diseases: Focus on recent advances. *Asian J. Pharm. Sci.* **2019**, *14*, 480–496. [CrossRef] [PubMed]
56. Dong, X. Current Strategies for Brain Drug Delivery. *Theranostics* **2018**, *8*, 1481–1493. [CrossRef] [PubMed]
57. Rueda, F.; Cruz, L.J. Targeting the Brain with Nanomedicine. *Curr. Pharm. Des.* **2017**, *23*, 1879–1896. [CrossRef]

58. Koog, L.; Gandek, T.B.; Nagelkerke, A. Liposomes and Extracellular Vesicles as Drug Delivery Systems: A Comparison of Composition, Pharmacokinetics, and Functionalization. *Adv. Healthc. Mater.* **2022**, *11*, 2100639. [CrossRef]
59. Eloy, J.O.; Petrilli, R.; Trevizan, L.N.F.; Chorilli, M. Immunoliposomes: A review on functionalization strategies and targets for drug delivery. *Colloids Surf. B Biointerfaces* **2017**, *159*, 454–467. [CrossRef]
60. Suk, J.S.; Xu, Q.; Kim, N.; Hanes, J.; Ensign, L.M. PEGylation as a strategy for improving nanoparticle-based drug and gene delivery. *Adv. Drug Deliv. Rev.* **2016**, *99*, 28–51. [CrossRef]
61. Smyth, T.; Kullberg, M.; Malik, N.; Smith-Jones, P.; Graner, M.W.; Anchordoquy, T.J. Biodistribution and delivery efficiency of unmodified tumor-derived exosomes. *J. Control Release* **2015**, *199*, 145–155. [CrossRef] [PubMed]
62. Szebeni, J.; Bedőcs, P.; Rozsnyay, Z.; Weiszhár, Z.; Urbanics, R.; Rosivall, L.; Cohen, R.; Garbuzenko, O.; Báthori, G.; Tóth, M.; et al. Liposome-induced complement activation and related cardiopulmonary distress in pigs: Factors promoting reactogenicity of Doxil and AmBisome. *Nanomed. Nanotechnol. Biol. Med.* **2012**, *8*, 176–184. [CrossRef] [PubMed]
63. Kowalski, P.S.; Rudra, A.; Miao, L.; Anderson, D.G. Delivering the Messenger: Advances in Technologies for Therapeutic mRNA Delivery. *Mol. Ther.* **2019**, *27*, 710–728. [CrossRef] [PubMed]
64. Hou, X.; Zaks, T.; Langer, R.; Dong, Y. Lipid nanoparticles for mRNA delivery. *Nat. Rev. Mater.* **2021**, *6*, 1078–1094. [CrossRef] [PubMed]
65. Makadia, H.K.; Siegel, S.J. Poly Lactic-co-Glycolic Acid (PLGA) as Biodegradable Controlled Drug Delivery Carrier. *Polymers* **2011**, *3*, 1377–1397. [CrossRef]
66. Song, E.; Gaudin, A.; King, A.R.; Seo, Y.E.; Suh, H.W.; Deng, Y.; Cui, J.; Tietjen, G.T.; Huttner, A.; Saltzman, W.M. Surface chemistry governs cellular tropism of nanoparticles in the brain. *Nat. Commun.* **2017**, *8*, 15322. [CrossRef]
67. Banstola, A.; Duwa, R.; Emami, F.; Jeong, J.-H.; Yook, S. Enhanced Caspase-Mediated Abrogation of Autophagy by Temozolomide-Loaded and Panitumumab-Conjugated Poly(lactic-co-glycolic acid) Nanoparticles in Epidermal Growth Factor Receptor Overexpressing Glioblastoma Cells. *Mol. Pharm.* **2020**, *17*, 4386–4400. [CrossRef]
68. Jackson, C.L.; Chanzy, H.D.; Booy, F.P.; Drake, B.J.; Tomalia, D.A.; Bauer, B.J.; Amis, E.J. Visualization of Dendrimer Molecules by Transmission Electron Microscopy (TEM): Staining Methods and Cryo-TEM of Vitrified Solutions. *Macromolecules* **1998**, *31*, 6259–6265. [CrossRef]
69. Zielińska, A.; Carreiró, F.; Oliveira, A.M.; Neves, A.; Pires, B.; Venkatesh, D.N.; Durazzo, A.; Lucarini, M.; Eder, P.; Silva, A.M.; et al. Polymeric Nanoparticles: Production, Characterization, Toxicology and Ecotoxicology. *Molecules* **2020**, *25*, 3731. [CrossRef]
70. Lim, J.-M.; Cai, T.; Mandaric, S.; Chopra, S.; Han, H.; Jang, S.; Il Choi, W.; Langer, R.; Farokhzad, O.C.; Karnik, R. Drug loading augmentation in polymeric nanoparticles using a coaxial turbulent jet mixer: Yong investigator perspective. *J. Colloid Interface Sci.* **2019**, *538*, 45–50. [CrossRef]
71. Gref, R.; Minamitake, Y.; Peracchia, M.T.; Trubetskoy, V.; Torchilin, V.; Langer, R. Biodegradable Long-Circulating Polymeric Nanospheres. *Science* **1994**, *263*, 1600–1603. [CrossRef]
72. Hu, X.; Zhang, Y.; Ding, T.; Liu, J.; Zhao, H. Multifunctional Gold Nanoparticles: A Novel Nanomaterial for Various Medical Applications and Biological Activities. *Front. Bioeng. Biotechnol.* **2020**, *8*, 990. [CrossRef] [PubMed]
73. Sababathy, M.; Ramanathan, G.; Tan, S.C. Targeted delivery of gold nanoparticles by neural stem cells to glioblastoma for enhanced radiation therapy: A review. *AIMS Neurosci.* **2022**, *9*, 303–319. [CrossRef] [PubMed]
74. Arias, L.; Pessan, J.; Vieira, A.; Lima, T.; Delbem, A.; Monteiro, D. Iron Oxide Nanoparticles for Biomedical Applications: A Perspective on Synthesis, Drugs, Antimicrobial Activity, and Toxicity. *Antibiotics* **2018**, *7*, 46. [CrossRef] [PubMed]
75. Najahi-Missaoui, W.; Arnold, R.D.; Cummings, B.S. Safe Nanoparticles: Are We There Yet? *Int. J. Mol. Sci.* **2020**, *22*, 385. [CrossRef]
76. Alshehri, R.; Ilyas, A.M.; Hasan, A.; Arnaout, A.; Ahmed, F.; Memic, A. Carbon Nanotubes in Biomedical Applications: Factors, Mechanisms, and Remedies of Toxicity. *J. Med. Chem.* **2016**, *59*, 8149–8167. [CrossRef]
77. Hoshino, A.; Costa-Silva, B.; Shen, T.L.; Rodrigues, G.; Hashimoto, A.; Tesic Mark, M.; Molina, H.; Kohsaka, S.; Di Giannatale, A.; Ceder, S.; et al. Tumour exosome integrins determine organotropic metastasis. *Nature* **2015**, *527*, 329–335. [CrossRef]
78. Antimisiaris, S.G.; Mourtas, S.; Marazioti, A. Exosomes and Exosome-Inspired Vesicles for Targeted Drug Delivery. *Pharmaceutics* **2018**, *10*, 218. [CrossRef]
79. Saleh, A.F.; Lázaro-Ibáñez, E.; Forsgard, M.A.-M.; Shatnyeva, O.; Osteikoetxea, X.; Karlsson, F.; Heath, N.; Ingelsten, M.; Rose, J.; Harris, J.; et al. Extracellular vesicles induce minimal hepatotoxicity and immunogenicity. *Nanoscale* **2019**, *11*, 6990–7001. [CrossRef]
80. Zhu, X.; Badawi, M.; Pomeroy, S.; Sutaria, D.S.; Xie, Z.; Baek, A.; Jiang, J.; Elgamal, O.A.; Mo, X.; Perle, K.L.; et al. Comprehensive toxicity and immunogenicity studies reveal minimal effects in mice following sustained dosing of extracellular vesicles derived from HEK293T cells. *J. Extracell. Vesicles* **2017**, *6*, 1324730. [CrossRef]
81. Imai, T.; Takahashi, Y.; Nishikawa, M.; Kato, K.; Morishita, M.; Yamashita, T.; Matsumoto, A.; Charoenviriyakul, C.; Takakura, Y. Macrophage-dependent clearance of systemically administered B16BL6-derived exosomes from the blood circulation in mice. *J. Extracell. Vesicles* **2015**, *4*, 26238. [CrossRef]
82. Mondal, J.; Pillarisetti, S.; Junnuthula, V.; Saha, M.; Hwang, S.R.; Park, I.K.; Lee, Y.K. Hybrid exosomes, exosome-like nanovesicles and engineered exosomes for therapeutic applications. *J. Control Release* **2022**, *353*, 1127–1149. [CrossRef] [PubMed]
83. Gurung, S.; Perocheau, D.; Touramanidou, L.; Baruteau, J. The exosome journey: From biogenesis to uptake and intracellular signalling. *Cell Commun. Signal.* **2021**, *19*, 47. [CrossRef] [PubMed]

84. Gauro, R.; Nandave, M.; Jain, V.K.; Jain, K. Advances in dendrimer-mediated targeted drug delivery to the brain. *J. Nanopart. Res.* **2021**, *23*, 76. [CrossRef]
85. Sajid, M.I.; Jamshaid, U.; Jamshaid, T.; Zafar, N.; Fessi, H.; Elaissari, A. Carbon nanotubes from synthesis to in vivo biomedical applications. *Int. J. Pharm.* **2016**, *501*, 278–299. [CrossRef] [PubMed]
86. Pednekar, P.P.; Godiyal, S.C.; Jadhav, K.R.; Kadam, V.J. Chapter 23—Mesoporous silica nanoparticles: A promising multifunctional drug delivery system. In *Nanostructures for Cancer Therapy*; Ficai, A., Grumezescu, A.M., Eds.; Elsevier: Amsterdam, The Netherlands, 2017; pp. 593–621.
87. Bharti, C.; Gulati, N.; Nagaich, U.; Pal, A. Mesoporous silica nanoparticles in target drug delivery system: A review. *Int. J. Pharm. Investig.* **2015**, *5*, 124. [CrossRef] [PubMed]
88. Akbarzadeh, A.; Rezaei-Sadabady, R.; Davaran, S.; Joo, S.W.; Zarghami, N.; Hanifehpour, Y.; Samiei, M.; Kouhi, M.; Nejati-Koshki, K. Liposome: Classification, preparation, and applications. *Nanoscale Res. Lett.* **2013**, *8*, 102. [CrossRef]
89. Gregoriadis, G.; Ryman, B.E. Fate of Protein-Containing Liposomes Injected into Rats. An Approach to the Treatment of Storage Diseases. *Eur. J. Biochem.* **1972**, *24*, 485–491. [CrossRef]
90. Mohamed, M.; Abu Lila, A.S.; Shimizu, T.; Alaaeldin, E.; Hussein, A.; Sarhan, H.A.; Szebeni, J.; Ishida, T. PEGylated liposomes: Immunological responses. *Sci. Technol. Adv. Mater.* **2019**, *20*, 710–724. [CrossRef]
91. Kulkarni, J.A.; Witzigmann, D.; Leung, J.; Tam, Y.Y.C.; Cullis, P.R. On the role of helper lipids in lipid nanoparticle formulations of siRNA. *Nanoscale* **2019**, *11*, 21733–21739. [CrossRef]
92. Natarajan, J.; Baskaran, M.; Humtsoe, L.C.; Vadivelan, R.; Justin, A. Enhanced brain targeting efficacy of Olanzapine through solid lipid nanoparticles. *Artif. Cells Nanomed. Biotechnol.* **2017**, *45*, 364–371. [CrossRef]
93. Pashirova, T.N.; Zueva, I.V.; Petrov, K.A.; Babaev, V.M.; Lukashenko, S.S.; Rizvanov, I.K.; Souto, E.B.; Nikolsky, E.E.; Zakharova, L.Y.; Masson, P.; et al. Nanoparticle-Delivered 2-PAM for Rat Brain Protection against Paraoxon Central Toxicity. *ACS Appl. Mater. Interfaces* **2017**, *9*, 16922–16932. [CrossRef] [PubMed]
94. Mitchell, M.J.; Billingsley, M.M.; Haley, R.M.; Wechsler, M.E.; Peppas, N.A.; Langer, R. Engineering precision nanoparticles for drug delivery. *Nat. Rev. Drug Discov.* **2021**, *20*, 101–124. [CrossRef] [PubMed]
95. Jaiswal, M.; Dudhe, R.; Sharma, P.K. Nanoemulsion: An advanced mode of drug delivery system. *3 Biotech* **2015**, *5*, 123–127. [CrossRef]
96. Carvalho, V.F.M.; Salata, G.C.; de Matos, J.K.R.; Costa-Fernandez, S.; Chorilli, M.; Steiner, A.A.; de Araujo, G.L.B.; Silveira, E.R.; Costa-Lotufo, L.V.; Lopes, L.B. Optimization of composition and obtainment parameters of biocompatible nanoemulsions intended for intraductal administration of piplartine (piperlongumine) and mammary tissue targeting. *Int. J. Pharm.* **2019**, *567*, 118460. [CrossRef] [PubMed]
97. Sánchez-López, E.; Guerra, M.; Dias-Ferreira, J.; Lopez-Machado, A.; Ettcheto, M.; Cano, A.; Espina, M.; Camins, A.; Garcia, M.L.; Souto, E.B. Current Applications of Nanoemulsions in Cancer Therapeutics. *Nanomaterials* **2019**, *9*, 821. [CrossRef] [PubMed]
98. Choudhury, H.; Gorain, B.; Karmakar, S.; Biswas, E.; Dey, G.; Barik, R.; Mandal, M.; Pal, T.K. Improvement of cellular uptake, in vitro antitumor activity and sustained release profile with increased bioavailability from a nanoemulsion platform. *Int. J. Pharm.* **2014**, *460*, 131–143. [CrossRef] [PubMed]
99. Gadhave, D.; Gorain, B.; Tagalpallewar, A.; Kokare, C. Intranasal teriflunomide microemulsion: An improved chemotherapeutic approach in glioblastoma. *J. Drug Deliv. Sci. Technol.* **2019**, *51*, 276–289. [CrossRef]
100. Shinde, R.L.; Devarajan, P.V. Docosahexaenoic acid–mediated, targeted and sustained brain delivery of curcumin microemulsion. *Drug Deliv.* **2017**, *24*, 152–161. [CrossRef]
101. Bonferoni, M.; Rossi, S.; Sandri, G.; Ferrari, F.; Gavini, E.; Rassu, G.; Giunchedi, P. Nanoemulsions for "Nose-to-Brain" Drug Delivery. *Pharmaceutics* **2019**, *11*, 84. [CrossRef]
102. Shieh, L.; Tamada, J.; Chen, I.; Pang, J.; Domb, A.; Langer, R. Erosion of a new family of biodegradable polyanhydrides. *J. Biomed. Mater. Res.* **1994**, *28*, 1465–1475. [CrossRef]
103. Tabata, Y.; Langer, R. Polyanhydride microspheres that display near-constant release of water-soluble model drug compounds. *Pharm. Res.* **1993**, *10*, 391–399. [CrossRef] [PubMed]
104. Jain, J.P.; Modi, S.; Kumar, N. Hydroxy fatty acid based polyanhydride as drug delivery system: Synthesis, characterization, in vitro degradation, drug release, and biocompatibility. *J. Biomed. Mater. Res. A* **2008**, *84*, 740–752. [CrossRef] [PubMed]
105. Deng, Y.; Saucier-Sawyer, J.K.; Hoimes, C.J.; Zhang, J.; Seo, Y.E.; Andrejecsk, J.W.; Saltzman, W.M. The effect of hyperbranched polyglycerol coatings on drug delivery using degradable polymer nanoparticles. *Biomaterials* **2014**, *35*, 6595–6602. [CrossRef] [PubMed]
106. Eivazi, N.; Rahmani, R.; Paknejad, M. Specific cellular internalization and pH-responsive behavior of doxorubicin loaded PLGA-PEG nanoparticles targeted with anti EGFRvIII antibody. *Life Sci.* **2020**, *261*, 118361. [CrossRef]
107. Gagliardi, A.; Giuliano, E.; Venkateswararao, E.; Fresta, M.; Bulotta, S.; Awasthi, V.; Cosco, D. Biodegradable Polymeric Nanoparticles for Drug Delivery to Solid Tumors. *Front. Pharmacol.* **2021**, *12*, 601626. [CrossRef]
108. Wang, W.; Meng, Q.; Li, Q.; Liu, J.; Zhou, M.; Jin, Z.; Zhao, K. Chitosan Derivatives and Their Application in Biomedicine. *Int. J. Mol. Sci.* **2020**, *21*, 487. [CrossRef]
109. Cheng, J.; Teply, B.; Sherifi, I.; Sung, J.; Luther, G.; Gu, F.; Levynissenbaum, E.; Radovicmoreno, A.; Langer, R.; Farokhzad, O. Formulation of functionalized PLGA–PEG nanoparticles for in vivo targeted drug delivery. *Biomaterials* **2007**, *28*, 869–876. [CrossRef]

110. Allyn, M.M.; Luo, R.H.; Hellwarth, E.B.; Swindle-Reilly, K.E. Considerations for Polymers Used in Ocular Drug Delivery. *Front. Med.* **2021**, *8*, 787644. [CrossRef]
111. Huntimer, L.; Ramer-Tait, A.E.; Petersen, L.K.; Ross, K.A.; Walz, K.A.; Wang, C.; Hostetter, J.; Narasimhan, B.; Wannemuehler, M.J. Evaluation of biocompatibility and administration site reactogenicity of polyanhydride-particle-based platform for vaccine delivery. *Adv. Healthc. Mater.* **2013**, *2*, 369–378. [CrossRef]
112. Vela-Ramirez, J.E.; Goodman, J.T.; Boggiatto, P.M.; Roychoudhury, R.; Pohl, N.L.B.; Hostetter, J.M.; Wannemuehler, M.J.; Narasimhan, B. Safety and Biocompatibility of Carbohydrate-Functionalized Polyanhydride Nanoparticles. *AAPS J.* **2015**, *17*, 256–267. [CrossRef] [PubMed]
113. Choi, J.; Rui, Y.; Kim, J.; Gorelick, N.; Wilson, D.R.; Kozielski, K.; Mangraviti, A.; Sankey, E.; Brem, H.; Tyler, B.; et al. Nonviral polymeric nanoparticles for gene therapy in pediatric CNS malignancies. *Nanomedicine* **2020**, *23*, 102115. [CrossRef] [PubMed]
114. Madej, M.; Kurowska, N.; Strzalka-Mrozik, B. Polymeric Nanoparticles—Tools in a Drug Delivery System in Selected Cancer Therapies. *Appl. Sci.* **2022**, *12*, 9479. [CrossRef]
115. Wang, Y.; Hu, A. Carbon quantum dots: Synthesis, properties and applications. *J. Mater. Chem. C* **2014**, *2*, 6921. [CrossRef]
116. Kushwaha, S.K.S.; Ghoshal, S.; Rai, A.K.; Singh, S. Carbon nanotubes as a novel drug delivery system for anticancer therapy: A review. *Braz. J. Pharm. Sci.* **2013**, *49*, 629–643. [CrossRef]
117. Valadi, H.; Ekström, K.; Bossios, A.; Sjöstrand, M.; Lee, J.J.; Lötvall, J.O. Exosome-mediated transfer of mRNAs and microRNAs is a novel mechanism of genetic exchange between cells. *Nat. Cell Biol.* **2007**, *9*, 654–659. [CrossRef]
118. Peters, P.J.; Geuze, H.J.; Van Donk, H.A.D.; Slot, J.W.; Griffith, J.M.; Stam, N.J.; Clevers, H.C.; Borst, J. Molecules relevant for T cell-target cell interaction are present in cytolytic granules of human T lymphocytes. *Eur. J. Immunol.* **1989**, *19*, 1469–1475. [CrossRef]
119. van Niel, G.; Raposo, G.; Candalh, C.; Boussac, M.; Hershberg, R.; Cerf-Bensussan, N.; Heyman, M. Intestinal epithelial cells secrete exosome-like vesicles. *Gastroenterology* **2001**, *121*, 337–349. [CrossRef]
120. Raposo, G.; Nijman, H.W.; Stoorvogel, W.; Liejendekker, R.; Harding, C.V.; Melief, C.J.; Geuze, H.J. B lymphocytes secrete antigen-presenting vesicles. *J. Exp. Med.* **1996**, *183*, 1161–1172. [CrossRef]
121. Raposo, G.; Tenza, D.; Mecheri, S.; Peronet, R.; Bonnerot, C.; Desaymard, C. Accumulation of Major Histocompatibility Complex Class II Molecules in Mast Cell Secretory Granules and Their Release upon Degranulation. *Mol. Biol. Cell* **1997**, *8*, 2631–2645. [CrossRef]
122. Wolfers, J.; Lozier, A.; Raposo, G.; Regnault, A.; Théry, C.; Masurier, C.; Flament, C.; Pouzieux, S.; Faure, F.; Tursz, T.; et al. Tumor-derived exosomes are a source of shared tumor rejection antigens for CTL cross-priming. *Nat. Med.* **2001**, *7*, 297–303. [CrossRef] [PubMed]
123. Zitvogel, L.; Regnault, A.; Lozier, A.; Wolfers, J.; Flament, C.; Tenza, D.; Ricciardi-Castagnoli, P.; Raposo, G.; Amigorena, S. Eradication of established murine tumors using a novel cell-free vaccine: Dendritic cell derived exosomes. *Nat. Med.* **1998**, *4*, 594–600. [CrossRef] [PubMed]
124. Heijnen, H.F.; Schiel, A.E.; Fijnheer, R.; Geuze, H.J.; Sixma, J.J. Activated platelets release two types of membrane vesicles: Microvesicles by surface shedding and exosomes derived from exocytosis of multivesicular bodies and alpha-granules. *Blood* **1999**, *94*, 3791–3799. [CrossRef] [PubMed]
125. Zheng, Y.; Tu, C.; Zhang, J.; Wang, J. Inhibition of multiple myeloma-derived exosomes uptake suppresses the functional response in bone marrow stromal cell. *Int. J. Oncol.* **2019**, *54*, 1061–1070. [CrossRef]
126. Wen, S.W.; Lima, L.G.; Lobb, R.J.; Norris, E.L.; Hastie, M.L.; Krumeich, S.; Moller, A. Breast Cancer-Derived Exosomes Reflect the Cell-of-Origin Phenotype. *Proteomics* **2019**, *19*, e1800180. [CrossRef] [PubMed]
127. Andriolo, G.; Provasi, E.; Lo Cicero, V.; Brambilla, A.; Soncin, S.; Torre, T.; Milano, G.; Biemmi, V.; Vassalli, G.; Turchetto, L.; et al. Exosomes From Human Cardiac Progenitor Cells for Therapeutic Applications: Development of a GMP-Grade Manufacturing Method. *Front. Physiol.* **2018**, *9*, 1169. [CrossRef] [PubMed]
128. Yuan, D.; Zhao, Y.; Banks, W.A.; Bullock, K.M.; Haney, M.; Batrakova, E.; Kabanov, A.V. Macrophage exosomes as natural nanocarriers for protein delivery to inflamed brain. *Biomaterials* **2017**, *142*, 1–12. [CrossRef] [PubMed]
129. Yu, B.; Zhang, X.; Li, X. Exosomes Derived from Mesenchymal Stem Cells. *Int. J. Mol. Sci.* **2014**, *15*, 4142–4157. [CrossRef]
130. Wan, R.; Hussain, A.; Behfar, A.; Moran, S.L.; Zhao, C. The Therapeutic Potential of Exosomes in Soft Tissue Repair and Regeneration. *Int. J. Mol. Sci.* **2022**, *23*, 3869. [CrossRef]
131. Liu, J.; Chen, Y.; Pei, F.; Zeng, C.; Yao, Y.; Liao, W.; Zhao, Z. Extracellular Vesicles in Liquid Biopsies: Potential for Disease Diagnosis. *BioMed Res. Int.* **2021**, *2021*, 6611244. [CrossRef]
132. García-Romero, N.; Carrión-Navarro, J.; Esteban-Rubio, S.; Lázaro-Ibáñez, E.; Peris-Celda, M.; Alonso, M.M.; Guzmán-De-Villoria, J.; Fernández-Carballal, C.; De Mendivil, A.O.; García-Duque, S.; et al. DNA sequences within glioma-derived extracellular vesicles can cross the intact blood-brain barrier and be detected in peripheral blood of patients. *Oncotarget* **2017**, *8*, 1416–1428. [CrossRef] [PubMed]
133. Théry, C.; Witwer, K.W.; Aikawa, E.; Alcaraz, M.J.; Anderson, J.D.; Andriantsitohaina, R.; Antoniou, A.; Arab, T.; Archer, F.; Atkin-Smith, G.K.; et al. Minimal information for studies of extracellular vesicles 2018 (MISEV2018): A position statement of the International Society for Extracellular Vesicles and update of the MISEV2014 guidelines. *J. Extracell. Vesicles* **2018**, *7*, 1535750. [CrossRef] [PubMed]

134. Johnstone, R.M.; Adam, M.; Hammond, J.R.; Orr, L.; Turbide, C. Vesicle formation during reticulocyte maturation. Association of plasma membrane activities with released vesicles (exosomes). *J. Biol. Chem.* **1987**, *262*, 9412–9420. [CrossRef] [PubMed]
135. Men, Y.; Yelick, J.; Jin, S.; Tian, Y.; Chiang, M.S.R.; Higashimori, H.; Brown, E.; Jarvis, R.; Yang, Y. Exosome reporter mice reveal the involvement of exosomes in mediating neuron to astroglia communication in the CNS. *Nat. Commun.* **2019**, *10*, 4136. [CrossRef]
136. Nolte-'t Hoen, E.N.; Buschow, S.I.; Anderton, S.M.; Stoorvogel, W.; Wauben, M.H. Activated T cells recruit exosomes secreted by dendritic cells via LFA-1. *Blood* **2009**, *113*, 1977–1981. [CrossRef]
137. Zhang, B.; Wang, M.; Gong, A.; Zhang, X.; Wu, X.; Zhu, Y.; Shi, H.; Wu, L.; Zhu, W.; Qian, H.; et al. HucMSC-Exosome Mediated-Wnt4 Signaling Is Required for Cutaneous Wound Healing. *Stem Cells* **2015**, *33*, 2158–2168. [CrossRef]
138. Osaki, M.; Okada, F. Exosomes and Their Role in Cancer Progression. *Yonago Acta Med.* **2019**, *62*, 182–190. [CrossRef]
139. Bang, C.; Batkai, S.; Dangwal, S.; Gupta, S.K.; Foinquinos, A.; Holzmann, A.; Just, A.; Remke, J.; Zimmer, K.; Zeug, A.; et al. Cardiac fibroblast–derived microRNA passenger strand-enriched exosomes mediate cardiomyocyte hypertrophy. *J. Clin. Investig.* **2014**, *124*, 2136–2146. [CrossRef]
140. Howitt, J.; Hill, A.F. Exosomes in the Pathology of Neurodegenerative Diseases. *J. Biol. Chem.* **2016**, *291*, 26589–26597. [CrossRef]
141. Al-Nedawi, K.; Meehan, B.; Micallef, J.; Lhotak, V.; May, L.; Guha, A.; Rak, J. Intercellular transfer of the oncogenic receptor EGFRvIII by microvesicles derived from tumour cells. *Nat. Cell Biol.* **2008**, *10*, 619–624. [CrossRef]
142. Thery, C.; Boussac, M.; Veron, P.; Ricciardi-Castagnoli, P.; Raposo, G.; Garin, J.; Amigorena, S. Proteomic analysis of dendritic cell-derived exosomes: A secreted subcellular compartment distinct from apoptotic vesicles. *J. Immunol.* **2001**, *166*, 7309–7318. [CrossRef] [PubMed]
143. Blanchard, N.; Lankar, D.; Faure, F.; Regnault, A.; Dumont, C.; Raposo, G.; Hivroz, C. TCR activation of human T cells induces the production of exosomes bearing the TCR/CD3/zeta complex. *J. Immunol.* **2002**, *168*, 3235–3241. [CrossRef] [PubMed]
144. Clayton, A.; Court, J.; Navabi, H.; Adams, M.; Mason, M.D.; Hobot, J.A.; Newman, G.R.; Jasani, B. Analysis of antigen presenting cell derived exosomes, based on immuno-magnetic isolation and flow cytometry. *J. Immunol. Methods* **2001**, *247*, 163–174. [CrossRef]
145. Théry, C.; Zitvogel, L.; Amigorena, S. Exosomes: Composition, biogenesis and function. *Nat. Rev. Immunol.* **2002**, *2*, 569–579. [CrossRef] [PubMed]
146. Skotland, T.; Sandvig, K.; Llorente, A. Lipids in exosomes: Current knowledge and the way forward. *Prog. Lipid Res.* **2017**, *66*, 30–41. [CrossRef]
147. Théry, C.; Duban, L.; Segura, E.; Véron, P.; Lantz, O.; Amigorena, S. Indirect activation of naïve CD4+ T cells by dendritic cell–derived exosomes. *Nat. Immunol.* **2002**, *3*, 1156–1162. [CrossRef]
148. Charoenviriyakul, C.; Takahashi, Y.; Morishita, M.; Nishikawa, M.; Takakura, Y. Role of Extracellular Vesicle Surface Proteins in the Pharmacokinetics of Extracellular Vesicles. *Mol. Pharm.* **2018**, *15*, 1073–1080. [CrossRef]
149. Huang, X.; Yuan, T.; Tschannen, M.; Sun, Z.; Jacob, H.; Du, M.; Liang, M.; Dittmar, R.L.; Liu, Y.; Liang, M.; et al. Characterization of human plasma-derived exosomal RNAs by deep sequencing. *BMC Genom.* **2013**, *14*, 319. [CrossRef]
150. Kooijmans, S.A.A.; Aleza, C.G.; Roffler, S.R.; Van Solinge, W.W.; Vader, P.; Schiffelers, R.M. Display of GPI-anchored anti-EGFR nanobodies on extracellular vesicles promotes tumour cell targeting. *J. Extracell. Vesicles* **2016**, *5*, 31053. [CrossRef]
151. Kooijmans, S.A.A.; Fliervoet, L.A.L.; van der Meel, R.; Fens, M.; Heijnen, H.F.G.; van Bergen En Henegouwen, P.M.P.; Vader, P.; Schiffelers, R.M. PEGylated and targeted extracellular vesicles display enhanced cell specificity and circulation time. *J. Control Release* **2016**, *224*, 77–85. [CrossRef]
152. Kamerkar, S.; Lebleu, V.S.; Sugimoto, H.; Yang, S.; Ruivo, C.F.; Melo, S.A.; Lee, J.J.; Kalluri, R. Exosomes facilitate therapeutic targeting of oncogenic KRAS in pancreatic cancer. *Nature* **2017**, *546*, 498–503. [CrossRef] [PubMed]
153. Murphy, D.E.; de Jong, O.G.; Brouwer, M.; Wood, M.J.; Lavieu, G.; Schiffelers, R.M.; Vader, P. Extracellular vesicle-based therapeutics: Natural versus engineered targeting and trafficking. *Exp. Mol. Med.* **2019**, *51*, 1–12. [CrossRef] [PubMed]
154. Lázaro Ibáñez, E.; Faruqu, F.N.; Saleh, A.F.; Silva, A.M.; Tzu-Wen Wang, J.; Rak, J.; Al-Jamal, K.T.; Dekker, N. Selection of Fluorescent, Bioluminescent, and Radioactive Tracers to Accurately Reflect Extracellular Vesicle Biodistribution in Vivo. *ACS Nano* **2021**, *15*, 3212–3227. [CrossRef] [PubMed]
155. Goh, W.J.; Zou, S.; Ong, W.Y.; Torta, F.; Alexandra, A.F.; Schiffelers, R.M.; Storm, G.; Wang, J.-W.; Czarny, B.; Pastorin, G. Bioinspired Cell-Derived Nanovesicles versus Exosomes as Drug Delivery Systems: A Cost-Effective Alternative. *Sci. Rep.* **2017**, *7*, 14322. [CrossRef] [PubMed]
156. Wen, Y.; Fu, Q.; Soliwoda, A.; Zhang, S.; Zheng, M.; Mao, W.; Wan, Y. Cell-derived nanovesicles prepared by membrane extrusion are good substitutes for natural extracellular vesicles. *Extracell. Vesicle* **2022**, *1*, 100004. [CrossRef]
157. Jang, S.C.; Kim, O.Y.; Yoon, C.M.; Choi, D.-S.; Roh, T.-Y.; Park, J.; Nilsson, J.; Lötvall, J.; Kim, Y.-K.; Gho, Y.S. Bioinspired Exosome-Mimetic Nanovesicles for Targeted Delivery of Chemotherapeutics to Malignant Tumors. *ACS Nano* **2013**, *7*, 7698–7710. [CrossRef]
158. Goh, W.J.; Lee, C.K.; Zou, S.; Woon, E.; Czarny, B.; Pastorin, G. Doxorubicin-loaded cell-derived nanovesicles: An alternative targeted approach for anti-tumor therapy. *Int. J. Nanomed.* **2017**, *12*, 2759–2767. [CrossRef]
159. Wilhelm, S.; Tavares, A.J.; Dai, Q.; Ohta, S.; Audet, J.; Dvorak, H.F.; Chan, W.C.W. Analysis of nanoparticle delivery to tumours. *Nat. Rev. Mater.* **2016**, *1*, 16014. [CrossRef]
160. Sun, C.; Ding, Y.; Zhou, L.; Shi, D.; Sun, L.; Webster, T.J.; Shen, Y. Noninvasive nanoparticle strategies for brain tumor targeting. *Nanomedicine* **2017**, *13*, 2605–2621. [CrossRef]

161. Li, J.; Zhao, J.; Tan, T.; Liu, M.; Zeng, Z.; Zeng, Y.; Zhang, L.; Fu, C.; Chen, D.; Xie, T. Nanoparticle Drug Delivery System for Glioma and Its Efficacy Improvement Strategies: A Comprehensive Review. *Int. J. Nanomed.* **2020**, *15*, 2563–2582. [CrossRef]
162. Hwang, D.W.; Choi, H.; Jang, S.C.; Yoo, M.Y.; Park, J.Y.; Choi, N.E.; Oh, H.J.; Ha, S.; Lee, Y.-S.; Jeong, J.M.; et al. Noninvasive imaging of radiolabeled exosome-mimetic nanovesicle using 99mTc-HMPAO. *Sci. Rep.* **2015**, *5*, 15636. [CrossRef] [PubMed]
163. Klibanov, A.L.; Maruyama, K.; Torchilin, V.P.; Huang, L. Amphipathic Polyethyleneglycols Effectively Prolong the Circulation Time of Liposomes. *FEBS Lett.* **1990**, *268*, 235–237. [CrossRef] [PubMed]
164. Hennig, R.; Pollinger, K.; Veser, A.; Breunig, M.; Goepferich, A. Nanoparticle multivalency counterbalances the ligand affinity loss upon PEGylation. *J. Control Release* **2014**, *194*, 20–27. [CrossRef] [PubMed]
165. Nunes, S.S.; De Oliveira Silva, J.; Fernandes, R.S.; Miranda, S.E.M.; Leite, E.A.; De Farias, M.A.; Portugal, R.V.; Cassali, G.D.; Townsend, D.M.; Oliveira, M.C.; et al. PEGylated versus Non-PEGylated pH-Sensitive Liposomes: New Insights from a Comparative Antitumor Activity Study. *Pharmaceutics* **2022**, *14*, 272. [CrossRef] [PubMed]
166. Frank, T.; Klinker, F.; Falkenburger, B.H.; Laage, R.; Lühder, F.; Göricke, B.; Schneider, A.; Neurath, H.; Desel, H.; Liebetanz, D.; et al. Pegylated granulocyte colony-stimulating factor conveys long-term neuroprotection and improves functional outcome in a model of Parkinson's disease. *Brain* **2012**, *135*, 1914–1925. [CrossRef] [PubMed]
167. Elinav, E.; Niv-Spector, L.; Katz, M.; Price, T.O.; Ali, M.; Yacobovitz, M.; Solomon, G.; Reicher, S.; Lynch, J.L.; Halpern, Z.; et al. Pegylated leptin antagonist is a potent orexigenic agent: Preparation and mechanism of activity. *Endocrinology* **2009**, *150*, 3083–3091. [CrossRef]
168. Yang, Q.; Lai, S.K. Anti-PEG immunity: Emergence, characteristics, and unaddressed questions. *Wiley Interdiscip. Rev. Nanomed. Nanobiotechnol.* **2015**, *7*, 655–677. [CrossRef]
169. Chao, M.P.; Weissman, I.L.; Majeti, R. The CD47–SIRPα pathway in cancer immune evasion and potential therapeutic implications. *Curr. Opin. Immunol.* **2012**, *24*, 225–232. [CrossRef]
170. Belhadj, Z.; He, B.; Deng, H.; Song, S.; Zhang, H.; Wang, X.; Dai, W.; Zhang, Q. A combined "eat me/don't eat me" strategy based on extracellular vesicles for anticancer nanomedicine. *J. Extracell. Vesicles* **2020**, *9*, 1806444. [CrossRef]
171. Rodriguez, P.L.; Harada, T.; Christian, D.A.; Pantano, D.A.; Tsai, R.K.; Discher, D.E. Minimal "Self" Peptides That Inhibit Phagocytic Clearance and Enhance Delivery of Nanoparticles. *Science* **2013**, *339*, 971–975. [CrossRef]
172. Hayat, S.M.G.; Jaafari, M.R.; Hatamipour, M.; Penson, P.E.; Sahebkar, A. Liposome Circulation Time is Prolonged by CD47 Coating. *Protein Pept. Lett.* **2020**, *27*, 1029–1037. [CrossRef] [PubMed]
173. Yu, M.; Zheng, J. Clearance Pathways and Tumor Targeting of Imaging Nanoparticles. *ACS Nano* **2015**, *9*, 6655–6674. [CrossRef] [PubMed]
174. Zhang, W.; Mehta, A.; Tong, Z.; Esser, L.; Voelcker, N.H. Development of Polymeric Nanoparticles for Blood–Brain Barrier Transfer—Strategies and Challenges. *Adv. Sci.* **2021**, *8*, 2003937. [CrossRef] [PubMed]
175. Juliano, R.L.; Stamp, D. The effect of particle size and charge on the clearance rates of liposomes and liposome encapsulated drugs. *Biochem. Biophys. Res. Commun.* **1975**, *63*, 651–658. [CrossRef] [PubMed]
176. Zhang, F.; Trent Magruder, J.; Lin, Y.-A.; Crawford, T.C.; Grimm, J.C.; Sciortino, C.M.; Wilson, M.A.; Blue, M.E.; Kannan, S.; Johnston, M.V.; et al. Generation-6 hydroxyl PAMAM dendrimers improve CNS penetration from intravenous administration in a large animal brain injury model. *J. Control Release* **2017**, *249*, 173–182. [CrossRef] [PubMed]
177. Sonavane, G.; Tomoda, K.; Makino, K. Biodistribution of colloidal gold nanoparticles after intravenous administration: Effect of particle size. *Colloids Surf. B Biointerfaces* **2008**, *66*, 274–280. [CrossRef]
178. Graham, D.K.; DeRyckere, D.; Davies, K.D.; Earp, H.S. The TAM family: Phosphatidylserine sensing receptor tyrosine kinases gone awry in cancer. *Nat. Rev. Cancer* **2014**, *14*, 769–785. [CrossRef]
179. Matsumoto, A.; Takahashi, Y.; Nishikawa, M.; Sano, K.; Morishita, M.; Charoenviriyakul, C.; Saji, H.; Takakura, Y. Role of Phosphatidylserine-Derived Negative Surface Charges in the Recognition and Uptake of Intravenously Injected B16BL6-Derived Exosomes by Macrophages. *J. Pharm. Sci.* **2017**, *106*, 168–175. [CrossRef]
180. Patel, H.M.; Tuzel, N.S.; Ryman, B.E. Inhibitory effect of cholesterol on the uptake of liposomes by liver and spleen. *Biochim. Biophys. Acta (BBA)—Gen. Subj.* **1983**, *761*, 142–151. [CrossRef]
181. Champion, J.A.; Mitragotri, S. Role of target geometry in phagocytosis. *Proc. Natl. Acad. Sci. USA* **2006**, *103*, 4930–4934. [CrossRef]
182. Huang, X.; Li, L.; Liu, T.; Hao, N.; Liu, H.; Chen, D.; Tang, F. The Shape Effect of Mesoporous Silica Nanoparticles on Biodistribution, Clearance, and Biocompatibility in Vivo. *ACS Nano* **2011**, *5*, 5390–5399. [CrossRef] [PubMed]
183. Arnida;Janát-Amsbury, M.M.; Ray, A.; Peterson, C.M.; Ghandehari, H. Geometry and surface characteristics of gold nanoparticles influence their biodistribution and uptake by macrophages. *Eur. J. Pharm. Biopharm.* **2011**, *77*, 417–423. [CrossRef] [PubMed]
184. Yang, T.; Martin, P.; Fogarty, B.; Brown, A.; Schurman, K.; Phipps, R.; Yin, V.P.; Lockman, P.; Bai, S. Exosome Delivered Anticancer Drugs Across the Blood-Brain Barrier for Brain Cancer Therapy in Danio Rerio. *Pharm. Res.* **2015**, *32*, 2003–2014. [CrossRef] [PubMed]
185. Na, J.H.; Koo, H.; Lee, S.; Min, K.H.; Park, K.; Yoo, H.; Lee, S.H.; Park, J.H.; Kwon, I.C.; Jeong, S.Y.; et al. Real-time and non-invasive optical imaging of tumor-targeting glycol chitosan nanoparticles in various tumor models. *Biomaterials* **2011**, *32*, 5252–5261. [CrossRef]
186. Maksimenko, O.; Malinovskaya, J.; Shipulo, E.; Osipova, N.; Razzhivina, V.; Arantseva, D.; Yarovaya, O.; Mostovaya, U.; Khalansky, A.; Fedoseeva, V.; et al. Doxorubicin-loaded PLGA nanoparticles for the chemotherapy of glioblastoma: Towards the pharmaceutical development. *Int. J. Pharm.* **2019**, *572*, 118733. [CrossRef]

187. Fang, C.; Wang, K.; Stephen, Z.R.; Mu, Q.; Kievit, F.M.; Chiu, D.T.; Press, O.W.; Zhang, M. Temozolomide Nanoparticles for Targeted Glioblastoma Therapy. *ACS Appl. Mater. Interfaces* **2015**, *7*, 6674–6682. [CrossRef]
188. Marchetti, L.; Engelhardt, B. Immune cell trafficking across the blood-brain barrier in the absence and presence of neuroinflammation. *Vasc. Biol.* **2020**, *2*, H1–H18. [CrossRef]
189. Liu, L.; Eckert, M.A.; Riazifar, H.; Kang, D.-K.; Agalliu, D.; Zhao, W. From Blood to the Brain: Can Systemically Transplanted Mesenchymal Stem Cells Cross the Blood-Brain Barrier? *Stem Cells Int.* **2013**, *2013*, 435093. [CrossRef]
190. Cao, M.; Mao, J.; Duan, X.; Lu, L.; Zhang, F.; Lin, B.; Chen, M.; Zheng, C.; Zhang, X.; Shen, J. In vivo tracking of the tropism of mesenchymal stem cells to malignant gliomas using reporter gene-based MR imaging. *Int. J. Cancer* **2018**, *142*, 1033–1046. [CrossRef]
191. Simionescu, M.; Ghinea, N.; Fixman, A.; Lasser, M.; Kukes, L.; Simionescu, N.; Palade, G.E. The cerebral microvasculature of the rat: Structure and luminal surface properties during early development. *J. Submicrosc. Cytol. Pathol.* **1988**, *20*, 243–261.
192. Azarmi, M.; Maleki, H.; Nikkam, N.; Malekinejad, H. Transcellular brain drug delivery: A review on recent advancements. *Int. J. Pharm.* **2020**, *586*, 119582. [CrossRef] [PubMed]
193. Moura, R.P.; Martins, C.; Pinto, S.; Sousa, F.; Sarmento, B. Blood-brain barrier receptors and transporters: An insight on their function and how to exploit them through nanotechnology. *Expert Opin. Drug Deliv.* **2019**, *16*, 271–285. [CrossRef]
194. Moscariello, P.; Ng, D.Y.W.; Jansen, M.; Weil, T.; Luhmann, H.J.; Hedrich, J. Brain Delivery of Multifunctional Dendrimer Protein Bioconjugates. *Adv. Sci.* **2018**, *5*, 1700897. [CrossRef] [PubMed]
195. Albertazzi, L.; Serresi, M.; Albanese, A.; Beltram, F. Dendrimer Internalization and Intracellular Trafficking in Living Cells. *Mol. Pharm.* **2010**, *7*, 680–688. [CrossRef] [PubMed]
196. Ordóñez-Gutiérrez, L.; Re, F.; Bereczki, E.; Ioja, E.; Gregori, M.; Andersen, A.J.; Antón, M.; Moghimi, S.M.; Pei, J.-J.; Masserini, M.; et al. Repeated intraperitoneal injections of liposomes containing phosphatidic acid and cardiolipin reduce amyloid-β levels in APP/PS1 transgenic mice. *Nanomed. Nanotechnol. Biol. Med.* **2015**, *11*, 421–430. [CrossRef]
197. Dehouck, B.; Fenart, L.; Dehouck, M.-P.; Pierce, A.; Torpier, G.; Cecchelli, R. A New Function for the LDL Receptor: Transcytosis of LDL across the Blood–Brain Barrier. *J. Cell Biol.* **1997**, *138*, 877–889. [CrossRef] [PubMed]
198. Jefferies, W.A.; Brandon, M.R.; Hunt, S.V.; Williams, A.F.; Gatter, K.C.; Mason, D.Y. Transferrin receptor on endothelium of brain capillaries. *Nature* **1984**, *312*, 162–163. [CrossRef]
199. Neves, A.R.; Queiroz, J.F.; Lima, S.A.C.; Reis, S. Apo E-Functionalization of Solid Lipid Nanoparticles Enhances Brain Drug Delivery: Uptake Mechanism and Transport Pathways. *Bioconj. Chem.* **2017**, *28*, 995–1004. [CrossRef]
200. Hu, K.; Shi, Y.; Jiang, W.; Han, J.; Huang, S.; Jiang, X. Lactoferrin conjugated PEG-PLGA nanoparticles for brain delivery: Preparation, characterization and efficacy in Parkinson's disease. *Int. J. Pharm.* **2011**, *415*, 273–283. [CrossRef]
201. Shilo, M.; Motiei, M.; Hana, P.; Popovtzer, R. Transport of nanoparticles through the blood-brain barrier for imaging and therapeutic applications. *Nanoscale* **2014**, *6*, 2146–2152. [CrossRef]
202. Xin, H.; Sha, X.; Jiang, X.; Zhang, W.; Chen, L.; Fang, X. Anti-glioblastoma efficacy and safety of paclitaxel-loading Angiopep-conjugated dual targeting PEG-PCL nanoparticles. *Biomaterials* **2012**, *33*, 8167–8176. [CrossRef] [PubMed]
203. Zhang, W.; Liu, Q.Y.; Haqqani, A.S.; Leclerc, S.; Liu, Z.; Fauteux, F.; Baumann, E.; Delaney, C.E.; Ly, D.; Star, A.T.; et al. Differential expression of receptors mediating receptor-mediated transcytosis (RMT) in brain microvessels, brain parenchyma and peripheral tissues of the mouse and the human. *Fluids Barriers CNS* **2020**, *17*, 47. [CrossRef] [PubMed]
204. Hawkins, B.T.; Egleton, R.D.; Davis, T.P. Modulation of cerebral microvascular permeability by endothelial nicotinic acetylcholine receptors. *Am. J. Physiol.-Heart Circ. Physiol.* **2005**, *289*, H212–H219. [CrossRef] [PubMed]
205. Ramalho, M.J.; Sevin, E.; Gosselet, F.; Lima, J.; Coelho, M.A.N.; Loureiro, J.A.; Pereira, M.C. Receptor-mediated PLGA nanoparticles for glioblastoma multiforme treatment. *Int. J. Pharm.* **2018**, *545*, 84–92. [CrossRef]
206. Kuang, Y.; Jiang, X.; Zhang, Y.; Lu, Y.; Ma, H.; Guo, Y.; Zhang, Y.; An, S.; Li, J.; Liu, L.; et al. Dual Functional Peptide-Driven Nanoparticles for Highly Efficient Glioma-Targeting and Drug Codelivery. *Mol. Pharm.* **2016**, *13*, 1599–1607. [CrossRef] [PubMed]
207. Johnsen, K.B.; Bak, M.; Melander, F.; Thomsen, M.S.; Burkhart, A.; Kempen, P.J.; Andresen, T.L.; Moos, T. Modulating the antibody density changes the uptake and transport at the blood-brain barrier of both transferrin receptor-targeted gold nanoparticles and liposomal cargo. *J. Control Release* **2019**, *295*, 237–249. [CrossRef]
208. Paris-Robidas, S.; Emond, V.; Tremblay, C.; Soulet, D.; Calon, F. In Vivo Labeling of Brain Capillary Endothelial Cells after Intravenous Injection of Monoclonal Antibodies Targeting the Transferrin Receptor. *Mol. Pharmacol.* **2011**, *80*, 32–39. [CrossRef]
209. Mao, J.; Meng, X.; Zhao, C.; Yang, Y.; Liu, G. Development of transferrin-modified poly(lactic-co-glycolic acid) nanoparticles for glioma therapy. *Anti-Cancer Drugs* **2019**, *30*, 604–610. [CrossRef]
210. Cabral Filho, P.E.; Cardoso, A.L.C.; Pereira, M.I.A.; Ramos, A.P.M.; Hallwass, F.; Castro, M.M.C.A.; Geraldes, C.F.G.C.; Santos, B.S.; Pedroso de Lima, M.C.; Pereira, G.A.L.; et al. CdTe quantum dots as fluorescent probes to study transferrin receptors in glioblastoma cells. *Biochim. Biophys. Acta (BBA)—Gen. Subj.* **2016**, *1860*, 28–35. [CrossRef]
211. Roberts, R.L.; Fine, R.E.; Sandra, A. Receptor-mediated endocytosis of transferrin at the blood-brain barrier. *J. Cell Sci.* **1993**, *104*, 521–532. [CrossRef]
212. Uchida, Y.; Ohtsuki, S.; Katsukura, Y.; Ikeda, C.; Suzuki, T.; Kamiie, J.; Terasaki, T. Quantitative targeted absolute proteomics of human blood-brain barrier transporters and receptors. *J. Neurochem.* **2011**, *117*, 333–345. [CrossRef] [PubMed]

213. Maussang, D.; Rip, J.; van Kregten, J.; van den Heuvel, A.; van der Pol, S.; van der Boom, B.; Reijerkerk, A.; Chen, L.; de Boer, M.; Gaillard, P.; et al. Glutathione conjugation dose-dependently increases brain-specific liposomal drug delivery in vitro and in vivo. *Drug Discov. Today Technol.* **2016**, *20*, 59–69. [CrossRef] [PubMed]
214. Da Silva-Candal, A.; Brown, T.; Krishnan, V.; Lopez-Loureiro, I.; Ávila-Gómez, P.; Pusuluri, A.; Pérez-Díaz, A.; Correa-Paz, C.; Hervella, P.; Castillo, J.; et al. Shape effect in active targeting of nanoparticles to inflamed cerebral endothelium under static and flow conditions. *J. Control Release* **2019**, *309*, 94–105. [CrossRef] [PubMed]
215. Kolhar, P.; Anselmo, A.C.; Gupta, V.; Pant, K.; Prabhakarpandian, B.; Ruoslahti, E.; Mitragotri, S. Using shape effects to target antibody-coated nanoparticles to lung and brain endothelium. *Proc. Natl. Acad. Sci. USA* **2013**, *110*, 10753–10758. [CrossRef] [PubMed]
216. Nowak, M.; Brown, T.D.; Graham, A.; Helgeson, M.E.; Mitragotri, S. Size, shape, and flexibility influence nanoparticle transport across brain endothelium under flow. *Bioeng. Transl. Med.* **2020**, *5*, e10153. [CrossRef]
217. Takeshita, Y.; Ransohoff, R.M. Inflammatory cell trafficking across the blood-brain barrier: Chemokine regulation and in vitro models. *Immunol. Rev.* **2012**, *248*, 228–239. [CrossRef]
218. Han, Y.; Li, X.; Zhang, Y.; Han, Y.; Chang, F.; Ding, J. Mesenchymal Stem Cells for Regenerative Medicine. *Cells* **2019**, *8*, 886. [CrossRef]
219. Roger, M.; Clavreul, A.; Venier-Julienne, M.C.; Passirani, C.; Sindji, L.; Schiller, P.; Montero-Menei, C.; Menei, P. Mesenchymal stem cells as cellular vehicles for delivery of nanoparticles to brain tumors. *Biomaterials* **2010**, *31*, 8393–8401. [CrossRef]
220. Li, L.; Guan, Y.; Liu, H.; Hao, N.; Liu, T.; Meng, X.; Fu, C.; Li, Y.; Qu, Q.; Zhang, Y.; et al. Silica Nanorattle–Doxorubicin-Anchored Mesenchymal Stem Cells for Tumor-Tropic Therapy. *ACS Nano* **2011**, *5*, 7462–7470. [CrossRef]
221. Choi, M.-R.; Stanton-Maxey, K.J.; Stanley, J.K.; Levin, C.S.; Bardhan, R.; Akin, D.; Badve, S.; Sturgis, J.; Robinson, J.P.; Bashir, R.; et al. A Cellular Trojan Horse for Delivery of Therapeutic Nanoparticles into Tumors. *Nano Lett.* **2007**, *7*, 3759–3765. [CrossRef]
222. Ibarra, L.E.; Beaugé, L.; Arias-Ramos, N.; Rivarola, V.A.; Chesta, C.A.; López-Larrubia, P.; Palacios, R.E. Trojan horse monocyte-mediated delivery of conjugated polymer nanoparticles for improved photodynamic therapy of glioblastoma. *Nanomedicine* **2020**, *15*, 1687–1707. [CrossRef] [PubMed]
223. Li, Z.; Huang, H.; Tang, S.; Li, Y.; Yu, X.F.; Wang, H.; Li, P.; Sun, Z.; Zhang, H.; Liu, C.; et al. Small gold nanorods laden macrophages for enhanced tumor coverage in photothermal therapy. *Biomaterials* **2016**, *74*, 144–154. [CrossRef] [PubMed]
224. Chu, D.; Gao, J.; Wang, Z. Neutrophil-Mediated Delivery of Therapeutic Nanoparticles across Blood Vessel Barrier for Treatment of Inflammation and Infection. *ACS Nano* **2015**, *9*, 11800–11811. [CrossRef] [PubMed]
225. Steinfeld, U.; Pauli, C.; Kaltz, N.; Bergemann, C.; Lee, H.H. T lymphocytes as potential therapeutic drug carrier for cancer treatment. *Int. J. Pharm.* **2006**, *311*, 229–236. [CrossRef]
226. Zhang, J.; Han, M.; Zhang, J.; Abdalla, M.; Sun, P.; Yang, Z.; Zhang, C.; Liu, Y.; Chen, C.; Jiang, X. Syphilis mimetic nanoparticles for cuproptosis-based synergistic cancer therapy via reprogramming copper metabolism. *Int. J. Pharm.* **2023**, *640*, 123025. [CrossRef]
227. Ji, J.; Lian, W.; Zhang, Y.; Lin, D.; Wang, J.; Mo, Y.; Xu, X.; Hou, C.; Ma, C.; Zheng, Y.; et al. Preoperative administration of a biomimetic platelet nanodrug enhances postoperative drug delivery by bypassing thrombus. *Int. J. Pharm.* **2023**, *636*, 122851. [CrossRef]
228. Zhuang, X.; Xiang, X.; Grizzle, W.; Sun, D.; Zhang, S.; Axtell, R.C.; Ju, S.; Mu, J.; Zhang, L.; Steinman, L.; et al. Treatment of Brain Inflammatory Diseases by Delivering Exosome Encapsulated Anti-inflammatory Drugs from the Nasal Region to the Brain. *Mol. Ther.* **2011**, *19*, 1769–1779. [CrossRef]
229. Sousa, F.; Dhaliwal, H.K.; Gattacceca, F.; Sarmento, B.; Amiji, M.M. Enhanced anti-angiogenic effects of bevacizumab in glioblastoma treatment upon intranasal administration in polymeric nanoparticles. *J. Control Release* **2019**, *309*, 37–47. [CrossRef]
230. Djupesland, P.G. Nasal drug delivery devices: Characteristics and performance in a clinical perspective—A review. *Drug Deliv. Transl. Res.* **2013**, *3*, 42–62. [CrossRef]
231. Bobo, R.H.; Laske, D.W.; Akbasak, A.; Morrison, P.F.; Dedrick, R.L.; Oldfield, E.H. Convection-enhanced delivery of macromolecules in the brain. *Proc. Natl. Acad. Sci. USA* **1994**, *91*, 2076–2080. [CrossRef]
232. Lonser, R.R.; Sarntinoranont, M.; Morrison, P.F.; Oldfield, E.H. Convection-enhanced delivery to the central nervous system. *J. Neurosurg.* **2015**, *122*, 697–706. [CrossRef] [PubMed]
233. Zhou, Z.; Singh, R.; Souweidane, M.M. Convection-Enhanced Delivery for Diffuse Intrinsic Pontine Glioma Treatment. *Curr. Neuropharmacol.* **2017**, *15*, 116–128. [CrossRef] [PubMed]
234. Souweidane, M.M.; Kramer, K.; Pandit-Taskar, N.; Zhou, Z.; Haque, S.; Zanzonico, P.; Carrasquillo, J.A.; Lyashchenko, S.K.; Thakur, S.B.; Donzelli, M.; et al. Convection-enhanced delivery for diffuse intrinsic pontine glioma: A single-centre, dose-escalation, phase 1 trial. *Lancet Oncol.* **2018**, *19*, 1040–1050. [CrossRef] [PubMed]
235. Bander, E.D.; Ramos, A.D.; Wembacher-Schroeder, E.; Ivasyk, I.; Thomson, R.; Morgenstern, P.F.; Souweidane, M.M. Repeat convection-enhanced delivery for diffuse intrinsic pontine glioma. *J. Neurosurg. Pediatr.* **2020**, *26*, 661–666. [CrossRef] [PubMed]
236. Mueller, S.; Kline, C.; Villanueva-Meyer, J.; Hoffman, C.; Raber, S.; Bonner, E.; Nazarian, J.; Lundy, S.; Molinaro, A.M.; Prados, M.; et al. EPCT-12. PNOC015: PHASE 1 STUDY OF MTX110 (AQUEOUS PANOBINOSTAT) DELIVERED BY CONVECTION ENHANCED DELIVERY (CED) IN CHILDREN WITH NEWLY DIAGNOSED DIFFUSE INTRINSIC PONTINE GLIOMA (DIPG) PREVIOUSLY TREATED WITH RADIATION THERAPY. *Neuro Oncol.* **2020**, *22*, iii306. [CrossRef]

237. Zacharoulis, S.; Szalontay, L.; CreveCoeur, T.; Neira, J.; Higgins, D.; Englander, Z.; Spinazzi, E.; Sethi, C.; Canoll, P.; Garvin, J. DDEL-07. A Phase I study examining the feasibility of intermittent convection-enhanced delivery (CED) of MTX110 for the treatment of children with newly diagnosed diffuse midline gliomas (DMGs). *Neuro Oncol.* **2022**, *24*, i35. [CrossRef]
238. Heiss, J.D.; Jamshidi, A.; Shah, S.; Martin, S.; Wolters, P.L.; Argersinger, D.P.; Warren, K.E.; Lonser, R.R. Phase I trial of convection-enhanced delivery of IL13-Pseudomonas toxin in children with diffuse intrinsic pontine glioma. *J. Neurosurg. Pediatr.* **2018**, *23*, 333–342. [CrossRef]
239. Kunwar, S.; Chang, S.; Westphal, M.; Vogelbaum, M.; Sampson, J.; Barnett, G.; Shaffrey, M.; Ram, Z.; Piepmeier, J.; Prados, M.; et al. Phase III randomized trial of CED of IL13-PE38QQR vs Gliadel wafers for recurrent glioblastoma. *Neuro Oncol.* **2010**, *12*, 871–881. [CrossRef]
240. Sampson, J.H.; Archer, G.; Pedain, C.; Wembacher-Schröder, E.; Westphal, M.; Kunwar, S.; Vogelbaum, M.A.; Coan, A.; Herndon, J.E.; Raghavan, R.; et al. Poor drug distribution as a possible explanation for the results of the PRECISE trial. *J. Neurosurg.* **2010**, *113*, 301–309. [CrossRef]
241. Mueller, S.; Polley, M.Y.; Lee, B.; Kunwar, S.; Pedain, C.; Wembacher-Schröder, E.; Mittermeyer, S.; Westphal, M.; Sampson, J.H.; Vogelbaum, M.A.; et al. Effect of imaging and catheter characteristics on clinical outcome for patients in the PRECISE study. *J. Neurooncol.* **2011**, *101*, 267–277. [CrossRef]
242. Bredlau, A.L.; Dixit, S.; Chen, C.; Broome, A.M. Nanotechnology Applications for Diffuse Intrinsic Pontine Glioma. *Curr. Neuropharmacol.* **2017**, *15*, 104–115. [CrossRef] [PubMed]
243. Zhang, R.; Saito, R.; Mano, Y.; Kanamori, M.; Sonoda, Y.; Kumabe, T.; Tominaga, T. Concentration rather than dose defines the local brain toxicity of agents that are effectively distributed by convection-enhanced delivery. *J. Neurosci. Methods* **2014**, *222*, 131–137. [CrossRef] [PubMed]
244. Zacharoulis, S.; Columbia University. CED of MTX110 Newly Diagnosed Diffuse Midline Gliomas. Available online: https://ClinicalTrials.gov/show/NCT04264143 (accessed on 30 October 2021).
245. Cheng, Z.; Zhang, J.; Liu, H.; Li, Y.; Zhao, Y.; Yang, E. Central Nervous System Penetration for Small Molecule Therapeutic Agents Does Not Increase in Multiple Sclerosis- and Alzheimer's Disease-Related Animal Models Despite Reported Blood-Brain Barrier Disruption. *Drug Metab. Dispos.* **2010**, *38*, 1355–1361. [CrossRef] [PubMed]
246. Somjen, G.; Segal, M.; Herreras, O. Osmotic-hypertensive opening of the blood-brain barrier in rats does not necessarily provide access for potassium to cerebral interstitial fluid. *Exp. Physiol.* **1991**, *76*, 507–514. [CrossRef]
247. Nance, E.; Timbie, K.; Miller, G.W.; Song, J.; Louttit, C.; Klibanov, A.L.; Shih, T.-Y.; Swaminathan, G.; Tamargo, R.J.; Woodworth, G.F.; et al. Non-invasive delivery of stealth, brain-penetrating nanoparticles across the blood − brain barrier using MRI-guided focused ultrasound. *J. Control Release* **2014**, *189*, 123–132. [CrossRef]
248. Nance, E.A.; Woodworth, G.F.; Sailor, K.A.; Shih, T.-Y.; Xu, Q.; Swaminathan, G.; Xiang, D.; Eberhart, C.; Hanes, J. A Dense Poly(Ethylene Glycol) Coating Improves Penetration of Large Polymeric Nanoparticles Within Brain Tissue. *Sci. Transl. Med.* **2012**, *4*, 149ra119. [CrossRef]
249. Schneider, C.S.; Perez, J.G.; Cheng, E.; Zhang, C.; Mastorakos, P.; Hanes, J.; Winkles, J.A.; Woodworth, G.F.; Kim, A.J. Minimizing the non-specific binding of nanoparticles to the brain enables active targeting of Fn14-positive glioblastoma cells. *Biomaterials* **2015**, *42*, 42–51. [CrossRef]
250. Matsumura, Y.; Maeda, H. A new concept for macromolecular therapeutics in cancer chemotherapy: Mechanism of tumoritropic accumulation of proteins and the antitumor agent smancs. *Cancer Res.* **1986**, *46*, 6387–6392.
251. Gabizon, A.; Shmeeda, H.; Barenholz, Y. Pharmacokinetics of Pegylated Liposomal Doxorubicin. *Clin. Pharmacokinet.* **2003**, *42*, 419–436. [CrossRef]
252. Mo, F.; Pellerino, A.; Soffietti, R.; Rudà, R. Blood–Brain Barrier in Brain Tumors: Biology and Clinical Relevance. *Int. J. Mol. Sci.* **2021**, *22*, 12654. [CrossRef]
253. Siegal, T.; Horowitz, A.; Gabizon, A. Doxorubicin encapsulated in sterically stabilized liposomes for the treatment of a brain tumor model: Biodistribution and therapeutic efficacy. *J. Neurosurg.* **1995**, *83*, 1029–1037. [CrossRef] [PubMed]
254. Sarin, H.; Kanevsky, A.S.; Wu, H.; Brimacombe, K.R.; Fung, S.H.; Sousa, A.A.; Auh, S.; Wilson, C.M.; Sharma, K.; Aronova, M.A.; et al. Effective transvascular delivery of nanoparticles across the blood-brain tumor barrier into malignant glioma cells. *J. Transl. Med.* **2008**, *6*, 80. [CrossRef] [PubMed]
255. Shein, S.A.; Kuznetsov, I.I.; Abakumova, T.O.; Chelushkin, P.S.; Melnikov, P.A.; Korchagina, A.A.; Bychkov, D.A.; Seregina, I.F.; Bolshov, M.A.; Kabanov, A.V.; et al. VEGF- and VEGFR2-Targeted Liposomes for Cisplatin Delivery to Glioma Cells. *Mol. Pharm.* **2016**, *13*, 3712–3723. [CrossRef] [PubMed]
256. Shein, S.A.; Nukolova, N.V.; Korchagina, A.A.; Abakumova, T.O.; Kiuznetsov, I.I.; Abakumov, M.A.; Baklaushev, V.P.; Gurina, O.I.; Chekhonin, V.P. Site-Directed Delivery of VEGF-Targeted Liposomes into Intracranial C6 Glioma. *Bull. Exp. Biol. Med.* **2015**, *158*, 371–376. [CrossRef] [PubMed]
257. Veiseh, M.; Gabikian, P.; Bahrami, S.B.; Veiseh, O.; Zhang, M.; Hackman, R.C.; Ravanpay, A.C.; Stroud, M.R.; Kusuma, Y.; Hansen, S.J.; et al. Tumor Paint: A Chlorotoxin:Cy5.5 Bioconjugate for Intraoperative Visualization of Cancer Foci. *Cancer Res.* **2007**, *67*, 6882–6888. [CrossRef] [PubMed]
258. Mortensen, J.H.; Jeppesen, M.; Pilgaard, L.; Agger, R.; Duroux, M.; Zachar, V.; Moos, T. Targeted Antiepidermal Growth Factor Receptor (Cetuximab) Immunoliposomes Enhance Cellular Uptake In Vitro and Exhibit Increased Accumulation in an Intracranial Model of Glioblastoma Multiforme. *J. Drug Deliv.* **2013**, *2013*, 209205. [CrossRef]

259. Greenall, S.A.; McKenzie, M.; Seminova, E.; Dolezal, O.; Pearce, L.; Bentley, J.; Kuchibhotla, M.; Chen, S.C.; McDonald, K.L.; Kornblum, H.I.; et al. Most clinical anti-EGFR antibodies do not neutralize both wtEGFR and EGFRvIII activation in glioma. *Neuro Oncol.* **2019**, *21*, 1016–1027. [CrossRef]
260. Pan, P.C.; Magge, R.S. Mechanisms of EGFR Resistance in Glioblastoma. *Int. J. Mol. Sci.* **2020**, *21*, 8471. [CrossRef]
261. Dhar, D.; Ghosh, S.; Das, S.; Chatterjee, J. A review of recent advances in magnetic nanoparticle-based theranostics of glioblastoma. *Nanomedicine* **2022**, *17*, 107–132. [CrossRef]
262. Ganipineni, L.P.; Ucakar, B.; Joudiou, N.; Bianco, J.; Danhier, P.; Zhao, M.; Bastiancich, C.; Gallez, B.; Danhier, F.; Préat, V. Magnetic targeting of paclitaxel-loaded poly(lactic-co-glycolic acid)-based nanoparticles for the treatment of glioblastoma. *Int. J. Nanomed.* **2018**, *13*, 4509–4521. [CrossRef]
263. Heggannavar, G.B.; Hiremath, C.G.; Achari, D.D.; Pangarkar, V.G.; Kariduraganavar, M.Y. Development of Doxorubicin-Loaded Magnetic Silica–Pluronic F-127 Nanocarriers Conjugated with Transferrin for Treating Glioblastoma across the Blood–Brain Barrier Using an in Vitro Model. *ACS Omega* **2018**, *3*, 8017–8026. [CrossRef] [PubMed]
264. Norouzi, M.; Yathindranath, V.; Thliveris, J.A.; Kopec, B.M.; Siahaan, T.J.; Miller, D.W. Doxorubicin-loaded iron oxide nanoparticles for glioblastoma therapy: A combinational approach for enhanced delivery of nanoparticles. *Sci. Rep.* **2020**, *10*, 11292. [CrossRef]
265. Li, B.; Chen, X.; Qiu, W.; Zhao, R.; Duan, J.; Zhang, S.; Pan, Z.; Zhao, S.; Guo, Q.; Qi, Y.; et al. Synchronous Disintegration of Ferroptosis Defense Axis via Engineered Exosome-Conjugated Magnetic Nanoparticles for Glioblastoma Therapy. *Adv. Sci.* **2022**, *9*, 2105451. [CrossRef] [PubMed]
266. Calatayud, M.P.; Soler, E.; Torres, T.E.; Campos-Gonzalez, E.; Junquera, C.; Ibarra, M.R.; Goya, G.F. Cell damage produced by magnetic fluid hyperthermia on microglial BV2 cells. *Sci. Rep.* **2017**, *7*, 8627. [CrossRef]
267. Shen, Z.; Liu, T.; Yang, Z.; Zhou, Z.; Tang, W.; Fan, W.; Liu, Y.; Mu, J.; Li, L.; Bregadze, V.I.; et al. Small-sized gadolinium oxide based nanoparticles for high-efficiency theranostics of orthotopic glioblastoma. *Biomaterials* **2020**, *235*, 119783. [CrossRef] [PubMed]
268. Kefayat, A.; Ghahremani, F.; Motaghi, H.; Amouheidari, A. Ultra-small but ultra-effective: Folic acid-targeted gold nanoclusters for enhancement of intracranial glioma tumors' radiation therapy efficacy. *Nanomed. Nanotechnol. Biol. Med.* **2019**, *16*, 173–184. [CrossRef]
269. Goubault, C.; Jarry, U.; Bostoen, M.; Eliat, P.A.; Kahn, M.L.; Pedeux, R.; Guillaudeux, T.; Gauffre, F.; Chevance, S. Radiosensitizing Fe-Au nanocapsules (hybridosomes(R)) increase survival of GL261 brain tumor-bearing mice treated by radiotherapy. *Nanomedicine* **2022**, *40*, 102499. [CrossRef]
270. Jing, Z.; Li, M.; Wang, H.; Yang, Z.; Zhou, S.; Ma, J.; Meng, E.; Zhang, H.; Liang, W.; Hu, W.; et al. Gallic acid-gold nanoparticles enhance radiation-induced cell death of human glioma U251 cells. *IUBMB Life* **2021**, *73*, 398–407. [CrossRef]
271. Hsieh, H.T.; Huang, H.C.; Chung, C.W.; Chiang, C.C.; Hsia, T.; Wu, H.F.; Huang, R.L.; Chiang, C.S.; Wang, J.; Lu, T.T.; et al. CXCR4-targeted nitric oxide nanoparticles deliver PD-L1 siRNA for immunotherapy against glioblastoma. *J. Control Release* **2022**, *352*, 920–930. [CrossRef]
272. Zhang, Y.; Ren, Y.; Xu, H.; Li, L.; Qian, F.; Wang, L.; Quan, A.; Ma, H.; Liu, H.; Yu, R. Cascade-Responsive 2-DG Nanocapsules Encapsulate aV-siCPT1C Conjugates to Inhibit Glioblastoma through Multiple Inhibition of Energy Metabolism. *ACS Appl. Mater. Interfaces* **2023**, *15*, 10356–10370. [CrossRef]
273. Rinaldi, A.; Caraffi, R.; Grazioli, M.V.; Oddone, N.; Giardino, L.; Tosi, G.; Vandelli, M.A.; Calzà, L.; Ruozi, B.; Duskey, J.T. Applications of the ROS-Responsive Thioketal Linker for the Production of Smart Nanomedicines. *Polymers* **2022**, *14*, 687. [CrossRef] [PubMed]
274. Oddone, N.; Boury, F.; Garcion, E.; Grabrucker, A.M.; Martinez, M.C.; Da Ros, F.; Janaszewska, A.; Forni, F.; Vandelli, M.A.; Tosi, G.; et al. Synthesis, Characterization, and In Vitro Studies of an Reactive Oxygen Species (ROS)-Responsive Methoxy Polyethylene Glycol-Thioketal-Melphalan Prodrug for Glioblastoma Treatment. *Front. Pharmacol.* **2020**, *11*, 574. [CrossRef] [PubMed]
275. Liu, Z.; Zhou, Z.; Dang, Q.; Xu, H.; Lv, J.; Li, H.; Han, X. Immunosuppression in tumor immune microenvironment and its optimization from CAR-T cell therapy. *Theranostics* **2022**, *12*, 6273–6290. [CrossRef]
276. Balakrishnan, P.B.; Sweeney, E.E. Nanoparticles for Enhanced Adoptive T Cell Therapies and Future Perspectives for CNS Tumors. *Front. Immunol.* **2021**, *12*, 600659. [CrossRef]
277. Chang, Y.; Cai, X.; Syahirah, R.; Yao, Y.; Xu, Y.; Jin, G.; Bhute, V.J.; Torregrosa-Allen, S.; Elzey, B.D.; Won, Y.-Y.; et al. CAR-neutrophil mediated delivery of tumor-microenvironment responsive nanodrugs for glioblastoma chemo-immunotherapy. *Nat. Commun.* **2023**, *14*, 2266. [CrossRef] [PubMed]
278. Zhang, F.; Stephan, S.B.; Ene, C.I.; Smith, T.T.; Holland, E.C.; Stephan, M.T. Nanoparticles That Reshape the Tumor Milieu Create a Therapeutic Window for Effective T-cell Therapy in Solid Malignancies. *Cancer Res.* **2018**, *78*, 3718–3730. [CrossRef] [PubMed]
279. Chen, Q.; Hu, Q.; Dukhovlinova, E.; Chen, G.; Ahn, S.; Wang, C.; Ogunnaike, E.A.; Ligler, F.S.; Dotti, G.; Gu, Z. Photothermal Therapy Promotes Tumor Infiltration and Antitumor Activity of CAR T Cells. *Adv. Mater.* **2019**, *31*, 1900192. [CrossRef] [PubMed]

pharmaceutics

Article

# Influence of Surface Ligand Density and Particle Size on the Penetration of the Blood–Brain Barrier by Porous Silicon Nanoparticles

**Weisen Zhang [1], Douer Zhu [1], Ziqiu Tong [1], Bo Peng [1,2], Xuan Cheng [3], Lars Esser [1,3,*] and Nicolas H. Voelcker [1,4,5,*]**

1 Drug Delivery, Disposition and Dynamics, Monash Institute of Pharmaceutical Sciences, Monash University, Parkville, VIC 3052, Australia; tommy.tong@monash.edu (Z.T.)
2 Frontiers Science Center for Flexible Electronics, Xi'an Institute of Flexible Electronics (IFE), Xi'an Institute of Biomedical Materials & Engineering (IBME), Northwestern Polytechnical University, Xi'an 710072, China
3 Commonwealth Scientific and Industrial Research Organisation (CSIRO), Clayton, VIC 3168, Australia; heidi.cheng@csiro.au
4 Melbourne Centre for Nanofabrication, Victorian Node of the Australian National Fabrication Facility, Clayton, VIC 3168, Australia
5 Department of Materials Science and Engineering, Monash University, Clayton, VIC 3800, Australia
* Correspondence: lars.esser@csiro.au (L.E.); nicolas.voelcker@monash.edu (N.H.V.)

**Abstract:** Overcoming the blood–brain barrier (BBB) remains a significant challenge with regard to drug delivery to the brain. By incorporating targeting ligands, and by carefully adjusting particle sizes, nanocarriers can be customized to improve drug delivery. Among these targeting ligands, transferrin stands out due to the high expression level of its receptor (i.e., transferrin receptor) on the BBB. Porous silicon nanoparticles (pSiNPs) are a promising drug nanocarrier to the brain due to their biodegradability, biocompatibility, and exceptional drug-loading capacity. However, an in-depth understanding of the optimal nanoparticle size and transferrin surface density, in order to maximize BBB penetration, is still lacking. To address this gap, a diverse library of pSiNPs was synthesized using bifunctional poly(ethylene glycol) linkers with methoxy or/and carboxyl terminal groups. These variations allowed us to explore different transferrin surface densities in addition to particle sizes. The effects of these parameters on the cellular association, uptake, and transcytosis in immortalized human brain microvascular endothelial cells (hCMEC/D3) were investigated using multiple in vitro systems of increasing degrees of complexity. These systems included the following: a 2D cell culture, a static Transwell model, and a dynamic BBB-on-a-chip model. Our results revealed the significant impact of both the ligand surface density and size of pSiNPs on their ability to penetrate the BBB, wherein intermediate-level transferrin densities and smaller pSiNPs exhibited the highest BBB transportation efficiency in vitro. Moreover, notable discrepancies emerged between the tested in vitro assays, further emphasizing the necessity of using more physiologically relevant assays, such as a microfluidic BBB-on-a-chip model, for nanocarrier testing and evaluation.

**Keywords:** blood–brain barrier; nanoparticles; porous silicon nanoparticles; BBB-on-a-chip; ligand density; organ-on-a-chip; nanomedicine; microfluidic model

**Citation:** Zhang, W.; Zhu, D.; Tong, Z.; Peng, B.; Cheng, X.; Esser, L.; Voelcker, N.H. Influence of Surface Ligand Density and Particle Size on the Penetration of the Blood–Brain Barrier by Porous Silicon Nanoparticles. *Pharmaceutics* **2023**, *15*, 2271. https://doi.org/10.3390/pharmaceutics15092271

Academic Editors: Nicolas Tournier and Toshihiko Tashima

Received: 25 June 2023
Revised: 23 July 2023
Accepted: 29 July 2023
Published: 3 September 2023



## 1. Introduction

Neurological disorders are a global health challenge and the second leading cause of mortality, with more than 10 million deaths reported globally in 2019 alone [1]. Diseases associated with neurological disorders, such as Alzheimer's disease, Parkinson's disease, and brain cancers currently affect over 349 million lives, sadly, with no effective treatments on hand [1–3]. Although pre-clinical research has resulted in the discovery of multiple promising drug candidates, clinical translation has trailed behind, as the presence of the blood–brain barrier (BBB) prevents the delivery of most drugs to the brain [4–6]. The BBB is a highly efficient physical barrier that consists of endothelial cells and other cells, such as pericytes and astrocytes [7]. The BBB functions as a vascular hurdle between the blood and the brain, blocking most blood constituents from entering the brain, as the BBB's tight junctions prevent paracellular transport; moreover, pinocytic activity is also very restricted [8,9].

Several strategies, such as focused ultrasounds [10], implantable reservoirs [11], and convection-enhanced injections [12], have been reported to help therapeutic molecules cross the BBB. Nevertheless, these technologies possess several limitations. For example, focused ultrasounds display limitations with regard to the reproducibility of clinical procedures, and brain implants are associated with infection risks due to invasive surgical procedures and the implant materials used [13,14]. On the other hand, nanoparticles are a promising technology as they promote BBB penetration, and they target diseased regions in the brain while limiting side effects [15–18]. For example, so-called "sequential targeting interlocking" nanoparticles were shown to cross the BBB and precisely target brain cancer [19]. This system was developed using a ligand for the glucose receptor, GLUT1, to promote BBB transcytosis, and it contained a pH-responsive linker to promote drug payload release in the acidic tumor microenvironment.

In more general terms, nanoparticles have the potential to cross the BBB when decorated with specific ligands, such as proteins and antibodies, that, upon binding to their respective receptor, follow the receptor-mediated transcytosis pathway [20]. This pathway enables more efficient and higher cargo transportation across the BBB compared with other transport pathways [7,21]. Among others, transferrin, apolipoprotein, lactoferrin, and rabies virus glycoproteins have been studied as BBB-crossing surface ligands due to the high expression levels of their respective receptors, which are as follows: transferrin receptor, low-density lipoprotein receptor, lipoprotein receptors, and acetylcholine receptors [22,23]. For example, transferrin receptors are expressed on the endothelial cells of brain capillaries, with an extracellular receptor concentration of 0.13 fmol/µg cell protein; they are involved in iron transport to the brain via receptor-mediated transcytosis [24]. This pathway has been successfully exploited by transferrin-coated nanoparticles [20]. Recent studies show that transferrin-decorated nanoparticles can also promote a higher cellular uptake in brain cancer cells [25,26]. However, the nanoparticle surface ligand density differs between published studies, and it is often not well characterized. For example, a study compared liposomes with different surface transferrin antibody densities (0.15, 0.3, and $0.6 \times 10^3$ antibodies $\mu m^{-2}$), and surprisingly, it was shown that the nanoparticles with the highest density limited BBB crossing capabilities [27].

In addition, BBB transportation efficiency can be associated with the size of nanoparticles, but the mechanism behind it remains ambiguous. Smaller nanoparticles generally have greater BBB penetration capabilities compared with larger nanoparticles [28–30]; for example, 100 nm poly-(lactic-co-glycolic acid) nanoparticles displayed longer blood circulation times and greater BBB penetration capabilities than the larger (i.e., 200 and 800 nm) nanoparticles in an in vivo mouse study [31]. In contrast, some other studies report that the size of nanoparticles does not influence their BBB penetration capabilities [27,32,33]. And one in vitro study showed exactly the opposite trend; larger polystyrene nanoparticles (500 nm) had greater BBB penetration capabilities than smaller nanoparticles (200 nm) [34].

pSiNPs nanoparticles exhibit immense potential as candidates for drug delivery purposes due to properties such as their biodegradability, large surface area for drug loading, and biocompatibility [35]. Recent studies have also demonstrated the potential of using pSiNPs for glioblastoma multiforme cancer targeting after crossing the BBB [26,36]. However, a clearer understanding of the optimal nanoparticle size and transferrin surface content, in order to maximize BBB penetration capabilities, is still required. Therefore, a systematic comparison of pSiNPs nanoparticular features, such as surface density and size, with regard to BBB penetration, using well-defined assays, is urgently needed to advance the development of this drug delivery platform for the treatment of central nervous system diseases. Herein, we investigate the optimal surface and size influence of this delivery system for BBB penetration. Using bifunctional poly(ethylene glycol)-(PEG) linkers (with either carboxyl or methoxy terminal group), we were able to tune the transferrin density on pSiNPs. In addition, different sizes of nanoparticles were prepared using a centrifugation-based size selection method. This pSiNP library was then assessed for their cell association and cellular uptake by means of flow cytometry and confocal microscopy in 2D cell culture. Afterward, the pSiNPs' transcytosis efficiency was investigated using both a static in vitro Transwell BBB model and a dynamic in vitro microfluidic BBB model (BBB-on-a-chip).

## 2. Materials and Methods

### 2.1. Materials

Silicon wafers used for the manufacturing of the nanoparticles were purchased from Siltronix (Archamps, France). Luminescent cell viability assay and VivoGlo$^{TM}$ Luciferin were purchased from Promega. Cyanine5 amine (Cy5) was purchased from Lumiprobe. Hydrofluoric acid (HF, 49%) was purchased from J. T. Baker (Center Valley, PA, USA). Human holo-transferrin, undecylenic acid (UA), 1-ethyl-3-(3-dimethylaminopropyl)carbodiimide (EDC) hydrochloride, *N*-hydroxysulfosuccinimide (NHS), 2-(*N*-morpholino)ethanesulfonic acid (MES) hydrate, ethanol (EtOH), dimethylformamide (DMF), dichloromethane (DCM), and triethylamine (TEA) were purchased from Merck (Macquarie Park, Australia). All solvents were of analytical grade. Water (HPLC grade) was obtained with a Milli-Q Advantage A10 water purification system (Merck Millipore, Bayswater, Australia). α-Carboxyl-ω-amino poly(ethylene glycol) 10 kDa ($NH_2$-PEG-COOH) and methoxy poly-(ethylene glycol)-amine 10 kDa (mPEG-$NH_2$) were purchased from Advanced BioChemicals (Lawrenceville, GA, USA). All other chemicals were purchased from Sigma-Aldrich (Macquarie Park, Australia) unless stated otherwise.

### 2.2. Methods

#### 2.2.1. Attenuated Total Reflection-Fourier Transform Infrared Spectroscopy (ATR-FTIR)

ATR-FTIR spectra of all nanomaterials were obtained using a Thermo Scientific Nicolet 6700. A diamond crystal was run in ATR configuration with a 2 mm diamond tip and a deuterium triglycine sulfate detector. The spectra collected were averaged from 64 recorded scans with a resolution of 8 $cm^{-1}$. Background spectra were blanked using air. The data were processed using OMNIC software (version 7.3).

#### 2.2.2. Transmission Electron Microscopy (TEM)

Bright Field (BF) TEM images were used to measure the nanoparticle size and visualize its morphological traits. TEM samples were prepared via drop casting the suspended sample of interest (in either ethanol or PBS) onto copper grids. The samples were examined using a Philips Tecnai 12 TEM at an operating voltage of 120 kV. Images were recorded using a FEI Eagle 4 k × 4 k CCD camera. Low dose conditions (<10 $e^-/Å^2$) were used to avoid damage to samples.

#### 2.2.3. Dynamic Light Scattering (DLS)

A Malvern Instruments Zetasizer Nano instrument ZEN3600 was employed with a 4 mW 633 nm HeNe gas laser. An Avalanche photodiode detector measured the back scatter light at an angle of 173° relative to the angle of the incident light beam. Samples were dissolved in ethanol or PBS (pH 7.41). A single-use folded capillary cell commercialized by Malvern Instruments (model DTS 1070) was used for measuring surface zeta potential.

#### 2.2.4. Electrochemical Etching of Silicon Wafer

A highly boron-doped p-type silicon wafer (0.00055–0.001 Ω cm resistivity, 6-inch) was anodically etched in a solution composed of 3:1 (*v:v*) of 49% aqueous HF: ethanol. The etching waveform consisted of a square wave in which a lower current pulse of 0.6 A for 20 s was followed by a higher current pulse of 24 A applied for 0.2 s (the latter used to form sacrificial layers). This waveform was repeated for 1000 cycles. The film was then lifted off from the silicon substrate by applying a current density of 24 A for 60 s in a solution containing 1:1 (*v:v*) of 49% aqueous HF: ethanol [37]. The film was then stored in a desiccator.

### 2.2.5. Thermal Hydrocarbonization of Porous Silicon Film

The freshly etched pSi film was placed in a ceramic boat into a quartz tube under a stream of constant $N_2$ flow at 2 L $min^{-1}$ for 45 min at room temperature (RT). Then a 1:1 $N_2$-acetylene mixture flow was introduced into the tube at RT for 15 min, with the quartz tube being placed into a preheated furnace at 525 °C for 14.5 min under a continuous flow of 1:1 $N_2$-acetylene, followed by 30 s with $N_2$ only. After that, the tube was allowed to cool down to RT under $N_2$ flow [36]. The thermal hydrocarbonized silicon film was stored in ethanol and analyzed by ATR-FTIR.

### 2.2.6. Fractioning of Silicon Wafer by Ultrasonication

The pSi film was shattered via shaking and then transferred into a 15 mm diameter Pyrex Quickfit glass test tube. The bottom of the test tube was filled with the shattered pSi film and then topped up with 6 mL ethanol. The mixture was then continuously ultrasonicated using a QSonica sonifier probe (Model CL-188) at 25% amplitude for 24 h in an ice bath with ice changed every 8 h. The thermal hydrocarbonized pSiNPs (THC-pSiNPs) were stored in ethanol [37].

### 2.2.7. Size Selection and Functionalization of pSiNPs with Undecylenic Acid (UDA)

Size selection was carried out using a bespoke centrifuge-based protocol. First, the dispersion of nanoparticles was centrifugated at 2000× *g* for 15 min, and the supernatant was collected. This step was repeated once to remove all large nanoparticles. Afterward, the combined supernatants were centrifugated at 19,000× *g* for 45 min to remove the remains of the sacrificial layers. The remaining precipitates were then redispersed in ethanol and centrifugated at 3500× *g* for 15 min to further narrow the size distribution, and supernatants were kept. The last two steps were repeated once respectively to improve the yield of selected medium-sized (170–180 nm in diameter) particles. These are referred to as the small (S) pSiNPs throughout the manuscript.

The larger pSiNPs (L, around 403 nm diameter) were selected by collecting the pellets from the first two centrifugation steps (i.e., 2000× *g* for 15 min), redispersing these in ethanol, and then collecting the supernatants after centrifugation at 1000× *g* for 15 min to remove very large particles.

Afterward, these two size-selected particles were divided into several Eppendorf tubes and centrifugated at 21,000× *g* for 10 min to remove ethanol. Pellets were then dispersed in 2% HF in ethanol for 5 min to remove any oxidation and washed thoroughly with ethanol three times. Next, the dispersion was transferred into a 20 mL glass vial, sealed with a rubber septum, and dried under $N_2$ flow. Next, 5 mL of undecylenic acid was prepared in another glass vial sealed with a rubber septum and sparged with $N_2$ for 30 min in a warm water bath. The deoxygenated undecylenic acid was then transferred to the dried particle-containing glass vial via a cannula under $N_2$ flow. The nanoparticles in undecylenic acid were sonicated to redisperse and reacted at 140 °C in an oil bath for 16 h [36]. Afterward, the unreacted undecylenic acid was removed by washing it with ethanol five times. The UDA-functionalized pSiNPs (UDA-pSiNPs) were stored in ethanol and analyzed via ATR-FTIR.

### 2.2.8. Preparation of Cy5-Labeled Transferrin and PEG-Conjugated Nanoparticles

Cy5, bifunctional PEG, and transferrin were all covalently conjugated to the carboxylic acid groups of the UDA-pSiNPs via EDC/NHS reaction. Briefly, pSiNPs were first washed three times with DMF to remove ethanol. Afterward, EDC and NHS (concentration of 10 mg/mL DMF) were added directly to UDA-pSiNPs (concentration of 4 mg/mL) with final concentrations of 10 mM and 5 mM, respectively. These reaction components were well mixed and allowed to react for 2 h at RT. After the NHS ester activation, the reaction mixture was washed with DMF and MES buffer to remove excess EDC and NHS. The activated UDA-pSiNPs were kept in low protein-binding tubes for direct surface conjugation.

For the two different sizes of $NH_2$-PEG-COOH and transferrin-coated pSiNPs, Tf-PEG-pSiNPs(S) and Tf-PEG-pSiNPs(L), 3 μL of Cy5-$NH_2$ (10 mg/mL in DMSO) and 500 μL of $NH_2$-PEG-COOH (10 mg/mL) in phosphate-buffered saline (PBS, pH 8) were added to 1 mg of two different sizes of activated UDA-pSiNPs. The mixtures were sonicated for 0.5 h and agitated for 1 h at RT. Afterward, the reaction mixture was washed three times in DMF and once in PBS (pH 7.4) to remove any free Cy5 and PEG linker. To conjugate transferrin to Cy5-labeled nanoparticles, these samples were reactivated with EDC (2.5 mM) and NHS (1.25 mM) in 500 μL of MES buffer for 20 min at RT followed by two times washing in MES buffer and once in PBS (pH 7.4). Afterward, 500 μL of transferrin (2 mg/mL) in PBS (pH 7.4) was added to 1 mg of the reactivated nanoparticles, followed by sonication for 0.5 h and agitation overnight at RT. The final products were washed four times in PBS (pH 7.4) to remove unreacted and non-covalently associated transferrin, where supernatants were collected and measured using a bicinchoninic acid assay (BCA) assay [38] to indirectly determine the amount of transferrin conjugated onto the nanoparticles.

For two different ratios of $NH_2$-PEG-COOH/mPEG-$NH_2$ and transferrin-coated pSiNPs (Tf-PEG/mPEG(1:9)-pSiNPs(S) and Tf-PEG/mPEG(1:50)-pSiNPs(S), 3 μL of Cy5-$NH_2$ (10 mg/mL in DMSO) and 50 μL or 5 μL $NH_2$-PEG-COOH (10 mg/mL in PBS (pH 8) and 450 μL or 495 μL of mPEG (10 mg/mL) in PBS (pH 8) were added to 1 mg of activated UDA-pSiNPs, respectively. The mixtures were sonicated for 0.5 h and agitated for 1 h at RT. Afterward, these samples were treated using the same procedure in terms of transferrin conjugation and washing steps as mentioned above in the Tf-PEG-pSiNPs(S) and Tf-PEG-pSiNPs(L).

Finally, for mPEG-coated pSiNPs, briefly, 3.6 μL of Cy5-$NH_2$ and 500 μL of mPEG-$NH_2$ (10 mg/mL) in PBS (pH 8) were added to 1 mg of activated UDA-pSiNPs followed by sonicating for 0.5 h and agitating for 1 h at RT. Constantly sonicating and mixing the sample is the key step to fabricating mPEG-pSiNPs(S). Afterward, the reaction mixture was washed three times in DMF and one time in PBS (pH 7.4) to remove any free Cy5 and mPEG-$NH_2$.

To prepare a positive control sample, transferrin-modified pSiNPs (Tf-pSiNPs), the procedure was followed from the previous report [36]. Briefly, 2.4 μL of Cy5-$NH_2$ (10 mg/mL in DMSO) was added to 1 mg of activated UDA-pSiNPs in 500 μL of PBS (pH 8), sonicating for 0.5 h and agitating for 1 h at RT. Afterward, these samples were treated using the same procedure in terms of transferrin conjugation and washing steps as mentioned above in Tf-PEG-pSiNPs(S) and Tf-PEG-pSiNPs(L).

#### 2.2.9. Cell Culture

Immortalized human brain microvascular endothelial cells (hCMEC/D3) were purchased from Merck. The hCMEC/D3 cell line was maintained with endothelial cell growth basal medium-2 (EBM-2, Lonza) with supplements of 5% fetal bovine serum (FBS) and growth factors as previously reported [39]. Cells were cultured on a collagen-coated (150 μg/mL) T-75 tissue culture flask at 37 °C in 5% $CO_2$ in the passage of 28 to 35 according to the supplier's protocol. The cell culture medium was changed every 2 to 3 days before reaching confluency. The cell culture procedure in the BBB-on-a-chip model was followed as previously reported [40].

#### 2.2.10. Cell Viability in Contact with pSiNPs

The biocompatibility of modified pSiNPs on the hCMEC/D3 cell line was determined using a CellTiter-Glo® luminescent cell viability assay (Promega, Alexandria, Australia). Briefly, hCMEC/D3 cells were seeded onto a 96-well white opaque polystyrene microplate (Sigma-Aldrich, Macquarie Park, Australia) at a density of 10,000 cells per well and maintained in the cell culture medium for 1 day. Subsequently, cells were treated with different concentrations (5, 10, 25, 50 µg/mL) of surface-modified pSiNPs. Cells without any treatment were used as control, and each condition was triplicated. After incubating cells for 48 h, a CellTiter-Glo® luminescent cell viability assay was used to evaluate the cell viability. Briefly, 100 µL of the solution of the assay kit was added to 100 µL of the medium in each well, and the plates were gently shaken at RT for 15 min. Finally, the luminescence intensity of each sample was obtained using a PerkinElmer EnSpire multimode plate reader, and data were expressed as the mean and standard deviation of 3 replicates.

#### 2.2.11. Cellular Association and Uptake of pSiNPs via Flow Cytometry and Confocal Microscopy

Flow cytometry was used to confirm the cellular association of pSiNPs in hCMEC/D3. Briefly, hCMEC/D3 was seeded onto a 24-well plate at the density of $1.2 \times 10^5$ cells per well and cultured overnight. The cells were then washed twice in PBS and incubated with 5 µg/mL of Cy5-labeled surface-modified pSiNPs for 1 h at 37 °C supplied with 5% $CO_2$. Afterward, the cells were washed 3× with PBS to remove any unattached pSiNPs, and the cells were harvested via trypsin and centrifugation for 3 min at 180× *g*. The resulting cell pellets were dispersed in cold PBS and stained with propidium iodide (PI) (5 µg/mL) for 5 min to assess cell viability. Samples were then analyzed using flow cytometry (BD FACS Canto II) for Cy5 and PI fluorescence signals. Cellular association percentage was calculated as the number of cells that displayed fluorescence signals compared to untreated cells (Cy5 negative).

For visualizing the cellular association and uptake, confocal microscopy was used. hCMEC/D3 cells were seeded onto an 8-well chamber (Ibidi) at the density of $1 \times 10^5$ cells per well and allowed to attach and were cultured for 1 day. The cells were washed twice in PBS and then treated with Cy5-labeled surface-modified pSiNPs (5 µg/mL). After 1 h, the wells were washed twice in PBS and fixed in 4% paraformaldehyde (PFA) for 15 min at RT followed by permeabilization with 0.1% Triton-X-100 in PBS for 5 min RT. The cells were then washed twice using PBS and incubated with Hoechst 33342 (5 µg/mL, Thermo Fisher Scientific, Scoresby, Australia) and Alexa Fluor™ 488 Phalloidin (5 µg/mL Thermo Fisher Scientific, Scoresby, Australia) for 30 min. Afterward, the cells were washed three times with PBS, and the images were taken using confocal microscopy (Leica TCS SP8, Leica Microsystems, Macquarie Park, Australia). Fluorophores were excited via 405, 561, and 647 nm laser lines. The laser powers and gains for each channel were adjusted against untreated controls to minimize sample autofluorescence.

#### 2.2.12. BBB Transwell Model Preparation for Nanoparticles Assessment

Transwell inserts (3 µm pore size, polyester membrane, Sigma-Aldrich, Macquarie Park, Australia) were first coated with 100 µL collagen-I (Sigma-Aldrich, Macquarie Park, Australia) in a concentration of 150 µg/mL in the incubator for 1 h and were seeded with hCMEC/D3 at a density of $1.65 \times 10^5$ cells/mL in 200 µL of cell medium. The bottom compartment was filled with 600 µL of cell medium. The cell culture medium was changed every two days until a monolayer formed. The transendothelial electrical resistance (TEER) was assessed every day for 7 to 10 days using a Millicell ERS-2 voltammeter EVOM2 and an STX02 chopstick electrode (Merck Millipore, Bayswater, Australia).

FITC-dextran (10 kDa) was used to confirm the BBB integrity formed on the Transwell culture insert after 7 days. Briefly, 200 µL of FITC-dextran (50 µg/mL) in complete cell culture media was added to the top compartment with a bottom compartment filled with 600 µL of complete culture media. Inserts were then incubated at 37 °C, 95% humidity, and 5% $CO_2$ for 6 h. A 200 µL aliquot was collected every hour to measure FITC fluorescence signals in the microplate reader, which was replaced with fresh 200 µL of complete cell culture medium. The concentration of dextran at each time point was calculated using a standard curve of dextran. The apparent permeability coefficients ($P_{app}$), as the indication of the integrity of BBB, were calculated according to the following equation [41]:

$$Papp = dC/dt \cdot Vr/(A \cdot C)$$

where *Vr* (mL) is the volume of the lower compartment, $dC/dt$ is the slope of the cumulative concentration of the dextran in the lower compartment over time, $A$ ($cm^2$) is the surface area of the inset and $C$ (μg/mL) is the initial concentration of dextran that was placed into the top compartment [34].

To investigate the BBB barrier integrity through examination of the cell surface protein expression levels, a confluent monolayer of brain endothelial cells was cultured in an 8-well Nunc Lab-Tek II Chamber Slide System. This confluent monolayer barrier was washed with PBS twice and incubated with 4% paraformaldehyde (PFA) at RT for 10 min. Fixed cells were then washed with PBS to remove PFA and permeabilized with 0.2% Triton X-100 in PBS for 10 min. Permeabilized cells were then washed with PBS three times and blocked with 2.5% BSA for 60 min at RT. After blocking, the cells were washed with PBS three times and incubated with anti ZO-1 (Cell Signaling Technology, Danvers, MA, USA D6L1E, rabbit mAb) (1:100 primary antibody diluted in 2.5% BSA PBS buffer) at 4 °C overnight. Cells were washed with PBS 2× before the secondary antibody goat anti-rabbit Alexa Fluor 488 antibody (Thermo Fisher, Scoresby, Australia) was added and incubated for 1 h at RT. Finally, the slides were rinsed with PBS 3×, and ProLong Diamond Antifade Mountant with DAPI (Thermo Fisher, Scoresby, Australia) was added. Samples were cured for 2 h at RT in the dark and tight junction expressions were imaged using a confocal fluorescence microscope (Leica TCS SP8, Leica Microsystems, Macquarie Park, Australia).

For assessment of nanoparticle performance in Transwells, on day 7 of monolayer culturing, diverse types of pSiNPs (50 μg/mL) were incubated at the top compartment (in 200 μL completed culture medium) and the lower compartment was filled with 600 μL of complete culture media and further incubated at 37 °C and 5% $CO_2$ for 48 h. After that, a 200 μL aliquot was collected from the bottom compartment and measured via the fluorescence microplate reader for the fluorescence intensity (assessing the Cy5 signal). The concentration was determined using a calibration curve of different concentrations of nanoparticles in the cell medium. The percentage of nanoparticles in the bottom compartment was calculated as the fluorescence intensity from the bottom compartment was divided by the original fluorescence intensity of nanoparticles that were placed in the top compartment.

#### 2.2.13. BBB-on-a-Chip Model Establishment and Nanoparticles Assessment

The BBB-on-a-chip models were prepared as described previously [40]. Briefly, the design includes three main channels (blood/brain/medium). Each channel is 500 μm wide, 100 μm high, and 2.0 cm in length. An array of microchannels (3 μm width, 80 μm length, and 3 μm height) connects the blood channel with the brain channel. Additional microchannels (50 μm in width, 80 μm length, and 3 μm height) are present between the brain channel and medium channel to facilitate the supply of nutrients.

After cells formed a monolayer in the blood channel, Matrigel (Corning, Mulgrave, Australia) was added to the brain channel to facilitate visualization of nanoparticles that cross the blood channel. Three control experiments were conducted before the nanoparticle assessment. Firstly, after forming a cell monolayer in the blood channel of BBB-on-a-chip, cells were subjected to immunofluorescence analysis (same procedures as mentioned before for the Transwell protein expression) using a confocal microscope (Leica TCS SP8, Leica Microsystems, Macquarie Park, Australia). Secondly, 10 kDa FITC-dextran (25 μg/mL) was diluted in EBM-2 medium and flowed through the blood channel in cell-seeded chips and blank chips (without cells seeded) at a flow rate of 5 μL/min using a programmable syringe pump (Harvard Apparatus, Inc, Holliston, MA, USA.). Afterward, these chips were subjected to the confocal microscope (Leica TCS SP8, Leica Microsystems, Macquarie

Park Australia) to quantify the permeation of FITC-dextran to the brain channel. Lastly, Tf-pSiNPs were diluted in EBM-2 medium to a concentration of 10 μg/Ml and flowed through chips in which the blood channel (previously seeded with cells or left empty). Afterward, these chips were rinsed with PBS and subjected to confocal microscopy.

To assess nanoparticles in BBB-on-a-chip, nanoparticles and 10 kDa FITC-dextran were diluted in EBM-2 medium to the concentrations of 10 μg/Ml and 25 μg/Ml, respectively, and flowed through the blood channel at a flow rate of 5 μL/min using a programmable syringe pump (Harvard Apparatus) for 4 h. The BBB-on-a-chip models were kept inside an incubator (37 °C supplied with 5% $CO_2$). After stopping the flow, the chips were detached from the syringe pump and carefully rinsed with PBS to remove any unbonded nanoparticles. Afterward, cells in the chips were fixed with 4% PFA, stained with DAPI, and subjected to confocal microscope (Leica TCS SP8, Leica Microsystems, Macquarie Park, Australia). FITC-dextran penetration in each sample was assessed. All experiments were triplicated using independent BBB-on-a-chip. The relative fluorescence intensity of nanoparticles in the microchannels of chips was further analyzed using ImageJ (NIH, Bethesda, MD, USA) and plotted using GraphPad Prism 7.

## 3. Results and Discussions

### 3.1. Preparation of pSiNPs with Various Ligand Surface Densities and Sizes

In brief, the pSiNPs were fabricated as followed. Initially, a multilayered porous silicon film was prepared through electrochemical etching of a silicon wafer in an ethanolic HF solution, followed by thermal hydrocarbonization (THC) [36,42]. This surface modification was conducted to enhance the stability of the pSiNPs and prevent any particle degradation during in vitro experiments which might complicate data analysis. ATR-FTIR spectroscopy confirmed the successful THC modification, as demonstrated by the existence of a C-H stretching absorption band from 2800 to 3000 $cm^{-1}$ and a Si-C band at 1063 $cm^{-1}$ (Figure S1). The THC-modified porous silicon film was then fractured into THC-pSiNPs through ultrasonication. Two different sizes of pSiNPs, referred to as small (S) and large (L), were subsequently prepared using a bespoke centrifuge-based size selection protocol.

Transmission electron microscope (TEM) images revealed that THC-pSiNPs(S) had an irregular, plate-like shape [37], with an average particle size of 199.8 ± 40.3 nm in length and 86.3 ± 12.6 nm in thickness, along with a pore size of 21.8 ± 5.3 nm. The average hydrodynamic diameter, as determined via dynamic light scattering (DLS), was 180.9 ± 63.2 nm, with a relatively low polydispersity index (PDI) of 0.11 (Figure S2). The larger porous silicon nanoparticles, THC-pSiNPs(L), exhibited an average particle size of 427.4 ± 144.2 nm in the x-y dimension, 177.6 ± 83.2 nm in the z dimension, and a pore size of 26.8 ± 7.5 nm. Their average hydrodynamic diameter was 291.6 ± 88.4 nm, with a PDI of 0.22 (Figure S2). The inconsistency between DLS and TEM measurements can be attributed to the plate-like shape of the particles.

The surface of the two types of nanoparticles was then modified with functional carboxyl groups through hydrosilylation of surface silicon hydride groups with 1-undecylenic acid (UDA) to generate UDA-pSiNPs (Figure S1) [43]. ATR-FTIR spectra confirmed this surface modification as demonstrated by the emergence of a C=O band at 1716 $cm^{-1}$ attributed to the carbonyl bond in UDA. Furthermore, more pronounced absorption bands emerged between 2800 $cm^{-1}$ and 3000 $cm^{-1}$ corresponding to C-H stretching vibrations from the aliphatic chains in UDA (Figure S1). The UDA modification did not significantly alter particle or pore size, as confirmed via TEM and DLS (Figure S2).

As shown in Figure 1, UDA-pSiNPs were conjugated with varying ratios of mPEG-$NH_2$ and $NH_2$-PEG-COOH (with an average molecular weight 10 kDa). This conjugation process aimed to fabricate pSiNPs with distinct surface densities of the functional carboxyl group. Simultaneously, the pSiNPs were co-labeled with Cy5 fluorophores to enable direct comparison between the nanoparticles in subsequent assays. Following activation of the carboxylic groups with NHS, an excess of transferrin was added to ensure maximal conjugation. This led to the creation of a library of Cy5-labeled PEGylated pSiNPs featuring diverse transferrin surface densities. Notably, the larger nanoparticle, pSiNP(L), was only modified with $NH_2$-PEG-COOH.

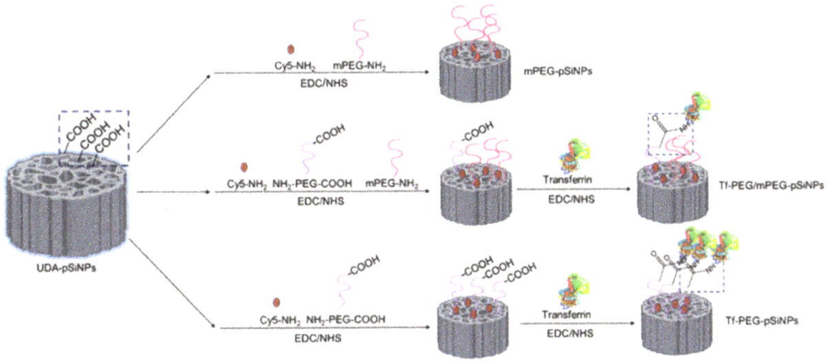


**Figure 1.** Schematic diagram of fabrication of a nanoparticle library with different transferrin ligand densities using different ratios of mPEG-$NH_2$ and $NH_2$-PEG-COOH.

ATR-FTIR was used to investigate the success of these modification steps (Figures 2C and S3). For ease of comparison, all spectra were normalized to the Si-C/Si-O signal (1000–1100 $cm^{-1}$). After modification with either mPEG-NH2 or NH2-PEG-COOH, a distinct vibration band appeared at 1100 $cm^{-1}$ (C-O) adjacent to the Si-C/Si-O signal (1000–1100 $cm^{-1}$). Moreover, stronger signals from C-H stretching bands in the 2800 to 3000 $cm^{-1}$ range were present too. Compared to mPEG-modified pSiNPs (mPEG-pSiNPs(S)), the transferrin-modified pSiNPs exhibited more pronounced C=O amide bands at 1657 $cm^{-1}$, indicating the successful conjugation of the amide-rich transferrin (Figure 2C). Moreover, the absence of the carboxyl C=O signal at 1716 $cm^{-1}$ from UDA indicated successful amidation of PEG-COOH with transferrin. After transferrin and mPEG-NH2 modification, the edges of these nanoparticles appeared less distinct—suggesting the presence of an organic coating, i.e., PEG and transferrin (Figures S4 and S5). DLS showed that the transferrin and PEG-modified pSiNPs(S) maintained a similar hydrodynamic diameter of around 170.1 ± 55.1 nm with low PDI values ranging from 0.07 to 0.11 (Figure 2A). Conversely, the larger nanoparticles (Tf-PEG-pSiNPs(L)) exhibited a hydrodynamic diameter of 299.3 ± 82.8 nm. Importantly, the PEG modification significantly improved the colloidal stability of the nanoparticles, as UDA-pSiNPs(S) precipitated immediately in water.

The amount of transferrin in different samples was determined indirectly using a BCA assay, measuring unconjugated transferrin present in the supernatant that was collected during the washing steps (Figure 2D). The amount of conjugated transferrin for the three different $NH_2$-PEG-COOH and mPEG-$NH_2$ ratios (1:50, 1:9, and 1:0)—represented as Tf-PEG/mPEG(1:50)-pSiNPs(S), Tf-PEG/mPEG(1:9)-pSiNPs(S), Tf-PEG-pSiNPs(S) and Tf-PEG-pSiNPs(L))—was determined, using the BCA assay, to be 2.10 ± 0.79, 3.83 ± 0.34, 4.92 ± 0.31, 5.03 ± 0.54 nmol per mg of nanoparticles, respectively. This unit (nmol per mg of nanoparticles) was used to express the ligand surface density, avoiding potential inaccuracies arising from attempting to convert it to a number of ligands per nanoparticle due to the porous and irregular morphology of the pSiNPs. These calculated transferrin amounts were as expected as the number of functional carboxyl groups available for transferrin conjugation increased for each sample. Notably, the larger transferrin-coated nanoparticles (Tf-PEG-pSiNPs(L) displayed a similar transferrin amount (around 5 nmol per mg of nanoparticles) compared to the smaller Tf-PEG pSiNPs(S), as both particles possess similar surface areas due to their inherent porosity. The ζ-potential of solely mPEG-coated pSiNPs was less negative than that of UDA-pSiNPs(S) (−20 mV) due to the neutral charge of the mPEG linker upon conjugation (Figure 2B). Some residual negative charge was expected as not all carboxyl groups can react, due to steric hindrance caused by the

PEG linker (10 kDa). All transferrin-PEG-modified samples also showed slightly negative surface charges, ranging range from −10 mV to −15 mV. These charges resulted from the combination of neutral mPEG, the slight negative charge of transferrin, and potentially remaining surface carboxyl groups, as described above.

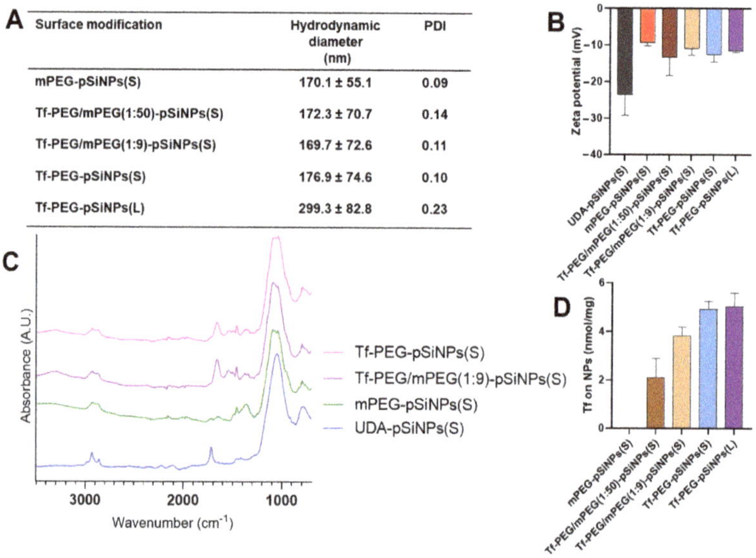


| Surface modification | Hydrodynamic diameter (nm) | PDI |
|---|---|---|
| mPEG-pSiNPs(S) | 170.1 ± 55.1 | 0.09 |
| Tf-PEG/mPEG(1:50)-pSiNPs(S) | 172.3 ± 70.7 | 0.14 |
| Tf-PEG/mPEG(1:9)-pSiNPs(S) | 169.7 ± 72.6 | 0.11 |
| Tf-PEG-pSiNPs(S) | 176.9 ± 74.6 | 0.10 |
| Tf-PEG-pSiNPs(L) | 299.3 ± 82.8 | 0.23 |

**Figure 2.** Physicochemical characterization of different surface-modified pSiNPs. (**A**) Particle hydrodynamic diameter (z-average) and PDI measurements by DLS; (**B**) ζ-potential; (**C**) ATR-FTIR spectra; and (**D**) transferrin quantification of pSiNPs based on BCA assay. Data in (**B**,**D**) are shown as mean ± standard deviation, N = 3. The two different sizes of pSiNPs are referred to as small (S) and large (L).

### *3.2. Evaluation of pSiNPs in Brain Microvascular Endothelial Cells*

The brain microvascular endothelial cells (hCMEC/D3) were incubated with varying concentrations of modified pSiNPs for 48 h, followed by assessment using an ATP activity-based luminescence assay (Figure S5). Across all samples, no significant toxicity was observed up to a concentration of 50 µg/mL. At the highest concentration of 50 µg/mL for some of the pSiNPs samples, a slight decrease in cell viability was noted, ranging from 83.6 ± 12.6% to 89.0 ± 1.7%. Furthermore, the permeability of the hCMEC/D3 monolayer in Transwell assays was not affected after incubation with 50 µg/mL of modified pSiNPs for 48 h, as determined by their TEER values (described in Section 3.3). Hence, we carried out all in vitro assays using concentrations no higher than 50 µg/mL.

Confocal microscopy and flow cytometry were used to investigate the interaction of different surface-modified nanoparticles with hCMEC/D3 cells. It is important to note that all pSiNP samples exhibited similar Cy5 intensities on a per mass basis, allowing for direct comparisons in subsequent measurements (Figure S6). The confocal images of particle association and uptake are presented in Figure 3A. Notably, all transferrin-conjugated nanoparticles showed higher Cy5 fluorescence signals within the cells compared to solely mPEG-modified particles. This finding is in alignment with previous reports illustrating the role of transferrin in nanoparticle association with brain endothelial cells. Our prior study, for instance, demonstrated that BSA-coated pSiNPs showed a lower cell association than Tf-coated pSiNPs and that Tf-coated pSiNPs were predominantly taken up via clathrin and caveolae-mediated endocytosis [44]. Nanoparticle internalization and uptake into the cells were confirmed by z-stack scanning confocal microscopy (Figure S7). These images showed that Tf-PEG-pSiNPs(S) were located within the cells, providing evidence of successful uptake and internalization.

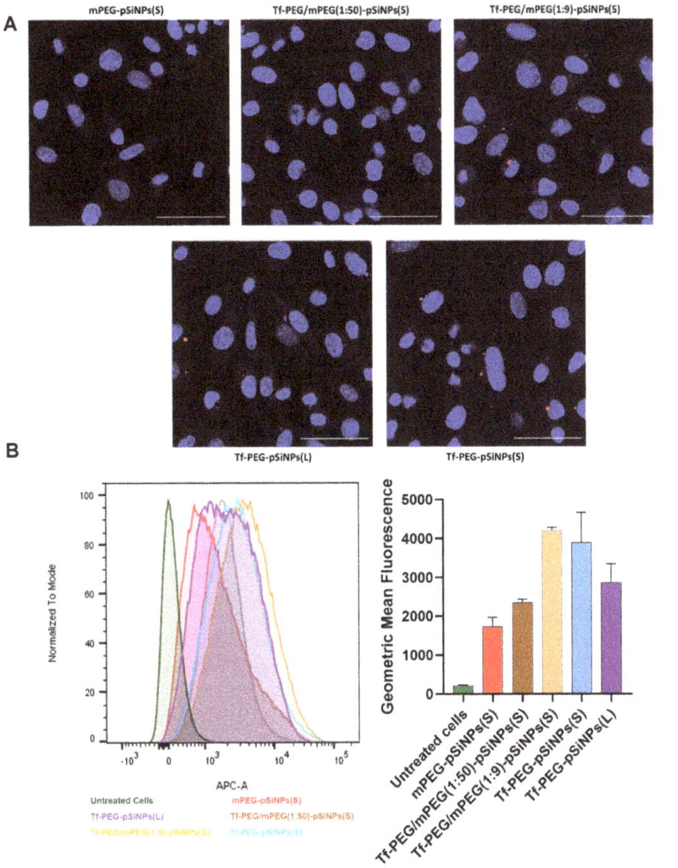


**Figure 3.** (**A**) Confocal fluorescence microscopy images of hCMEC/D3 cells after incubation with mPEG-pSiNPs(S), Tf-PEG/mPEG(1:50)-pSiNPs(S), Tf-PEG/mPEG(1:9)-pSiNPs(S), Tf-PEG-pSiNPs(L) and Tf-PEG-pSiNPs(S) (blue = nucleus, green = F-actin, red = Cy5 in nanoparticles, scale bars = 50 μm); (**B**) flow cytometry analysis of hCMEC/D3 cellular association of different modified pSiNPs. Histogram and the geometric mean of Cy5 positive hCMEC/D3 cells by treating different modified samples. The geometric mean values are shown by mean ± sd, N = 3.

Flow cytometry was employed to quantitatively assess the impact of transferrin surface density on cell association in hCMEC/D3 cells (Figure 3B). All transferrin-modified nanoparticles presented higher geometric fluorescence mean intensity (GMF) in comparison to the mPEG-pSiNPs(S) sample, consistent with the observations from confocal imaging. Furthermore, differences in cell association were discernable among nanoparticles with varying transferrin surface densities. Although the lowest transferrin surface density, Tf-PEG/mPEG(1:50)-pSiNPs(S), displayed only a slightly higher cellular association than mPEG-pSiNPs(S), Tf-PEG/mPEG(1:9)-pSiNPs(S) (boasting a higher ligand density) showed a significant increase, approximately doubling the GMF compared to Tf-PEG/mPEG(1:50)-pSiNPs(S) and mPEG-pSiNPs(S). Interestingly, no further increase in cell association was observed with the highest transferrin ligand density (Tf-PEG-pSiNPs(S)). This suggests a non-monotonic positive relationship between the range of transferrin surface density and its relative association and uptake for our pSiNP system. It is important to note that this phenomenon extends beyond pSiNPs; for example, Song et al. reported that higher ligand densities did not necessarily lead to increased uptake for transferrin-decorated micelles [45]. In addition, the larger Tf-PEG-pSiNPs(L) exhibited a notably lower GMF than Tf-PEG-pSiNPs(S) despite a similar transferrin coverage. This difference in GMF indicates that the size of nanoparticles also plays a critical role in the cellular association and uptake.

### 3.3. Assessment of pSiNPs Using Transwell Assay

The hCMEC/D3 transcytosis of the pSiNPs was first investigated using a Transwell model (Figure 4A). This model comprises two compartments, with an hCMEC/D3 monolayer cultured on an insert that separates the two compartments. The TEER value, a marker for BBB barrier tightness, was measured daily to confirm the presence of a confluent monolayer (Figure 4B). TEER values reached approximately 10 $\Omega \times cm^2$ on day 4, increasing to around 26 $\Omega \times cm^2$ by day 6. Afterward, TEER values remained stable, ranging between 25 and 27 $\Omega \times cm^2$, comparable to literature values [34]. We also confirmed the presence of the tight-junction-associated protein, ZO-1, which is mostly expressed at the interface of cell-to-cell contact [34] (Figure 4C). The integrity of the BBB in the Transwell model was further assessed using 10 kDa FITC-labeled dextran. This yielded an apparent permeability value of $2.37 \pm 0.38 \times 10^{-6}$ cm/s (N = 3) on day 6, consistent with findings in other studies [46]. The TEER values obtained, the expression of ZO-1 protein, and the low permeability of FITC-dextran collectively affirm the integrity of the BBB formed on the Transwell inserts. As a control experiment, blank Transwells with inserts devoid of an hCMEC/D3 monolayer were treated with transferrin-coated pSiNPs to examine nanoparticle diffusion through the porous membrane without a functional BBB. This control revealed that 69–74% of the nanoparticles accumulated in the bottom compartment after 48 h, consistent with free diffusion of pSiNPs across both compartments, considering the volume of the bottom compartment accounted for 75% of the total volume. This control experiment also confirmed that the nanoparticles did not interact with the insert. Consequently, this Transwell model proved suitable for evaluating the permeability and thus transcytosis potential of the Cy-5 labeled nanoparticle library in an hCMEC/D3 monolayer.

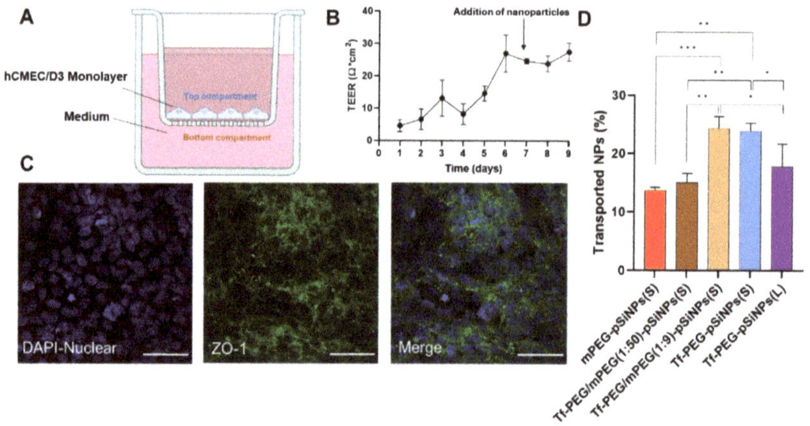


**Figure 4.** (**A**) Schematic representation of a BBB Transwell model that was formed by a monolayer of hCMEC/D3 cells over an insert with 3 μm sized pores; (**B**) TEER value of hCMEC/D3 monolayer over 9 days of culture, N = 3. The TEER value increased over time and reached a plateau on day 6. pSiNPs were applied to the Transwell insert on day 7; (**C**) Characterization of ZO-1 expression by the hCMEC/D3 monolayer (scale bar = 50 μm); and (**D**) percentage of accumulated nanoparticles in the bottom compartment of the Transwell after applying nanoparticles in the top compartment for 48 h, N = 3, one-way ANOVA test, * $p < 0.1$, ** $p < 0.01$, *** $p < 0.001$. All data are shown by mean ± sd.

All five nanoparticle types (mPEG-pSiNPs(S), Tf-PEG/mPEG(1:50)-pSiNPs(S), Tf-PEG/mPEG(1:9)-pSiNPs(S), Tf-PEG-pSiNPs(S), and Tf-PEG-pSiNPs(L)) were evaluated using the Transwell assay, and each experiment was done in triplicate. Among these, mPEG-pSiNPs(S) and Tf-PEG/mPEG(1:50)-pSiNPs(S) displayed the lowest average transport percentage (13.7% and 15.0%) to the bottom compartment. This is in accordance with them displaying their lowest association in the previous flow cytometry experiment. Tf-PEG/mPEG(1:9)-pSiNPs(S) and Tf-PEG-pSiNPs(S) both showed higher average accumulations of 24.4% and 23.6%, respectively, with no significant differences between them.

Transferrin-modified nanoparticles can cross the BBB by binding to transferrin receptors on endothelial cells. This binding initiates a process known as receptor-mediated transcytosis, which involves three key steps: (i) attachment of protein-coated nanoparticles to receptors on the endothelial cells, (ii) internalization and sorting of the nanoparticles within the cell, and (iii) release of the nanoparticles on the other side of the endothelial cells. Intuitively, one might expect that higher levels of transferrin on the nanoparticle surface would lead to a greater likelihood of attachment to the cells and BBB crossing. However, in the Transwell assay, nanoparticles with varying transferrin amounts, specifically, $3.83 \pm 0.34$ nmol per mg (Tf-PEG/mPEG(1:9)-pSiNPs(S)) and $4.92 \pm 0.31$ nmol per mg (Tf-PEG-pSiNPs(S)) presented similar transport levels. This reveals that there may be an optimal surface ligand density on pSiNPs, and an increase in transferrin surface density on the nanoparticles might not necessarily increase or could even diminish their penetration ability across the BBB. This could be caused by several factors: a higher transferrin density might result in an overly strong affinity to transferrin receptors, potentially preventing release [47] or possibly inducing lysosomal sorting and degradation, thus preventing transportation [48]. Interestingly, similar trends have been reported in nanoparticle delivery systems, where an excessively high ligand density hindered BBB penetration [27,49]. For example, gold nanoparticles with excessively high transferrin density exhibited reduced entry into the brain parenchyma in mice [49]. Similarly, liposomes with the lowest density of antibody exhibited comparable low levels of BBB transport as nanoparticles with the highest density of antibody, while the intermediate-density antibody nanoparticles exhibited the highest accumulation [27]. Our result demonstrated that the pSiNP delivery system shares some universal characteristics with other nanoparticles system. Specifically, an optimal surface ligand density appears crucial for efficient BBB penetration of pSiNPs.

The effect of the pSiNP size on BBB penetration was investigated by comparing two different sized nanoparticles with comparable ligand density, i.e., Tf-PEG-pSiNPs(L) (around 420 nm) and Tf-PEG-pSiNPs(S) (around 203 nm). Tf-PEG-pSiNPs(L) presented an average transport percentage of $17.5 \pm 3.9\%$, while the smaller Tf-PEG-pSiNPs(S) showed a significantly higher average transport percentage of $23.6 \pm 1.4\%$. This result aligns with their performance in cellular association and uptake in 2D cell culture experiments, suggesting that an increase in pSiNP size, while maintaining the same surface ligand density, can have a detrimental effect on BBB transport. Despite the unique physical structure of pSiNPs (porous and irregular), this outcome is consistent with observations in other nanoparticle systems [30,50].

### 3.4. Assessment of pSiNPs Using BBB-on-a-Chip Model

Although the Transwell assay is commonly used to assess nanoparticle transcytosis potential, it lacks the presence of hemodynamic shear stress that plays an essential role in endothelial cell phenotype and function. This factor is essential for achieving a more accurate physiological representation [51,52]. Moreover, flow conditions also influence the binding of nanoparticles to receptors and, consequently, cellular uptake [53]. Hence, we wanted to investigate if this factor would affect the trends observed for our set of pSiNPs. To address this, a dynamic model known as a BBB-on-a-chip was used to examine how flow affects the ability of nanoparticles to penetrate the BBB (Figure 5A) [40]. In the model, two main channels were constructed, representing the "brain" and "blood" compartments. The blood channel was constructed as a simplified version of the BBB, while the brain channel was used to assess nanoparticle penetration. Several validation experiments were performed to confirm the presence of a confluent physical monolayer on the chip. First, like the Transwell model, clear protein expression of ZO-1 was observed at the intercellular junctions of the seeded hCMEC/D3 chips, indicating the presence of tight connections in the monolayer (Figure 5B). Second, the integrity of the formed BBB layer was examined using 10 kDa FITC-labeled dextran, with a characteristic permeability value of $5.61 \pm 1.48 \times 10^{-6}$ cm/s (N = 3) [40]. Confocal microscopy further confirmed these findings as a much lower dextran fluorescence intensity was observed in the brain channel of the chips where the blood channel was seeded with cells compared to blank chips (Figure S8A,B). The average relative fluorescence intensity value (RFU) of randomly selected regions of interest in the brain channel was four times lower in seeded chips compared to blank chips (Figure S8C). In addition, we compared the penetration of nanoparticles in seeded BBB-on-a-chip versus blank chips, and as expected, significantly fewer nanoparticles were able to cross to the brain compartment in a seeded BBB-on-a-chip (Figure S9).

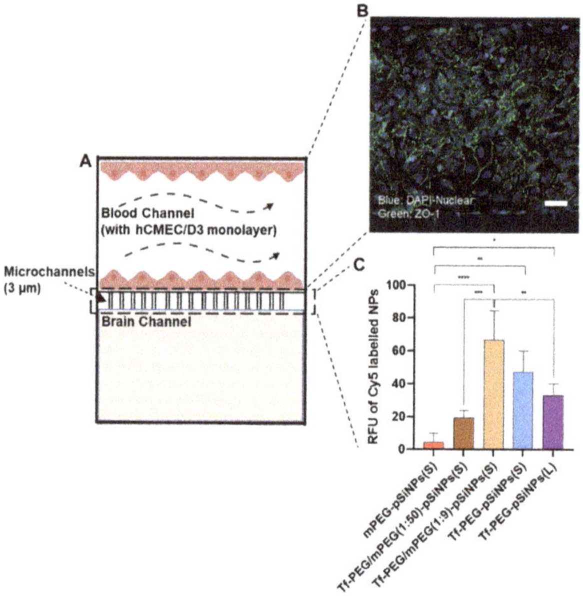


**Figure 5.** (**A**) Schematic of the BBB-on-a-chip model consisting of two channels. The blood channel was formed by a monolayer of hCMEC/D3 cells over 3 μm microchannels under a fluidic environment. (**B**) Characterization of ZO-1 expression by the hCMEC/D3 monolayer (scale bar = 50 μm). (**C**) Corresponding RFU of pSiNPs crossing blood channel in BBB-on-a-chip. N > 3, one-way ANOVA test, * $p < 0.1$, ** $p < 0.01$, *** $p < 0.001$, **** $p < 0.0001$. The values are shown by mean ± sd.

As a quality control measure, all microfluidic chips used for the assessment of the nanoparticle library were treated with FITC-dextran to ensure the presence of a functional barrier before experimentation (Figure S8D). Although the overall trend for the nanoparticle penetration remained consistent with the results from the Transwell assay, some intriguing differences emerged. mPEG-pSiNPs(S) and Tf-PEG/mPEG(1:50)-pSiNPs(S) again showed the lowest and second-lowest RFU (i.e., BBB crossing potential) (Figure 5C). In contrast, Tf-PEG/mPEG(1:9)-pSiNPs(S) presented the highest RFU, followed by Tf-PEG-pSiNPs(S) and Tf-PEG-pSiNPs(L).

The impact of the various transferrin surface densities was more pronounced in the BBB-on-a-chip model compared to the Transwell assay. For example, a clear increase in BBB penetration could be observed for nanoparticles with the lowest transferrin ligand density

(Tf-PEG/mPEG(1:50)-pSiNPs(S)) when compared to mPEG-pSiNPs(S). This increase was not as apparent in the Transwell assay. Moreover, whereas the Transwell assay showed a 67% improvement in BBB crossing for nanoparticles with intermediate transferrin ligand density (Tf-PEG/mPEG(1:9)-pSiNPs(S)) when compared to those with low transferrin ligand density (Tf-PEG/mPEG(1:50)-pSiNPs(S)), the BBB-on-a-chip model demonstrated a much higher increase of approximately 300%. Of particular interest, in the BBB-on-a-chip model, nanoparticles with the highest transferrin density, Tf-PEG-pSiNPs(S), showed nearly a 40% lower BBB crossing potential compared to those with intermediate transferrin density (Tf-PEG/mPEG(1:9)-pSiNPs(S)). In contrast, these two variants had a similar BBB penetration in the Transwell assay. This confirms that the highest transferrin density on the pSiNPs does not necessarily translate to the highest BBB penetration. Notably, this observation becomes more prominent under the physiologically relevant conditions of the BBB-on-a-chip model. The observed differences between the Transwell and BBB-on-a-chip assays may be attributed to the influence of fluid flow on nanoparticle association and consequent transcytosis. Lin et al. investigated the difference in human aortic endothelial cellular association with nanoparticles, comparing those with targeted moieties (i.e., platelet glycoprotein Ib$\alpha$), to those without, under both flow and static environments [54]. In their study, the cellular uptake of nanoparticles with targeting moieties was significantly higher under flow conditions than those without targeting moieties. Similarly, Zukerman et al. demonstrated that under shear stress, nanoparticles with higher ligand surface coating density exhibited significantly increased adhesion when compared to nanoparticles with lower ligand surface densities [55]. However, it is noted that the range of ligand densities on nanoparticles plays an important role in their cellular association. In some cases, an excessive number of ligands on the nanoparticle surfaces can hinder their selectivity and adhesion [56].

The BBB crossing efficacy of the two differently sized pSiNPs (Tf-PEG-pSiNPs(S) and Tf-PEG-pSiNPs(L)) showed a consistent pattern in both assays (Figure 5C) where the smaller nanoparticle size exhibited slightly higher BBB penetration than their larger counterparts. The reason why we did not observe more significant differences between these two pSiNP sizes in the chips, may be the higher cytoadhesion of larger nanoparticles under flow conditions [31,57]. Larger nanoparticles tend to adhere and marginate closer to the channel wall than smaller nanoparticles due to their larger contact area [31,58,59]. However, it must be noted that size also affects biodistribution. For example, larger nanoparticles are more likely to be cleared by the spleen and liver, a factor that is currently not replicable in a dynamic BBB-on-a-chip model [60]. In addition, in vitro models lack other intricate complexities present in in vivo situations, such as the mononuclear phagocyte system and the wider immune system. On the other hand, ex vivo models allow a personalized medicine approach, allowing the study of cells from human pathologies. In general, ex vivo and humanized in vitro models hold superiority over rodent models [61].

In summary, the BBB-on-a-chip model revealed notable differences in the BBB crossing efficacy between pSiNPs with varying transferrin surface densities. Specifically, in this assay, pSiNPs with intermediate transferrin density exhibited the highest penetration efficacy, suggesting an optimal transferrin level for maximizing the BBB penetration performance for pSiNPs. The BBB results of the two sizes of pSiNPs are in agreement with the Transwell, indicating that smaller pSiNPs had a better BBB transportation.

## 4. Conclusions

PSiNPs were synthesized with two different sizes (average size of 203 and 420 nm) and decorated with different densities of transferrin by adjusting the ratio of bifunctional PEG linkers. We evaluated the effect of transferrin density and size on the hCMEC/D3 cell association and BBB transport of pSiNPs in both static and dynamic models. The results revealed that the surface density of transferrin on pSiNPs affects their hCMEC/D3 cell association, where increasing transferrin content from 0 nmol/mg to 3.8 nmol/mg enhances hCMEC/D3 association. The surface density of transferrin also affects the BBB transport of pSiNPs in the static Transwell assay. Here, the intermediate transferrin surface density showed the highest BBB transport. The use of a dynamic BBB-on-a-chip model resulted in more pronounced differences between the various surface ligand densities, where the intermediate transferrin surface density again showed the highest level of BBB crossing. These findings indicate that there is an optimal transferrin ligand density to maximize pSiNP delivery across the BBB, which could be influenced by their affinity to the transferrin receptor and underscore the role of flow in nanoparticle assessment. Furthermore, the smaller pSiNPs showed a consistently higher BBB penetration potential than the larger pSiNPs in all tested models, indicating that the size of pSiNPs significantly affects their BBB performance. Overall, our study demonstrated that surface density and size are important parameters in designing pSiNPs for crossing the BBB. Further in vivo experiments may provide additional validation of the BBB-on-a-chip results. In addition, the designed Tf-coated pSiNPs may have potential applications for the improved delivery of hydrophobic anti-cancer drugs such as doxorubicin and camptothecin to brain cancers like glioblastoma multiforme.

**Supplementary Materials:** The following supporting information can be downloaded at: https://www.mdpi.com/article/10.3390/pharmaceutics15092271/s1, Figure S1: ATR-FTIR spectra of THC-pSiNPs and the subsequent hydrosilylation with undecylenic acid (UDA-pSiNPs). Figure S2: Characterization of THC-pSiNPs(S), UDA-pSiNPs(S), THC-pSiNPs(L) and UDA-pSiNPs(L). Figure S3: ATR-FTIR spectra of mPEG-$NH_2$ and $NH_2$-PEG-COOH in comparison with UDA-pSiNPs(S) and Tf-PEG/mPEG(1:50)-pSiNPs(S). Figure S4: BFTEM images Tf-PEG-pSiNPs(S) and Tf-PEG-pSiNPs(L) and their length (x-y dimension), thickness (z-dimension), and pore size. Figure S5: Cell viability results for hCMEC/D3 cells treated with different concentrations (5, 10, 25, 50 μg/mL) of modified pSiNPs for 48 h. Figure S6: Cy5 intensity of all modified pSiNPs on a per mass basis. Figure S7: Cellular uptake of Tf-PEG-pSiNPs(S) in hCMEC/D3 with z-stack scan. Figure S8: Validation of BBB-on-a-chip model. Figure S9: Transportation of Tf-pSiNPs from blood to brain channels after flowing for 4 h.

**Author Contributions:** Conceptualization, L.E., Z.T. and N.H.V.; methodology, W.Z., L.E, Z.T., B.P. and N.H.V.; validation, W.Z., L.E. and B.P.; formal analysis, W.Z. and X.C.; investigation, W.Z., D.Z., B.P. and L.E.; resources, L.E. and N.H.V.; data curation, W.Z.; writing—original draft preparation, W.Z.; writing—review and editing, L.E., X.C., Z.T. and N.H.V.; visualization, W.Z.; supervision, L.E, Z.T. and N.H.V.; project administration, W.Z., L.E., Z.T. and N.H.V.; funding acquisition, L.E. and N.H.V. All authors have read and agreed to the published version of the manuscript.

**Funding:** This research was co-funded by a Commonwealth Scientific and Industrial Research Organisation (CSIRO) PhD top-up scholarship.

**Institutional Review Board Statement:** Not applicable.

**Informed Consent Statement:** Not applicable.

**Data Availability Statement:** Data are contained within the paper or supplementary information.

**Acknowledgments:** This work was performed in part at the Melbourne Centre for Nanofabrication (MCN) in the Victorian Node of the Australian National Fabrication Facility (ANFF).

**Conflicts of Interest:** The authors declare no conflict of interest.

## References

1. Ding, C.; Wu, Y.; Chen, X.; Chen, Y.; Wu, Z.; Lin, Z.; Kang, D.; Fang, W.; Chen, F. Global, regional, and national burden and attributable risk factors of neurological disorders: The Global Burden of Disease study 1990–2019. *Front. Public Health* **2022**, *10*, 952161. [CrossRef]
2. Iqbal, K.; Liu, F.; Gong, C.-X. Tau and neurodegenerative disease: The story so far. *Nat. Rev. Neurol.* **2016**, *12*, 15–27. [CrossRef] [PubMed]
3. Omuro, A.; DeAngelis, L.M. Glioblastoma and other malignant gliomas: A clinical review. *JAMA* **2013**, *310*, 1842–1850. [CrossRef]
4. Chu, C.; Jablonska, A.; Lesniak, W.G.; Thomas, A.M.; Lan, X.; Linville, R.M.; Li, S.; Searson, P.C.; Liu, G.; Pearl, M.; et al. Optimization of osmotic blood-brain barrier opening to enable intravital microscopy studies on drug delivery in mouse cortex. *J. Control. Release* **2020**, *317*, 312–321. [CrossRef] [PubMed]

5. Huang, L.-K.; Chao, S.-P.; Hu, C.-J. Clinical trials of new drugs for Alzheimer disease. *J. Biomed. Sci.* **2020**, *27*, 18. [CrossRef]
6. Cirotti, C.; Contadini, C.; Barilà, D. SRC Kinase in Glioblastoma: News from an Old Acquaintance. *Cancers* **2020**, *12*, 1558. [CrossRef]
7. Anthony, D.P.; Hegde, M.; Shetty, S.S.; Rafic, T.; Mutalik, S.; Rao, B.S.S. Targeting receptor-ligand chemistry for drug delivery across blood-brain barrier in brain diseases. *Life Sci.* **2021**, *274*, 119326. [CrossRef]
8. Pardridge, W.M. The blood-brain barrier: Bottleneck in brain drug development. *NeuroRx* **2005**, *2*, 3–14. [CrossRef] [PubMed]
9. Swissa, E.; Serlin, Y.; Vazana, U.; Prager, O.; Friedman, A. Blood–brain barrier dysfunction in status epileptics: Mechanisms and role in epileptogenesis. *Epilepsy Behav.* **2019**, *101*, 106285. [CrossRef]
10. Burgess, A.; Shah, K.; Hough, O.; Hynynen, K. Focused ultrasound-mediated drug delivery through the blood–brain barrier. *Expert Rev. Neurother.* **2015**, *15*, 477–491. [CrossRef]
11. Hersh, D.S.; Wadajkar, A.S.; Roberts, N.; Perez, J.G.; Connolly, N.P.; Frenkel, V.; Winkles, J.A.; Woodworth, G.F.; Kim, A.J. Evolving Drug Delivery Strategies to Overcome the Blood Brain Barrier. *Curr. Pharm. Des.* **2016**, *22*, 1177–1193. [CrossRef]
12. Furtado, D.; Björnmalm, M.; Ayton, S.; Bush, A.I.; Kempe, K.; Caruso, F. Overcoming the blood–brain barrier: The role of nanomaterials in treating neurological diseases. *Adv. Mater.* **2018**, *30*, 1801362. [CrossRef]
13. Conen, A.; Raabe, A.; Schaller, K.; Fux, C.A.; Vajkoczy, P.; Trampuz, A. Management of neurosurgical implant-associated infections. *Swiss Med. Wkly.* **2020**, *150*, w20208. [CrossRef] [PubMed]
14. Gandhi, K.; Barzegar-Fallah, A.; Banstola, A.; Rizwan, S.B.; Reynolds, J.N.J. Ultrasound-Mediated Blood–Brain Barrier Disruption for Drug Delivery: A Systematic Review of Protocols, Efficacy, and Safety Outcomes from Preclinical and Clinical Studies. *Pharmaceutics* **2022**, *14*, 833. [CrossRef] [PubMed]
15. Bastiancich, C.; Danhier, P.; Préat, V.; Danhier, F. Anticancer drug-loaded hydrogels as drug delivery systems for the local treatment of glioblastoma. *J. Control. Release* **2016**, *243*, 29–42. [CrossRef] [PubMed]
16. Saraiva, C.; Praça, C.; Ferreira, R.; Santos, T.; Ferreira, L.; Bernardino, L. Nanoparticle-mediated brain drug delivery: Overcoming blood–brain barrier to treat neurodegenerative diseases. *J. Control. Release* **2016**, *235*, 34–47. [CrossRef]
17. Anselmo, A.C.; Mitragotri, S. Nanoparticles in the clinic: An update. *Bioeng. Transl. Med.* **2019**, *4*, e10143. [CrossRef]
18. Portioli, C.; Bovi, M.; Benati, D.; Donini, M.; Perduca, M.; Romeo, A.; Dusi, S.; Monaco, H.L.; Bentivoglio, M. Novel functionalization strategies of polymeric nanoparticles as carriers for brain medications. *J. Biomed. Mater. Res. Part A* **2017**, *105*, 847–858. [CrossRef]
19. Wu, H.; Lu, H.; Xiao, W.; Yang, J.; Du, H.; Shen, Y.; Qu, H.; Jia, B.; Manna, S.K.; Ramachandran, M. Sequential targeting in crosslinking nanotheranostics for tackling the multibarriers of brain tumors. *Adv. Mater.* **2020**, *32*, 1903759. [CrossRef]
20. Zhang, W.; Mehta, A.; Tong, Z.; Esser, L.; Voelcker, N.H. Development of Polymeric Nanoparticles for Blood-Brain Barrier Transfer-Strategies and Challenges. *Adv. Sci.* **2021**, *8*, 2003937. [CrossRef]
21. Pulgar, V.M. Transcytosis to Cross the Blood Brain Barrier, New Advancements and Challenges. *Front. Neurosci.* **2019**, *12*, 1019. [CrossRef] [PubMed]
22. Mi, P.; Cabral, H.; Kataoka, K. Ligand-Installed Nanocarriers toward Precision Therapy. *Adv. Mater.* **2020**, *32*, 1902604. [CrossRef] [PubMed]
23. Zhou, A.L.; Swaminathan, S.K.; Curran, G.L.; Poduslo, J.F.; Lowe, V.J.; Li, L.; Kandimalla, K.K. Apolipoprotein A-I Crosses the Blood-Brain Barrier through Clathrin-Independent and Cholesterol-Mediated Endocytosis. *J. Pharmacol. Exp. Ther.* **2019**, *369*, 481–488. [CrossRef] [PubMed]
24. Visser, C.C.; Voorwinden, L.H.; Crommelin, D.J.A.; Danhof, M.; de Boer, A.G. Characterization and Modulation of the Transferrin Receptor on Brain Capillary Endothelial Cells. *Pharm. Res.* **2004**, *21*, 761–769. [CrossRef] [PubMed]
25. Abdalla, Y.; Luo, M.; Mäkilä, E.; Day, B.W.; Voelcker, N.H.; Tong, W.Y. Effectiveness of porous silicon nanoparticle treatment at inhibiting the migration of a heterogeneous glioma cell population. *J. Nanobiotechnol.* **2021**, *19*, 60. [CrossRef] [PubMed]
26. Sheykhzadeh, S.; Luo, M.; Peng, B.; White, J.; Abdalla, Y.; Tang, T.; Mäkilä, E.; Voelcker, N.H.; Tong, W.Y. Transferrin-targeted porous silicon nanoparticles reduce glioblastoma cell migration across tight extracellular space. *Sci. Rep.* **2020**, *10*, 2320. [CrossRef]
27. Johnsen, K.B.; Bak, M.; Melander, F.; Thomsen, M.S.; Burkhart, A.; Kempen, P.J.; Andresen, T.L.; Moos, T. Modulating the antibody density changes the uptake and transport at the blood-brain barrier of both transferrin receptor-targeted gold nanoparticles and liposomal cargo. *J. Control. Release* **2019**, *295*, 237–249. [CrossRef]
28. Kulkarni, S.A.; Feng, S.-S. Effects of Particle Size and Surface Modification on Cellular Uptake and Biodistribution of Polymeric Nanoparticles for Drug Delivery. *Pharm. Res.* **2013**, *30*, 2512–2522. [CrossRef]
29. Chen, Y.P.; Chou, C.M.; Chang, T.Y.; Ting, H.; Dembélé, J.; Chu, Y.T.; Liu, T.P.; Changou, C.A.; Liu, C.W.; Chen, C.T. Bridging Size and Charge Effects of Mesoporous Silica Nanoparticles for Crossing the Blood-Brain Barrier. *Front. Chem.* **2022**, *10*, 931584. [CrossRef]
30. Meng, Q.; Meng, H.; Pan, Y.; Liu, J.; Li, J.; Qi, Y.; Huang, Y. Influence of nanoparticle size on blood–brain barrier penetration and the accumulation of anti-seizure medicines in the brain. *J. Mater. Chem. B* **2022**, *10*, 271–281. [CrossRef]
31. Nowak, M.; Brown, T.D.; Graham, A.; Helgeson, M.E.; Mitragotri, S. Size, shape, and flexibility influence nanoparticle transport across brain endothelium under flow. *Bioeng. Transl. Med.* **2020**, *5*, e10153. [CrossRef] [PubMed]
32. Talamini, L.; Violatto, M.B.; Cai, Q.; Monopoli, M.P.; Kantner, K.; Krpetić, Ž.; Perez-Potti, A.; Cookman, J.; Garry, D.; Silveira, C.P.; et al. Influence of Size and Shape on the Anatomical Distribution of Endotoxin-Free Gold Nanoparticles. *ACS Nano* **2017**, *11*, 5519–5529. [CrossRef] [PubMed]

33. Voigt, N.; Henrich-Noack, P.; Kockentiedt, S.; Hintz, W.; Tomas, J.; Sabel, B.A. Surfactants, not size or zeta-potential influence blood–brain barrier passage of polymeric nanoparticles. *Eur. J. Pharm. Biopharm.* **2014**, *87*, 19–29. [CrossRef] [PubMed]
34. Brown, T.D.; Habibi, N.; Wu, D.; Lahann, J.; Mitragotri, S. Effect of Nanoparticle Composition, Size, Shape, and Stiffness on Penetration Across the Blood–Brain Barrier. *ACS Biomater. Sci. Eng.* **2020**, *6*, 4916–4928. [CrossRef]
35. Li, W.; Liu, Z.; Fontana, F.; Ding, Y.; Liu, D.; Hirvonen, J.T.; Santos, H.A. Tailoring porous silicon for biomedical applications: From drug delivery to cancer immunotherapy. *Adv. Mater.* **2018**, *30*, 1703740. [CrossRef]
36. Luo, M.; Lewik, G.; Ratcliffe, J.C.; Choi, C.H.J.; Mäkilä, E.; Tong, W.Y.; Voelcker, N.H. Systematic Evaluation of Transferrin-Modified Porous Silicon Nanoparticles for Targeted Delivery of Doxorubicin to Glioblastoma. *ACS Appl. Mater. Interfaces* **2019**, *11*, 33637–33649. [CrossRef]
37. Zhang, D.-X.; Tieu, T.; Esser, L.; Wojnilowicz, M.; Lee, C.-H.; Cifuentes-Rius, A.; Thissen, H.; Voelcker, N.H. Differential Surface Engineering Generates Core–Shell Porous Silicon Nanoparticles for Controlled and Targeted Delivery of an Anticancer Drug. *ACS Appl. Mater. Interfaces* **2022**, *14*, 54539–54549. [CrossRef]
38. Cortés-Ríos, J.; Zárate, A.M.; Figueroa, J.D.; Medina, J.; Fuentes-Lemus, E.; Rodríguez-Fernández, M.; Aliaga, M.; López-Alarcón, C. Protein quantification by bicinchoninic acid (BCA) assay follows complex kinetics and can be performed at short incubation times. *Anal. Biochem.* **2020**, *608*, 113904. [CrossRef]
39. Weksler, B.; Subileau, E.; Perriere, N.; Charneau, P.; Holloway, K.; Leveque, M.; Tricoire-Leignel, H.; Nicotra, A.; Bourdoulous, S.; Turowski, P. Blood-brain barrier-specific properties of a human adult brain endothelial cell line. *FASEB J.* **2005**, *19*, 1872–1874. [CrossRef]
40. Peng, B.; Tong, Z.; Tong, W.Y.; Pasic, P.J.; Oddo, A.; Dai, Y.; Luo, M.; Frescene, J.; Welch, N.G.; Easton, C.D. In situ surface modification of microfluidic blood–brain-barriers for improved screening of small molecules and nanoparticles. *ACS Appl. Mater. Interfaces* **2020**, *12*, 56753–56766. [CrossRef]
41. Hubatsch, I.; Ragnarsson, E.G.; Artursson, P. Determination of drug permeability and prediction of drug absorption in Caco-2 monolayers. *Nat. Protoc.* **2007**, *2*, 2111–2119. [CrossRef]
42. Bimbo, L.M.; Mäkilä, E.M.; Raula, J.; Laaksonen, T.; Laaksonen, P.; Strommer, K.; Kauppinen, E.I.; Salonen, J.J.; Linder, M.B.; Hirvonen, J.; et al. Functional hydrophobin-coating of thermally hydrocarbonized porous silicon microparticles. *Biomaterials* **2011**, *32*, 9089–9099. [CrossRef] [PubMed]
43. Riikonen, J.; Nissinen, T.; Alanne, A.; Thapa, R.; Fioux, P.; Bonne, M.; Rigolet, S.; Morlet-Savary, F.; Aussenac, F.; Marichal, C.; et al. Stable surface functionalization of carbonized mesoporous silicon. *Inorg. Chem. Front.* **2020**, *7*, 631–641. [CrossRef]
44. Chang, J.; Jallouli, Y.; Kroubi, M.; Yuan, X.-B.; Feng, W.; Kang, C.-S.; Pu, P.-Y.; Betbeder, D. Characterization of endocytosis of transferrin-coated PLGA nanoparticles by the blood–brain barrier. *Int. J. Pharm.* **2009**, *379*, 285–292. [CrossRef] [PubMed]
45. Song, X.; Li, R.; Deng, H.; Li, Y.; Cui, Y.; Zhang, H.; Dai, W.; He, B.; Zheng, Y.; Wang, X.; et al. Receptor mediated transcytosis in biological barrier: The influence of receptor character and their ligand density on the transmembrane pathway of active-targeting nanocarriers. *Biomaterials* **2018**, *180*, 78–90. [CrossRef]
46. Li, G.; Simon, M.J.; Cancel, L.M.; Shi, Z.-D.; Ji, X.; Tarbell, J.M.; Morrison, B.; Fu, B.M. Permeability of endothelial and astrocyte cocultures: In vitro blood–brain barrier models for drug delivery studies. *Ann. Biomed. Eng.* **2010**, *38*, 2499–2511. [CrossRef]
47. Yu, Y.J.; Zhang, Y.; Kenrick, M.; Hoyte, K.; Luk, W.; Lu, Y.; Atwal, J.; Elliott, J.M.; Prabhu, S.; Watts, R.J.; et al. Boosting brain uptake of a therapeutic antibody by reducing its affinity for a transcytosis target. *Sci. Transl. Med.* **2011**, *3*, 84ra44. [CrossRef]
48. Niewoehner, J.; Bohrmann, B.; Collin, L.; Urich, E.; Sade, H.; Maier, P.; Rueger, P.; Stracke, J.O.; Lau, W.; Tissot, A.C.; et al. Increased brain penetration and potency of a therapeutic antibody using a monovalent molecular shuttle. *Neuron* **2014**, *81*, 49–60. [CrossRef]
49. Wiley, D.T.; Webster, P.; Gale, A.; Davis, M.E. Transcytosis and brain uptake of transferrin-containing nanoparticles by tuning avidity to transferrin receptor. *Proc. Natl. Acad. Sci. USA* **2013**, *110*, 8662–8667. [CrossRef]
50. Betzer, O.; Shilo, M.; Opochinsky, R.; Barnoy, E.; Motiei, M.; Okun, E.; Yadid, G.; Popovtzer, R. The effect of nanoparticle size on the ability to cross the blood–brain barrier: An in vivo study. *Nanomedicine* **2017**, *12*, 1533–1546. [CrossRef]
51. Davies, P.F. Hemodynamic shear stress and the endothelium in cardiovascular pathophysiology. *Nat. Clin. Pract. Cardiovasc. Med.* **2009**, *6*, 16–26. [CrossRef]
52. Dessalles, C.A.; Leclech, C.; Castagnino, A.; Barakat, A.I. Integration of substrate- and flow-derived stresses in endothelial cell mechanobiology. *Commun. Biol.* **2021**, *4*, 764. [CrossRef]
53. Shurbaji, S.; Anlar, G.G.; Hussein, E.A.; Elzatahry, A.; Yalcin, H.C. Effect of Flow-Induced Shear Stress in Nanomaterial Uptake by Cells: Focus on Targeted Anti-Cancer Therapy. *Cancers* **2020**, *12*, 1916. [CrossRef] [PubMed]
54. Lin, A.; Sabnis, A.; Kona, S.; Nattama, S.; Patel, H.; Dong, J.-F.; Nguyen, K.T. Shear-regulated uptake of nanoparticles by endothelial cells and development of endothelial-targeting nanoparticles. *J. Biomed. Mater. Res. Part A* **2010**, *93*, 833–842. [CrossRef] [PubMed]
55. Zukerman, H.; Khoury, M.; Shammay, Y.; Sznitman, J.; Lotan, N.; Korin, N. Targeting functionalized nanoparticles to activated endothelial cells under high wall shear stress. *Bioeng. Transl. Med.* **2020**, *5*, e10151. [CrossRef] [PubMed]
56. Zern, B.J.; Chacko, A.-M.; Liu, J.; Greineder, C.F.; Blankemeyer, E.R.; Radhakrishnan, R.; Muzykantov, V. Reduction of Nanoparticle Avidity Enhances the Selectivity of Vascular Targeting and PET Detection of Pulmonary Inflammation. *ACS Nano* **2013**, *7*, 2461–2469. [CrossRef] [PubMed]

57. Doshi, N.; Prabhakarpandian, B.; Rea-Ramsey, A.; Pant, K.; Sundaram, S.; Mitragotri, S. Flow and adhesion of drug carriers in blood vessels depend on their shape: A study using model synthetic microvascular networks. *J. Control. Release* **2010**, *146*, 196–200. [CrossRef]
58. Tan, J.; Shah, S.; Thomas, A.; Ou-Yang, H.D.; Liu, Y. The influence of size, shape and vessel geometry on nanoparticle distribution. *Microfluid. Nanofluidics* **2013**, *14*, 77–87. [CrossRef]
59. Cooley, M.; Sarode, A.; Hoore, M.; Fedosov, D.A.; Mitragotri, S.; Sen Gupta, A. Influence of particle size and shape on their margination and wall-adhesion: Implications in drug delivery vehicle design across nano-to-micro scale. *Nanoscale* **2018**, *10*, 15350–15364. [CrossRef]
60. Blanco, E.; Shen, H.; Ferrari, M. Principles of nanoparticle design for overcoming biological barriers to drug delivery. *Nat. Biotechnol.* **2015**, *33*, 941–951. [CrossRef]
61. Williams-Medina, A.; Deblock, M.; Janigro, D. In vitro Models of the Blood-Brain Barrier: Tools in Translational Medicine. *Front. Med. Technol.* **2020**, *2*, 623950. [CrossRef] [PubMed]

*pharmaceutics*

*Review*

# Nose-to-Brain (N2B) Delivery: An Alternative Route for the Delivery of Biologics in the Management and Treatment of Central Nervous System Disorders

**Elizabeth J. Patharapankal [1], Adejumoke Lara Ajiboye [1], Claudia Mattern [2] and Vivek Trivedi [1,*]**

1 Medway School of Pharmacy, University of Kent, Central Avenue, Chatham Maritime, Canterbury ME4 4TB, UK; e.j.pathrapankal@kent.ac.uk (E.J.P.); l.ajiboye@kent.ac.uk (A.L.A.)
2 MetP Pharma AG, Schynweg 7, 6376 Emmetten, Switzerland; info@mattern-pharma.com
* Correspondence: v.trivedi@kent.ac.uk

**Abstract:** In recent years, there have been a growing number of small and large molecules that could be used to treat diseases of the central nervous system (CNS). Nose-to-brain delivery can be a potential option for the direct transport of molecules from the nasal cavity to different brain areas. This review aims to provide a compilation of current approaches regarding drug delivery to the CNS via the nose, with a focus on biologics. The review also includes a discussion on the key benefits of nasal delivery as a promising alternative route for drug administration and the involved pathways or mechanisms. This article reviews how the application of various auxiliary agents, such as permeation enhancers, mucolytics, in situ gelling/mucoadhesive agents, enzyme inhibitors, and polymeric and lipid-based systems, can promote the delivery of large molecules in the CNS. The article also includes a discussion on the current state of intranasal formulation development and summarizes the biologics currently in clinical trials. It was noted that significant progress has been made in this field, and these are currently being applied to successfully transport large molecules to the CNS via the nose. However, a deep mechanistic understanding of this route, along with the intimate knowledge of various excipients and their interactions with the drug and nasal physiology, is still necessary to bring us one step closer to developing effective formulations for nasal–brain drug delivery.

**Keywords:** CNS disorders; nasal delivery; biologics; nose-to-brain

**Citation:** Patharapankal, E.J.; Ajiboye, A.L.; Mattern, C.; Trivedi, V. Nose-to-Brain (N2B) Delivery: An Alternative Route for the Delivery of Biologics in the Management and Treatment of Central Nervous System Disorders. *Pharmaceutics* **2024**, *16*, 66. https://doi.org/10.3390/pharmaceutics16010066

Academic Editors: Nicolas Tournier and Toshihiko Tashima

Received: 8 November 2023
Revised: 21 December 2023
Accepted: 26 December 2023
Published: 31 December 2023



## 1. Introduction

A growing number of central nervous system (CNS) disorders (e.g., caused by infection, injury, blood clots, age-related degeneration, cancer, autoimmune dysfunction, birth defects, multiple sclerosis, Alzheimer's disease, Parkinson's disease, meningitis, cerebral ischemia, etc.) are becoming more prevalent due to population growth and increased life expectancy. This poses a huge threat to patients and their families, as well as to society and the economy. These disorders require comprehensive treatment, which involves delivering therapeutics to the brain at appropriate levels to elicit a pharmacological response. However, despite the major advancements both in neuroscience and drug delivery research, the administration of drugs to the CNS remains challenging. In general, effectiveness-related issues arise when drugs cannot cross the blood–brain barrier (BBB). Therefore, currently, drugs with a low central bioavailability are applied by heavily invasive methods such as intrathecal and intracerebroventricular injection or by sensitive galenic approaches in oral dosage forms. Intranasal (IN) administration, on the other hand, serves as an alternative route for effective delivery to the CNS. It is non-invasive and can use nerve pathways for nose-to-brain drug transport to provide a fast onset of action, a possible reduction in systemic adverse effects, and higher bioavailability in the brain. Furthermore, the intranasal application is convenient for the patients, easier to apply in emergencies, and can save costs (e.g., reduced burden on trained medical and care staff).

Over the past decades, there has been significant progress in drug delivery and design by the pharmaceutical industry. However, areas focusing on the management of CNS disorders have considerably lagged [1]. The analysis conducted by Kesselheim, Hwang, and Franklin indicated a decline in CNS drug development since 1990, both in early and late-stage clinical trials [2]. Several factors, including an inadequate understanding of requirements for targeted CNS delivery, the complexity of both CNS physiology and diseases, increased drug development times and costs, and the higher risk of clinical failures, have severely limited the growth of new treatment possibilities for CNS disorders [1,3]. Moreover, the difficulty of poor drug transport across the BBB has been identified as the primary issue for the under-development of CNS pharmaceuticals [4–6]. It is widely accepted that most CNS disorders are unmanageable by non-invasive drug therapies because more than 98% of all potential CNS drugs do not cross the BBB. Therefore, researchers are now focusing on enhancing the delivery of potential therapeutics, including biomolecules, to the brain. This review provides a summary of challenges and specific approaches used to enhance both BBB permeability and drug bioavailability in the brain, with a specific interest in the use of large molecules (e.g., proteins, peptides, oligonucleotides, antibodies, steroids, and vaccines) via the possibility of direct nose-to-brain (N2B) drug delivery.

## 2. Potential of Biologics for the Management of CNS Disorders

The scope of therapeutic biologics to serve as an established first-line treatment of CNS disorders has rapidly evolved over the last few years because of their vast potential in managing these diseases. Table 1 highlights some of the biologics and their therapeutic applications in the treatment/management of CNS disorders.

**Table 1.** List of biologics for the treatment of CNS disorders.

| Therapeutic Moiety | Applications in CNS Diseases | Ref. |
|---|---|---|
| ***Peptides:*** *Modulate neurotransmitter function, regulate signalling pathways, prevent protein misfolding and aggregation* | | |
| Insulin | Alzheimer's disease | [7] |
| NAP neuropeptide | Alzheimer's disease | [8] |
| Vasoactive intestinal peptide | Neuroprotection | [9] |
| Urocortin | Alzheimer's disease | [10] |
| Leucine-enkephalin | CNS disorders | [11] |
| MS-1 (amino acid sequence CRGGKRSSC) novel peptide ligand | Multiple sclerosis | [12] |
| Gly14-humanin | Alzheimer's disease | [13] |
| Oxytocin | Autism spectrum disorders | [14] |
| ***Proteins:*** *Target specific receptors, enzymes, and transporters in the CNS, regulate synaptic transmission, promote cell survival and differentiation* | | |
| Neurotrophic factors (NGF, BDNF, CNTF, NT-4) | Focal ischemia, neuronal death, traumatic brain injury | [15] |
| Growth factors (IGF-1, TGF-α, FGF, HNGF, VEGF, BFGF) | Alzheimer's disease, stroke, Parkinson's disease, epilepsy, traumatic brain injury | [15,16] |
| Erythropoietin | Traumatic brain injury | [15] |
| Ovalbumin | Neurodegenerative disorders | [17] |
| ***Nucleic acid-based drugs:*** *Regulate gene expression, modulate RNA splicing, and translation* | | |
| Mac-1 siRNA | CNS disorders | [18] |
| GFP-mRNA luciferase mRNA | CNS disorders | [19] |
| Plasmid DNA | Neurodegenerative disorders | [20] |

**Table 1.** *Cont.*

| Therapeutic Moiety | Applications in CNS Diseases | Ref. |
|---|---|---|
| 499-siRNA or 233-ASO | Parkinson's disease | [21] |
| anti-eGFP siRNA and dsDNA | Alzheimer's disease | [22] |
| anti-ITCH siRNA | CNS disorders | [23] |
| siRNA or dsDNA | Neurodegenerative disorders | [24] |
| ***Steroids:*** *Regulate inflammation, protect against oxidative stress, promote cell survival and differentiation* | | |
| Sex hormone (progesterone, testosterone, oestradiol) | CNS disorders | [25] |
| Thyrotropin-releasing hormone (TRH)-peptide | Epilepsy | [26] |
| Melanocortin-4 receptor antagonist | Neuropathic pain | [27] |
| ***Antibodies:*** *Target pathogenic proteins, modulate immune responses, promote cell clearance and phagocytosis* | | |
| Antibody fragment (TNF-a inhibitory single-chain Fv antibody fragment) | Parkinson's disease Alzheimer's disease, MS | [28] |
| RNA based aptamers | CNS disorders | [29] |
| Full-length anti-Nogo-A antibody | Ischemic stroke | [30] |

## 3. Limitations Associated with Drug Delivery to the Brain

In contrast to other organs in the human body, the functioning of the CNS is distinctly defined by the presence of physiological barriers known as the BBB and blood–cerebrospinal fluid barrier (BCSFB) [31]. These physical, metabolic, and transporter-regulated barriers act to separate the CNS from the peripheral system by protecting it from any external toxins, stimuli, and foreign substances, including active pharmaceutical ingredients (APIs). Furthermore, the BBB maintains the homeostasis of the brain by selectively regulating the entry/exit of important nutrients, proteins, ions, and metabolites [32,33]. The limited permeability of the BBB is mainly attributed to its structure, which consists of brain capillary endothelial cells that are interconnected by tight junctions [34]. Typically, access to the brain via transcellular or paracellular mechanisms across the BBB is restricted to lipid-soluble small molecules with a molecular weight of <500 Da [4]. On the other hand, water-soluble substances with a larger size and positive charge could be transferred to the brain through alternative pathways such as receptor-mediated/adsorptive endocytosis or via transporter proteins. However, particularly for APIs, the active efflux transporters in the BBB, such as P-glycoprotein (P-gp), still pose a major obstacle to their delivery to the brain [35,36]. Also, the BBB comprises a metabolic barrier containing several enzymes (e.g., cytochrome p450) with the capacity to alter endogenous and exogenous molecules that could otherwise evade the physical barrier [37]. Therefore, a proper understanding of the physiological features of the BBB is important to be able to achieve effective brain transport of therapeutic agents.

As a result, several approaches have been attempted to either bypass or facilitate drug access across the BBB. These explorative strategies involve:

i. BBB disruption that includes the temporary opening of tight junctions to enable passage through the BBB by optimizing the physio-chemical properties of therapeutic molecules [38–45].
ii. The use of drug delivery systems (DDS) and brain transport vectors for targeted BBB passage [46–49].
iii. Developing approaches to exploit various endogenous transport systems present at the BBB [50–53].
iv. Formulations to utilize alternative transport routes for direct brain delivery that can exclude the BBB [54–56].

Overall, it is important to develop novel approaches to enhance the delivery of APIs to the CNS and revolutionize the treatment of CNS disorders to improve patient outcomes.

Amongst various approaches, intranasal delivery of drugs can be a promising approach to bypassing the BBB and delivering therapeutics directly to the brain.

## 4. Intranasal Drug Delivery

Several invasive techniques, including intraparenchymal, intraventricular, and intrathecal delivery, have been investigated to establish the direct transport of drug molecules to the brain [57]. However, these procedures may not be suitable for patients with chronic illnesses who require long-term treatment due to associated discomfort and the possibility of reduced effectiveness of the drug. The IN route of administration can provide a fast, pain-free, and non-invasive option for the delivery of drug substances to the CNS [58]. The large surface area of the nasal cavity and high vascularization of its mucosa can facilitate rapid drug absorption and fast onset [59]. Not to mention that the IN route also avoids harsh environmental conditions of the gastrointestinal (GI) tract and the first-pass metabolism. The possibility to exploit the nerve pathways after nasal administration also offers the unique opportunity of targeting drugs directly to the brain, making it highly attractive for the delivery of sensitive biotherapeutics [59].

IN drug delivery is based on the unique physiology of the nasal cavity, which provides a direct connection between the external environment and the CNS. A simple illustration of the anatomy of the human nasal cavity is presented in Figure 1.

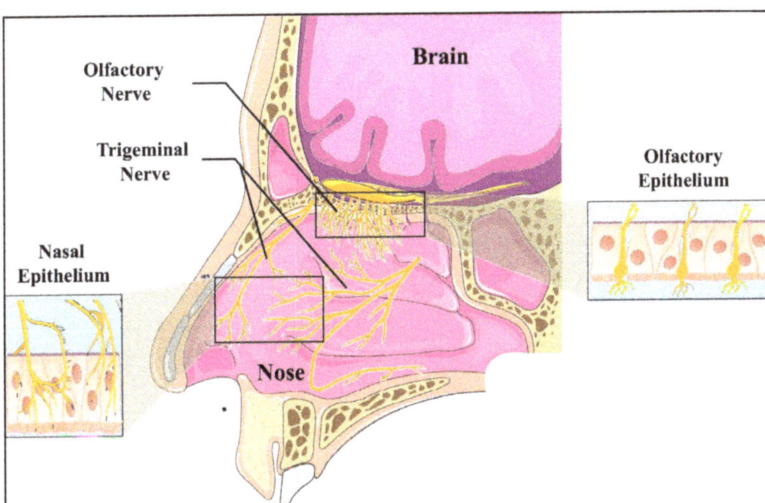


**Figure 1.** Illustration of the anatomy of the human nasal cavity (reprinted with permission from Elsevier) [60].

The details of nasal physiology have been comprehensively covered by various authors [61–66]. Nonetheless, features including the highly vascularized and permeable mucosal lining of the nasal cavity to allow for the rapid and efficient absorption of drugs and the availability of the olfactory and trigeminal nerve pathways are important to mention in this context. The olfactory area is directly connected to the brain (especially the olfactory bulb) via olfactory nerves. Along with this, the respiratory region is supplied with trigeminal sensory neurons and blood vessels [67]. Through a direct neuronal pathway, drugs may enter into different regions of the brain, providing a strategy to overcome the BBB. The exact mechanism of drug transport from the nasal cavity to the brain is still a topic of discussion, but some authors describe that the presence of transporters both in the olfactory bulb and respiratory mucosa of the nasal cavity may play an important role [68–70].

### 4.1. Challenges Associated with IN Delivery

There are various challenges associated with the IN delivery of drugs that include limited size of the nasal cavity, nasal mucus, mucociliary clearance (MCC), and enzymatic degradation but also changes in the nasal anatomy, e.g., polyps. The mean volumes of the nasal septum left/right nasal cavity, left/right inferior nasal conchae, and left/right middle nasal conchae are about 5 $cm^3$, 7.6 $cm^3$, 3.1 $cm^3$ and 1.3 $cm^3$, respectively, but gender and age differences can be statistically significant [71]. Therefore, nasal drug delivery is limited by the applicable volume of about 150 μL per nostril for adults and is potentially mainly suitable for high-potency drugs. If the instilled volumes exceed the limited capacity of the nose, the administered preparations are partially swallowed, or they simply run out of the nose.

Nasal mucus consists of a lower, liquid layer ("periciliary liquid") that is covered by a more viscous gel phase and includes a thin layer of surfactant that spreads mucus all over the epithelial surface. Mucus contains inorganic salts, antimicrobial enzymes, immunoglobulins, and glycoproteins [72]. It is slightly acidic (pH 5.5–6.5), required for optimal ciliary clearance, and has limited buffering capacity [73]. The nasal mucus plays an important role in mediating immune responses to allergens and infectious particles by trapping them as they enter the respiratory passage [74–81]. MCC is the self-cleaning mechanism of the airways and a protective process for the lungs in removing inhaled particles, including pathogens. Within the thin periciliary liquid layer, the cilia (tiny hairs) beat in a coordinated fashion directed to the pharynx and create motions that drain mucus from the nasal passage to the throat, where it is swallowed and digested by stomach juices or removed by blowing the nose. Effective MCC depends on factors such as the number of cilia, their structure (particularly their height), and especially the quality of the mucus. On the other hand, particle transport by MCC may restrict the absorption of medication in aqueous formulations to an estimated 20–30 min. If the formulation irritates the nasal mucosa, this causes the irritant to be rapidly diluted, followed by increased clearance.

The in vivo clinical or pre-clinical (animal) experiments are particularly challenging when it comes to IN delivery. For example, the application of mild anesthetics is very common during IN studies that, in some instances, could result in different brain delivery and pharmacokinetics due to the activation of the glymphatic system [82,83]. Therefore, in vivo microdialysis experiments in freely moving animals could be considered in such cases [84]. Other options, such as laser scanning fluorescence microscopy, positron emission tomography (PET), and nuclear magnetic resonance spectroscopy (MRS), provide an elegant option for the evaluation of the distribution of nasally applied drugs with systemic/brain activity [85,86]. In contrast, traditional immunolabeling procedures require cutting the sample into thin sections, which restricts the ability to label and examine intact structures.

It is often difficult to estimate the results from publications since the exact galenical formulation is rarely apparent, information on the duration of the experiment (stability of the API over time, dosage regimen), and sampling of blood and tissue are limited [87]. Sometimes the test set-up also plays a role if unrealistically large volumes are applied or the IN formulation is not comparable to that of the oral/IP/SC applications.

The bioavailability of intranasally administered drugs can be greatly affected by enzymatic degradation, as the nasal mucosa contains a wide spectrum of xenobiotic-metabolizing enzymes [80,81]. Aldehyde dehydrogenases, cytochrome P450-dependent monooxygenases, rhodanese, glutathione transferases, epoxide hydrolases, flavin-containing monooxygenases, and carboxyl esterases have all been reported to occur in substantial amounts in the nasal cavity. These play a major role in the decomposition of actives in the nasal cavity. For example, oestradiol, testosterone, and decongestants are enzymatically degraded by cytochrome P450-dependent monooxygenases [26,80]. Although the impact of enzymatic degradation in the nasal mucosa remains inconclusive, it can be reduced to some extent either by enzyme inhibitors or by the saturation of enzymes.

### 4.2. Strategies to Enhance in Drug Delivery to the CNS

The selection of suitable excipients or formulations is critical for the effective IN delivery of actives, which becomes paramount for biologics. The hostile environment of nasal tissue, which is designed to protect the body from pathogens, makes delivery of complex biologics difficult. However, applications of agents such as permeation enhancers, mucoadhesive compounds, enzyme inhibitors, and vasoconstrictors can aid in increasing the efficacy of the IN formulations. As a general requirement, it is a must that an aqueous IN formulation is safe to deliver with respect to the nasal pH and osmolality. The pH of the healthy nasal epithelium is 5.5–6.5; a pH lower than 5.5 or higher than 6.5 may cause local adverse effects and affect drug permeation. The osmolality of the nasal solution should be 290–500 mOsm/kg; higher values are tolerable for emergencies or single applications, but isotonic formulations are important for chronic use, and hypotonic solutions should be avoided [88]. The section below briefly discusses existing strategies for promoting the absorption of therapeutics through the nasal cavity.

The selective IN permeation of small hydrophilic and lipophilic molecules is usually achievable, but the same cannot be said for high-molecular-weight actives as the nasal epithelia serves as a robust barrier for N2B transportation. This limitation can be addressed by increasing the nasal permeability with a permeation enhancer that can aid the transfer of biologics via neural or cellular pathways [89,90]. Permeation enhancers open up the tight junctions of the nasal epithelium either by swelling or by temporarily dissolving the membrane protein [64]. Furthermore, these are also known to improve drug solubilisation, reduce mucociliary clearance, limit enzymatic degradation, and increase the contact time of the drug with the nasal mucosa [91]. In general, they are classified according to their molecular weight, with linear or cyclic structures such as thiolated polymers. Low-molecular-weight compounds such as phospholipids, surfactants, bile salts, and their derivatives, as well as cyclodextrin, polymers (e.g., chitosan and carbopol), and cell-penetrating peptides (CPP), referred to as high-molecular-weight compounds, are commonly utilized as permeation enhancers [92–94].

The use of CPPs in particular has gained a lot of attention lately. The permeation enhancement mechanisms associated with CPPs are still debated in the literature, but electrostatic interactions between the positively charged CPPs and the plasma membrane are considered a possible first step to promote drug permeation [95,96]. The research by Ziegler et al. provided a complete overview of the cellular absorption efficiency of CPPs [97]. There is also evidence that CPPs containing unconventional stereochemical forms (D-from instead of L-form) can, on occasion, provide greater resistance to enzymatic degradation [98]. Therefore, CPPs in such cases can act as a permeability enhancer and also prevent the drug from enzymatic degradation. Low-molecular-weight permeation enhancers, on the other hand, are effective owing to their structural resemblance to the endothelial membrane. These agents can interfere with lipophilic as well as hydrophilic fractions due to their bipolar structures, thereby disrupting membrane bilayer integrity and promoting drug absorption [99].

Mucins are a prominent component of nasal mucus, and mucolytics (e.g., N-acetyl-cysteine) are needed to reduce the viscosity of the bronchial secretions and facilitate penetration of the drug by breaking disulphide crosslinks between mucin monomers [100–102]. With an average thickness of 10–15 μm, the nasal mucus layer is the upper respiratory tract's first-line defensive barrier, hence maintaining a healthy airway and safeguarding the epithelium [103]. Thiol-containing fatty acids such as N-dodecyl-4-mercaptobutanimidamide and 2-mercapto-N-octylacetamide are reported to increase the mucus-penetrating capabilities of formulations such as self-emulsifying drug delivery systems (SEDDS) [103]. These formulations were shown to outperform equivalent SEDDS without thiols in terms of mucus permeation.

Mucoadhesive agents such as pectin, chitosan, and hydroxypropyl methylcellulose (HPMC) retain the therapeutic agent close to the site of absorption, resulting in a larger drug concentration gradient at the nasal epithelial membrane and hence increased absorption [104]. Depending on the functional groups present on the polymer backbone, mucoadhesives can improve absorption via enhanced nasal drug retention and/or decrease nasomucosal clearance [105]. Mucoadhesion primarily occurs through hydrogen bonding between the mucoadhesive polymer's carboxylic acid groups and the hydroxyl groups that characterize mucus glycoproteins in the case of negatively charged polymers such as polyacrylic acid [106–108]. In addition, cationic polymers with a high density of positive charges (e.g., chitosan) can also interact with negatively charged mucus glycoproteins via electrostatic interactions, resulting in enhanced retention of the formulation at the delivery site. The use of vasoconstrictors (either in conjunction with a nasal formulation or as an excipient in the formulation) while targeting the olfactory region can also ensure increased drug concentration in the brain and limit systemic absorption [64].

Nasal mucosa includes a range of enzymes, including monooxygenase, reductase, transferase, and proteolytic enzymes, which can induce the degradation of drugs and limit their absorption. Incorporation of appropriate nanocarrier systems, such as polymeric nanoparticles or lipid-based nanocarriers (e.g., liposomes, solid-lipid nanoparticles (SLNs), nanostructured-lipid carriers (NLCs), nanoemulsions, lipid drug conjugates (LDCs), self-emulsifying drug delivery systems (SEDDS), etc.), is known to prevent the enzymatic degradation of drugs in the nasal cavity [109,110]. Other approaches, including PEGylation, have also been shown to protect biologics from degradation and can increase the half-life of a drug [111]. However, it should be noted that sometimes PEGylation might result in unexpected alterations in the biological activity of biologics. For example, the substrate selectivity of cholesterol oxidase was noted to change from total cholesterol to high-density lipoprotein (HDL) cholesterol following PEGylation. Similarly, the PEGylated growth hormone (pegvisomant) exhibited agonistic rather than antagonistic action compared to the non-PEGylated hormone [112]. So, in these cases, the protective effect of PEGylation was minimal; hence, this approach requires further investigation for the nasal administration of biologics.

Polymer-based drug carrier systems include polymeric nanoparticles, colloidal carrier systems, polymer–drug conjugates, and the application of a smart polymer-based system such as stimuli-sensitive hydrogels or in situ nasal gels, etc. [113,114]. In recent years, a number of biodegradable and biocompatible natural (e.g., alginate, chitosan) and synthetic (poly (lactic-co-glycolic acid) (PLGA), poly (acrylamide), poly (lactic acid) (PLA), poly (lysine), poly (caprolactone), and poly (acryl cyanoacrylate), etc.) polymers have been investigated to develop novel carrier systems for controlled and targeted CNS delivery via the nasal route [115–118].

Liposomes, nanoemulsions, lipid nanoparticles, SLNs, LDCs, and NLCs are also extensively utilized for nasal drug administration due to their biocompatibility and biodegradability [119]. Liposomes have been extensively investigated as carrier systems for therapeutic drug delivery to the brain. Salade et al. showed the use of chitosan-modified anionic liposomes for ghrelin nasal administration [120]. Similarly, the application of cationic liposomes instead of a typical solution for IN administration of a model protein (ovalbumin) showed increased bioavailability and activity in the brain at a substantially lower dosage [121]. Nanoemulsion can also be a promising system for N2B delivery because of its small droplet size, lipophilicity, biocompatibility, low toxicity, and greater permeability. The nanoemulsions containing zolmitriptan and quetiapine fumarate showed high brain targeting efficiency when delivered intranasally [122,123]. SLNs are considered more stable than liposomes, and because of their smaller size, they can be a viable option for N2B drug delivery [124]. For example, in one study, levofloxacin and doxycycline SLNs showed improved AUC and brain concentration compared to the simple nasal solution [124,125]. NLCs are second-generation SLNs that are characterized by higher drug encapsulation and improved stability. Chitosan-modified NLCs containing glial cell-derived neurotrophic factor (GDNF) showed improved therapeutic efficacy and resulted in considerable improvement in the 6-OHDA-lesioned rat model's behavioral function, indicating a successful delivery of GDNF to the brain [126]. Efavirenz containing NLCs, when delivered intranasally as treatment for neuroAIDS, revealed a significant improvement in the drug distribution in the brain [127]. It is also worth mentioning that devices play a very important role in the IN delivery and targeting of APIs, but discussion on devices was considered out of scope for this review. Table 2 outlines the application of various approaches/excipients used in the IN delivery of APIs to target them to the brain.

**Table 2.** Examples of various approaches and excipients used in the IN delivery of APIs for brain targeting.

| Enhancer | Drug | Species/In Vitro/In Vivo | Comments | Ref. |
|---|---|---|---|---|
| ***Surfactants*** | | | | |
| Laurate sucrose ester | Sumatriptan succinate | Rat | Promising IN absorption enhancer for poorly permeable drugs | [128] |
| Pluronic F-127 | Donepezil | In vitro<br>Ex vivo<br>In vivo (pig) | Adequate mucoadhesive properties; improved drug permeation through nasal mucosa | [129] |
| Rhamnolipids (biosurfactant) | Dextran | In vitro | Safe and effective excipient for the improvement of mucosal absorption of macromolecules<br>Concentration-dependent permeability effect; higher permeability observed for lower MW dextran | [130] |
| ***Cell-penetrating peptides (CPP)*** | | | | |
| Low-molecular-weight protamine (LMWP) | Bovine serum albumin<br>Peroxidase<br>β-galactosidase | Mouse | Successful nose-to-brain delivery with selected enzymes retaining their biological function after delivery | [131] |
| Penetratin | Insulin | Rat | Efficient intranasal absorption of insulin up to deeper regions of the brain such as the hippocampus and cerebellum, reduced systemic exposure with D-penetratin | [7,132] |
| Polyethylene glycol–polycaprolactone copolymers conjugated with Tat peptide (MPEG–PCL–Tat) | siRNA<br>Dextran | Rat | The CPP-modified nanomicelles improved transport along the olfactory and trigeminal nerve pathway due to their high nasal mucosa permeability | [133] |
| L-penetratin | Leptin | Rat | Improved nasal absorption with co-administration of L-penetratin; increased plasma concentrations and brain distribution (particularly in the olfactory bulb and hypothalamus); no toxic effect on epithelial cells | [134] |
| Exendin-4–CPP conjugate | Exendin-4, a glucagon-like protein-1 | Mouse | Improved the scope for treatment of progressive cognitive dysfunction | [135] |
| ***Bile salts*** | | | | |
| Sodium-ursodeoxycolate/ Sodium taurocholate | Zidovudine | In vitro<br>In vivo (rat) | Results indicating antiviral drug targeting of macrophages in CSF using nano-systems coated with these bile salts | [136] |
| ***Polymeric system*** | | | | |
| Chitosan nanoparticles | Bromocriptine | Mouse | Significant improvement of bromocriptine bioavailability in the brain following IN administration of drug-loaded chitosan nanoparticles | [137] |
| Chitosan glutamate microspheres | Rokitamycin | In vitro<br>In vivo (rat) | Improved dissolution rate and successful nose-to-CSF delivery of the drug molecules | [138] |

**Table 2.** *Cont.*

| Enhancer | Drug | Species/In Vitro/In Vivo | Comments | Ref. |
|---|---|---|---|---|
| Chitosan nanoparticles | Venlafaxine | Ex vivo<br>In vivo (rat) | Higher drug transport efficiency and direct brain transport percentage with these nanosystems in comparison to other formulations | [57] |
| Chitosan glutamate (CG)/chitosan base (CB)/hydroxypropyl methylcellulose (HPMC) microparticles | Zolmitriptan | In vitro<br>Ex vivo<br>In vivo (rat) | Among the investigated nasal formulations, CG-based microparticles showed the best efficacy in promoting the central uptake of zolmitriptan | [139] |
| Chitosan + glycerophosphate + magnesium chloride hydrogels | Exenatide | In vivo (rat) | Presence of $MgCl_2$ led to improved exenatide stability, extended gelling time, improved transepithelial transport, biodistribution and bioavailability | [140] |
| PEG-PCL- or stearate-modified arginine-rich-CH2R4H2C peptide | Dextran | In vivo (rat) | Effective N2B delivery with less distribution to other peripheral tissues than that with IV administration; stearate-CH2R4H2C is more suitable for drug transport to the forebrain while PEG-PCL-CH2R4H2C allows for targeted transport to the hindbrain | [141] |
| Poly (lactic-co-glycolic acid) (PLGA) nanoparticles conjugated with glutathione | Paclitaxel | In vitro<br>Ex vivo<br>In vivo (rat) | Efficient brain delivery following nasal administration of drug-loaded- conjugated carrier; glutathione shows to be a suitable vector for the successful transport of poorly bioavailable drug to the brain | [142] |
| Alginate–chitosan nanoparticles | Venlafaxine | Ex vivo<br>In vivo<br>(rat) | Improved drug's pharmacodynamics when compared to IN solution and oral tablet. Also, greater brain/blood drug ratios with nanoparticles | [143] |
| Polycaprolactone nanoparticles | Aripiprazole | In vitro<br>Ex vivo<br>In vivo (rat) | Better drug distribution in the brain than IV. Nasal toxicity study indicated the safety of the developed nanoparticle formulation | [144] |
| Glycol chitosan-coated nanostructured lipid carrier | Asenapine | In vitro<br>In vivo (rat) | Promising delivery system for the brain transport via the IN route, with better pharmacokinetic and safety profile; approximately, 2.3- and 4-fold higher systemic and brain bioavailability respectively for the drug-loaded carrier. | [145] |
| Chitosan-coated solid lipid nanoparticles | BACE1 siRNA + RVG-9R (cell-penetrating peptide) complex | In vitro | Mucoadhesive properties and prolonged residence time in the nasal cavity; improved siRNA epithelial cell (Caco-2) permeation after release from coated particles | [146] |
| PLGA nanoparticles embedded in in situ poloxamer 407® (P407) gel | Rivastigmine hydrogen tartrate (RHT) | In vitro<br>Ex vivo | Nanocomposites showed higher amounts of drug permeation through sheep nasal mucosa than plain drug gel | [147] |

**Table 2.** *Cont.*

| Enhancer | Drug | Species/In Vitro/In Vivo | Comments | Ref. |
|---|---|---|---|---|
| Chitosan nanoemulsions | Kaempferol | In vitro<br>Ex vivo<br>In vivo (rat) | Higher permeation, brain bioavailability, and efficacy of the drug when compared to free drug or non-mucoadhesive nanoemulsions; histopathological examination showed safety of nanoemulsion for nasal mucosal and ability to preserve drug antioxidant capability | [148] |
| Polycarbonate nanoparticles | Apomorphine | In-vitro<br>In-vivo (Rat) | Improved brain bioavailability | [149] |
| Lectin-modified PEG–PLGA nanoparticles | Basic fibroblast growth factor | In vitro<br>In vivo (rat) | Enhanced spatial memory, bioavailability, therapeutic activity, and reduced side effects | [150] |
| N-trimethyl chitosan nanoparticles | Leucine-enkephalin | In vitro<br>Ex vivo<br>In vivo (rat) | Improved brain uptake, antinociceptive effect and therapeutic activity | [151] |
| Chitosan based nanoemulsion gel | Naringenin | In vitro<br>Ex vivo<br>In vivo (rat) | Increased brain bioavailability and showed no toxicological or inflammatory response | [152] |
| Gelatin nanoparticles | Osteopontin | Rat | Gelatin microspheres enhanced the neuroprotective effects of osteopontin | [153] |
| ***Lipid-based systems*** | | | | |
| Chitosan-coated nanostructured lipid carrier. | hIGF-I | In vitro | Enhanced biodistribution and facilitated efficient drug delivery | [154] |
| | Glial cell-derived neurotrophic factor (hGDNF) | Ex vivo<br>In vivo (rat)<br>In vivo (rat) | Improved behavioral patterns and neuroprotection | [155] |
| Gelatin-NLCs | Basic fibroblast growth factor | In vitro (mouse) | Improved brain bioavailability, target efficiency and therapeutic effects | [156] |
| Oil-in-water nanoemulsion | Cyclosporine-A | In vivo (rat) | Improved targeted drug delivery and bioavailability | [157] |
| Chitosan NLCs | Glial cell-derived neurotrophic factor | Rat | Enhanced brain distribution in the PD model | [126] |
| Cationic liposomes | GFP-mRNA luciferase mRNA | Rat | Higher expression of GFP-mRNA expression post 24 h compared to naked mRNA | [21] |
| ***Miscellaneous*** | | | | |
| Capmul MCM (oil) + labrasol (surfactant) + transcutol P (co-surfactant) + Carbopol 934P (mucoadhesive agent) + Pluronic F127, F68 (gelling excipient) | Nimodipine | Rat | A combination of Pluronics and Carbopol 934P can significantly increase the N2B delivery of nimodipine | [114] |

**Table 2.** *Cont.*

| Enhancer | Drug | Species/In Vitro/In Vivo | Comments | Ref. |
|---|---|---|---|---|
| Human serum albumin + chitosan | Sulforhodamine B sodium salt | Ex vivo | Confirmation of mucoadhesive properties of chitosan; added advantage of opening of tight junctions | [158] |
| Cationic liposomes | Ovalbumin | Rat | Brain delivery of model protein via the nasal olfactory route and extended brain residence time of the delivered biomolecule | [121] |
| Chitosan + hydroxypropyl-b-cyclodextrin microemulsions | Buspirone hydrochloride | In vivo (rat)<br>Ex vivo | Direct N2B transport of 88% buspirone following IN administration | [159] |
| *Delonix regia* gum-coated nanostructured lipid carriers (DRG-NLCs) [NLCs comprising of glycerol monostearate (solid lipid); Capryol 90 (liquid lipid); soya lecithin (surfactant); poloxamer 188 (cosurfactant)] | Ondansetron | In vitro<br>Ex vivo<br>In vivo (rat) | Rapid drug transport and improved bioavailability to the brain by IN administration of DRG-NLCs | [160] |
| Liposomes (cholesterol + egg phosphatidylcholine) | Quetiapine | In vitro<br>Ex vivo<br>In vivo (mouse) | Better potential for quetiapine N2B delivery with formulated liposomes in comparison to simple drug dispersions | [161] |
| Flexible liposomes (soya phosphatidylcholine + cholesterol + propylene glycol + water) | Galanthamine hydrobromide | In vivo (rat) | Improved efficiency of drug activity in the brain after IN administration in comparison to oral. Increased $C_{max}$ and $AUC_{0\rightarrow10}$, and reduced drug cell cytotoxicity with nasal delivery using liposome carrier | [162] |
| Ion-activated deacetylated gellan gum (DGG) in situ gel incorporating resveratrol nanosuspensions | Resveratrol | In vitro<br>In vivo (mouse) | Direct transport of drug (78%) to the brain via the nasal cavity | [163] |
| Flaxseed oil containing cationic DOTAP nanoemulsions | Anti-TNFa siRNA | In vitro<br>In vivo<br>(rat) | Enhanced cell (J774A.1 murine macrophage) uptake by endocytosis of siRNA in comparison to Lipofectamine® formulations; higher relative gene silencing effect in lipopolysaccharide (LPS)—stimulated macrophages | [164] |
| Agomelatine-nanoemulsion in situ poloxamer-407 gel (Ag-NE-gel) + 0.5% chitosan | Agomelatine | In vitro<br>Ex vivo<br>In vivo (Rat) | Improved drug bioavailability in the brain following IN administration; rapid gel erosion, faster drug release from NE and better drug permeation through the olfactory epithelial layer | [165] |
| Nanoliposomes (phospholipon 90G + cholesterol + Tween 80) | Lamotrigine | In vitro<br>Ex vivo | High drug release; enhanced drug permeation across the nasal mucosa | [166] |
| PGLA Nanoparticles | | In vivo (rat)<br>In vitro | Increased bioavailability and permeation in the brain | [115] |
| Poly (lactic-co-glycolic acid) nanoparticles (NPs) | Diazepam | In vivo (sheep)<br>In vivo (rat) | Potential carrier for N2B delivery of outpatient management of status epilepticus | [116] |
| Thiolated chitosan nanoparticles | Galantamine | In vivo (mouse) | Significantly improved efficacy ($p < 0.05$) compared to oral administration. | [117] |

**Table 2.** *Cont.*

| Enhancer | Drug | Species/In Vitro/In Vivo | Comments | Ref. |
|---|---|---|---|---|
| Polycaprolactone nanoparticles | Melatonin | In vitro<br>In vivo (rat) | Increased apparent solubility (~35 fold), effective treatment for glioblastoma | [118] |
| Nanoemulsion [triacetin (oil phase) + Tween 80 (surfactant) + PEG-400 (co-surfactant)] | Letrozole | In vitro ex vivo<br>In vivo (mouse) | Enhanced release compared to drug suspension. Higher bioavailability in the brain and improved anticonvulsant drug effect with the IN nanoemulsion in comparison to intraperitoneal route | [167] |
| Pluronic F-127 + Carbopol 974P thermoreversible gel | Levetiracetam | In vitro<br>In vivo (mouse) | Higher cerebral concentrations following IN administration and, similar plasma PK profile to IV. No change in cell viability in nasal and lung cells in the presence of drug–gel formulation | [168] |
| Pluronic F-127 + Carbopol 934 thermoreversible gel | Naratriptan | In vitro<br>Ex vivo | Carbopol acts as both a mucoadhesive agent and a penetration enhancer | [169] |
| Microemulsion of Capmul MCM EP (oil) + surfactant mix (labrasol + Tween 80 + transcutol-P) + DW or mucoadhesive ME with chitosan or methyl-b-cyclodextrin | Quetiapine | Ex vivo<br>In vivo (rat) | Superiority of chitosan ME formulation; enhanced brain uptake following IN administration | [170] |

## 5. In Delivery of Biologics to the CNS

A significant amount of work has been conducted on the suitability of the IN route for delivering high-molecular-weight therapeutics (e.g., peptides, proteins, nucleic acids etc) and various neurosteroids [171]. The susceptibility of biologics to enzymatic breakdown and their limited permeability through the epithelium via transcellular and paracellular pathways result in poor absorption of biologics from a mucosal site. As a result, they are often delivered through invasive and painful injections to boost their bioavailability. However, novel formulations and delivery techniques are being continuously developed to improve the administration of both small molecules and macromolecular therapeutics [172]. As previously noted, unlike parenteral administration, IN delivery is extremely easy and convenient for patients, making it particularly appealing for chronic treatments. The following sections discuss the formulation strategies used in the delivery of biologics in the treatment of CNS disorders.

The delivery of peptides to the brain has received growing interest in recent decades due to its pharmacological significance in the treatment of various CNS ailments, including neurodegenerative diseases, cancer, and ischemic strokes [173–175]. Insulin is one of the most extensively researched biologics in terms of its effects on the CNS after IN delivery. One of the earliest studies on peptide delivery to the brain involved the IN administration of an aqueous solution of insulin that showed pharmacological efficacy but also provided information on its limited transportation into the brain [176]. Since then, IN administration of insulin aqueous solutions has been extensively studied in various preclinical and clinical trials for the treatment of Alzheimer's disease, mild cognitive impairment, diabetes, insulin resistance, and Parkinson's disease, among other conditions.

The impact of excipients and formulation types is very important while developing an IN-drug delivery system. For example, Kamei et al. studied IN delivery of insulin solution using L-penetratin and D-penetratin (cell-penetrating, 16 mer peptide). They reported that the IN administration of radio-labeled insulin with L-penetratin in rats resulted in higher levels of insulin in the anterior region [177]. This finding was further confirmed in Alzheimer's disease model mice, where co-administration of insulin with L-penetratin resulted in slower memory loss progression than co-administration of insulin with D-penetratin or with the administration of insulin alone [178]. In another study, Picone et al. developed negatively charged nanogels constructed of polyvinylpyrrolidone (PVP) that resulted in enhanced insulin delivery to the brain [179]. Maitani et al. investigated the permeability of insulin-entrapped liposomes through rabbit nasal mucosa and compared it with the permeability of insulin solution with/without pre-treatment with sodium glycocholate (GC) [180]. They reported a positive outcome of pre-treatment with GC, especially for insulin-containing liposomes (i.e., the liposomes penetrated more efficiently following pre-treatment with GC). Similarly, Morimoto et al. developed polyacrylic acid (PLA) gel using insulin and calcitonin for IN delivery to the brain [181]. They reported higher insulin absorption from 0.15 $w/v$ PLA gel than that from 1% $w/v$ gel after nasal delivery in rats, which could be related to the gel viscosity [181]. A similar study investigated the effects of putative bioadhesive polymer gels on nasal mucociliary clearance in rat models. The results showed that all formulations reduced IN mucociliary clearance, increasing the formulations' resident duration in the nasal cavity [182].

Pringles et al. used dry insulin powder in deposition trials in rabbits to assess the effect of deposition patterns utilising different spray devices on insulin bioavailability [183]. The authors concluded that anterior deposition of the formulation in the nasal cavity results in maximum insulin bioavailability due to the high degree of surface coverage over the nasal epithelium. In another study, Nagai et al. investigated the absorption of dry powder insulin combined with microcrystalline cellulose (MCC) and other cellulosic derivatives, where MCC was shown to have the largest permeability-boosting impact [184]. It is understood that MCC could be able to bind with the calcium ions in the nasal epithelium to open up the tight junctions while temporarily hindering mucociliary clearance due to its mucoadhesive nature [185].

In a study conducted by During et al., where they dispersed [Ser(2)] exendin (1–9) [a glucagon-like peptide-1 (GLP-1R) receptor agonist] in a 10% β-cyclodextrin solution that is believed to act as a permeation enhancer, peptide solubilizer and stabilizer [186], an increase in learning and diminished kainic acid-induced apoptosis were observed in mice, most likely mediated by GLP-1R expression in the hippocampus. Similarly, Banks et al. investigated the brain distribution of the radioactively labeled GLP-1 antagonist exendin (9–39) (I-Ex) after IN and IV administrations [187]. An I-Ex solution in phosphate buffer or normal saline with or without cyclodextrin was utilized in this study. After IN administration, the results showed that olfactory bulb absorption of I-Ex was substantially faster than after IV administration, and it increased by roughly 60% when cyclodextrin was added. Kamei et al. prepared a formulation of exendin-4 with L-penetratin that resulted in the delivery of the peptide to the hypothalamus and hippocampus after the IN delivery [135]. These findings indicated that the IN exendin-4/CPP combined with the supplementary insulin resulted in a therapeutic response against severe cognitive deterioration in a senescence-accelerated animal model of cognitive dysfunction as tested via the Morris water maze test [135].

The IN delivery of proteins is equally gathering substantial interest amongst pharmaceutical scientists. For example, neurotrophic factors have enormous potential as protein therapeutics in the CNS, but their use has been severely limited due to delivery issues and systemic adverse effects. Insulin-like growth factor-1 (IGF-1) is one of the most effective proteins delivered to the brain via the IN route. Thorne et al. demonstrated that the IN administration of recombinant human IGF-1, wherein [$^{125}$I]-IGF-1 was dispersed in PBS containing 0.25% BSA, resulted in substantially higher CNS concentrations of the drug than the equivalent IV dosage [188]. These studies were among the first to indicate widespread distribution of a protein inside the CNS, possibly by utilising the olfactory and trigeminal nerve pathways. Lin et al. [189] demonstrated that IN administration of recombinant human IGF-1 enhanced neurobehavioral functions, decreased apoptotic cell death, and boosted the proliferation of neuronal and oligodendroglial progenitors in neonatal rats 1 h after hypoxic-ischemic brain injury.

The 18 kDa polypeptide growth factor basic fibroblast growth factor (bFGF) exhibits neuroprotective effects in a variety of brain-related illnesses. In a study conducted by Zhang et al., bFGF coupled with functionalized Solanum tuberosum lectin NPs (STL–PEG–PLGA NPs) (120 nm and negative surface charge) was delivered intranasally in an AD mouse model. The results revealed that the IN administration of NPs increased the AUC of radio-labeled-bFGF by 1.5 times when compared to the free protein, and the modification with the targeting ligand enhanced the value of the AUC by up to 3 times more [150]. In an ischemic rat model, bFGF encapsulated in gelatine NLC (128 nm and negatively charged) comprising phospholipids, cholesterol, and Poloxamer 118, was evaluated. As compared to IV, the results showed 1.5 times more protein accumulation in different brain areas, as well as an improved therapeutic response [190]. The same nanocarrier was employed to deliver bFGF for PD treatment. The findings revealed high protein levels in various areas of the brain, including the olfactory bulb and striatum, as well as an improvement in their therapeutic effect after IN administration in a PD rat model, when compared to free protein and IV administration of the nanoencapsulated protein [156].

Monoclonal antibodies (mAbs) have received special attention among biologics recently, resulting in a rising number of therapeutic antibodies in clinical trials and even on the market [191,192]. As of 2021, the FDA had approved 103 therapeutic antibody drugs including the use of aducanumab (marketed as Aduhelm®) for the treatment of Alzheimer's, clearing the path for future research into antibody-based treatments for other CNS diseases [193,194]. Nevertheless, only a few researchers have looked into IN delivery of an antibody to the CNS since their high molecular mass (~150 kDa) and polarity prevent BBB penetration. In a study, a TNF-α inhibitory single-chain Fv antibody fragment (scFv) (ESBA105) was delivered intranasally through Pz-peptide (4-phenylazobenzoxycarbonyl-Pro-Leu-Gly-Pro-DArg) in mice [195]. The addition of a penetration-enhancing peptide to the formulation increased the antibody distribution to the olfactory bulb and cerebrum while reducing systemic exposure. Similarly, anti-TRAIL antibodies adsorbed onto the surface of PLGA and NLC NPs were shown to swiftly and efficiently reach the CNS in mice following IN delivery. Another example includes the delivery of active-containing PLGA NPs coupled with mAb anti-EPH3 and trimethyl chitosan coating [196]. This strategy is based on the anti-EPH3 antibodies' ability to target a membrane receptor that is overexpressed in the stroma and vasculature of gliomas. In a glioma rat model, the NPs were loaded with temozolomide and delivered intranasally. Although the antibody in this case is effectively used as an excipient, it still suggests that the nasal route can be suitable for the delivery of large molecules. Fluorescence imaging revealed that NPs functionalized with anti-EPH3 antibodies accumulated in the brain more than non-functionalized NPs. These results suggest that the IN route can be an excellent, simple, and effective non-invasive method in the treatment of CNS disorders such as AD [197].

The IN route has been similarly studied for the delivery of nucleotide-based drugs. The importance of oligonucleotide therapy in the treatment of chronic inflammatory respiratory diseases is comprehensively discussed in a review published by Mehta et al where they also emphasised the importance of delivery routes including nasal administration [198]. Many investigations have employed the olfactory pathway to transport oligonucleotides or oligonucleotide-loaded nanoparticles [199–207] to the brain. Current research has concentrated on cell-penetrating peptide (CPP)-based delivery methods for the treatment of neurodegenerative illnesses, which have significant transmembrane capabilities and tremendous therapeutic potential [208]. For example, CPP Tat linked to ethylene glycol-polycaprolactone copolymers (mPEG-PCLTat/siRNA nanomicelles) when delivered intranasally showed superior siRNA targeting to the brain while reducing systemic toxicity [199]. The findings suggested that mPEGPCL-Tat has a role in delivering greater levels of siRNA to the brain via a non-invasive IN route using the trigeminal and olfactory nerve pathways. The results also indicated that the findings might be used in the treatment of persistent neuropsychiatric illnesses, brain tumors, and cerebral infarction. Similarly, in a study by Yang et al., a cell-penetrating peptide (DP7-C) encapsulated with hyaluronic acid (HA) was developed to create multifunctional core-shell structure nanomicelles (HA/DP7-C) [200]. To test its efficacy in glioma, siRNA was encapsulated within the nanomicelles and delivered intranasally to rats. In the in vitro studies, the nanomicelles demonstrated high cell uptake and minimal cytotoxicity. In vivo investigations revealed that IN delivery of the HA/DP7-C siRNA reached the CNS via the trigeminal nerve route within hours. Moreover, higher accumulation was seen near the tumor site, which might be explained by the interaction of HA with the hyaluronate receptor (CD44). The effective administration of an anti-glioma siRNA in GL261 tumor-bearing mice resulted in tumor growth suppression and increased survival time. Moreover, toxicology testing on rats revealed no harmful effects on the trigeminal nerves or nasal mucosa; hence, it could be concluded that the HA/DP7-C could be a potential delivery system for siRNA delivery via the IN route for glioma treatment.

Nowadays, antisense nucleotides (ASOs) have gained prominence in the treatment of a variety of illnesses, including neurodegenerative and neuromuscular disorders [201]. But still, the clinical effectiveness of ASOs is limited by their fast clearance and vulnerability to nucleases [202]. In a study, using the emulsification solvent evaporation process, nasal mucoadhesive microparticles were formulated for the delivery of phosphorothioate ASO (PTO-ODNs) [209]. PTO-ODN microparticles were either coated with the mucoadhesive polymer polycarbophil–cysteine (PCP–Cys) or with unmodified PCP and reduced glutathione (GSH). They showed slower clearance from the nasal cavity, a longer contact time with the nasal mucosa, high stability, better ASO penetration, and controlled release. The nano/microparticles resulted in a 2.2-fold increased absorption from the nasal mucosa, suggesting their suitability as carriers for IN delivery of ASOs. Vetter et al. investigated the role of thiolated polycarbophil as a multifunctional adjuvant in the IN administration of ASOs [210]. They found that the ASO uptake from the nasal mucosa increased by 1.7-fold in the presence of 0.45% thiolated polycarbophil and 0.5% glutathione. These findings suggested that thiolated polycarbophil/GSH might also be a viable excipient for nasal delivery of ASOs and useful in enhancing transport across the nasal mucosa without affecting its morphology.

Neurosteroids, generated in the glial cells and neurons in the CNS, are powerful endogenous neuromodulators and have been found to have diverse functions in the CNS [211,212]. Sex hormones such as progesterone, testosterone, and oestradiol have been reported to have specialized functions in normal or pathological brain function, such as impacts on cognition, anxiety, depression, appetite management, emotion, motivation, and motor abilities [25,213–223]. There is substantial evidence that these steroids are absorbed into nasal mucosal capillaries and subsequently transferred from venous circulation through the BBB into the brain, but a portion of the dose is delivered straight to the brain, circumventing the BBB upon IN administration. As a result, after deposition into the nose, the relative concentrations of these steroids in particular brain areas (e.g., olfactory bulb) closer to the nasal cavity were found to be greater [213,214].

Pregnenolone, the precursor of neuronal progesterone, is acquired from the circulation or by local de novo synthesis from cholesterol and is then converted to progesterone by 3-hydroxysteroid dehydrogenase [25,213,214]. In research conducted by Ducharme et al., radio-labeled pregnenolone and progesterone administered intranasally in an oleogel formulation (a viscous castor oil mixture, MetP Pharma AG, Emmetten, Switzerland) appeared to target the brain more efficiently than IV treatment in CD-1 mice [215]. Pregnenolone-induced memory improvement and anxiety reduction associated with progesterone indicated that therapeutic amounts of neurosteroids were achieved in the brain following IN administration using these formulations. Similarly, IN administration of progesterone (0.5, 1.0, or 2.0 mg/kg) using proprietary MetP Pharma oleogel, to male Wistar rats (5 µL each) resulted in an immediate substantial rise in dopamine levels in the basolateral amygdala and a delayed significant increase in the neostriatum. Based on the findings, the authors concluded the potential of progesterone in increasing dopamine levels in the brain. Another study developed oestradiol and progesterone formulations by dissolving them in ethanol with randomly methylated β-cyclodextrin (RAMEB) (molar ratio 1:2) to form inclusion complexes to improve their solubility [217,218]. To achieve the final oestradiol and progesterone formulations, ethanol was evaporated under a moderate nitrogen stream (50 °C), and the inclusion complexes were dissolved in sterile saline. Two percent (*w*/*v*) of oestradiol and 9% (*w*/*v*) of progesterone formulations attained $C_{max}$ levels in plasma and CSF within 15 min after IN administration in rats. Similarly, Wang et al. used the microdialysis method to investigate the absorption of oestradiol in rats using formulations based on RAMEB inclusion complexes [219]. The results showed that oestradiol was carried into CSF via olfactory neurons, indicating a direct transport pathway from the nose to CSF.

Testosterone is an endogenous steroid that has essential functions in both peripheral tissues and the CNS. IN administration of testosterone in CD-1 mice using Noseafix® (patented gel formulation) resulted in brain targeting, especially in the olfactory bulb, hypothalamus, striatum, and hippocampus [220]. Silva et al. delivered testosterone intranasally to anesthetized male rats, and its effects on the activity of dopaminergic and serotonergic neurons were examined. Testosterone treatment using proprietary MetP Pharma oleogel in both nostrils of Wister rats resulted in increased levels of dopamine and serotonin in the neostriatum and nucleus accumbens. Based on these findings, the authors concluded that IN testosterone delivery is more effective in reaching the brain than the subcutaneous route and may be used to activate the central dopaminergic and serotonergic systems. In addition, Zang et al. reported that IN administration of testosterone dissolved in sesame oil enhances mobility, exploratory activity, and motor and grooming behavior in rats. In rats, intranasally delivered allopregnanolone at a concentration of 16 mg/mL in an aqueous solution containing 0.9% NaCl and 40% sulfobutylether-β-cyclodextrin protected rats against seizures without inducing behavioral adverse effects, indicating direct N2B transport with preferential transport to seizure-relevant brain regions [223]. Table 3 summarizes various biologics used for direct N2B delivery.

**Table 3.** Intranasal delivery of biologics for CNS delivery.

| Active | Mol wt. (kDa) | Carrier System | Formulation Type | Species | Observations | Potential Treatment/Application | Ref |
|---|---|---|---|---|---|---|---|
| Arginine-vasopressin (AVP) | 1.1 | -- | AVP (10 IU) in 10 µL sterile water was administered via Rhintile (Ferring, Germany) (0.2 mL per nostril) | Human | Amplified P3 component of event-related potentials (ERPs) in brain | Increased brain activity | [224] |
| Angiotensin II (ANG II) | 1.0 | ANG II diluted in sterile 0.9% NaCl solution | Spray-single intranasal puffs of 100 µL (dose of 400 µg ANGII) within 1 min | Human | Acutely increased blood pressure by directly influencing the CNS; maintained plasma norepinephrine levels | Regulation in blood pressure in CNS | [225] |
| Activin A and Serpin B2 | 26.2<br>45–47 | Tetradecyl-β-D-maltoside (TDM) | 1 µg each of Activin A, SerpinB2, GFP, ΔNpas4, or 1 µg Activin A + 1 µg SerpinB2 in 20 µL, with or without TDM | Mouse | Maintains the structural and functional integrity of neurons, slows down the progressive cognitive disease | Alzheimer's disease, Huntington's disease, and amyotrophic lateral sclerosis, Parkinson's disease, brain damage and stroke | [226] |
| Apomorphine | 0.285 | Polycarbonate nanoparticles | Free AMP/polymer conjugated AMP in PBS | Mouse | Improved bioavailability | Parkinson's disease | [149] |
| Anti-trail monoclonal antibody | 40 | PLGA nanoparticles and NLCs | Solution | Mouse | Reduced neuroinflammation | Alzheimer's disease, Parkinson's disease, Epilepsy | [197] |
| Brain-derived neurotrophic factor (BDNF) with co-delivery of simvastatin | 14 | PEG-PLA polymersomes and pluronic F127 | Polymersome formulations: prepared at 1 µg/mL BDNF loading, simvastatin concentration varied at 5, 10, and 20 µg/mL | Mouse | Maintains and protects neurons. Attenuates lipopolysaccharide-induced inflammation | Alzheimer's disease, Parkinson's disease, Huntington's disease, Multiple sclerosis | [227] |
| BDNF | 26.9 | --- | 70 µg of neurotrophic factor in 70 µL sterile PBS | Rat | Neuroprotective improvement | Parkinson's disease, Multiple sclerosis | [15] |
| Basic fibroblast growth factor (BFGF) | 18 | Gelatin NLCs | Suspension (2 mg/mL) | Rat | Neuroprotective improvement | Parkinson's disease | [156] |

**Table 3.** *Cont.*

| Active | Mol wt. (kDa) | Carrier System | Formulation Type | Species | Observations | Potential Treatment/Application | Ref |
|---|---|---|---|---|---|---|---|
| Calcitonin gene-related peptide | 3.8 | -- | 1 μg CGRP in 50 μL water, 10 injections (5 μL each), alternating nostrils, 2 min interval | Rat | Reduced vasospasm, improved cerebral blood flow, reduced cell death, and stimulated angiogenesis following subarachnoid haemorrhage | Cerebral vasospasm | [228] |
| | | Acidic and basic gelatin | Salmon calcitonin gelatin microspheres (swelling in pH 7 PBS) and sCT solution (0.1 mL/kg, pH 7.0 PBS) via intranasal route at 15.0 U/kg | Rat | Improved nasal absorption of the drug | Improved nasal absorption of the drug | [229] |
| | | Pheroid™ | Pheroid vesicles and microsponges loaded with salmon calcitonin, *N*-trimethyl chitosan chloride (TMC) saline solution | Rat | Improved nasal absorption of the drug | --- | [230] |
| Cholecystokinin-8 | 1.1 | --- | CCK8 dissolved in sterile water and dose of 5 μg was sprayed in each nostril (solution) | Human | Amplified P3 component of auditory evoked potentials as well as plasma corticotropin levels. | Increased brain activity | [231] |
| Cystatin C-peptide | 13 | --- | 20 μg of CysC-AβBP and scrambled peptide (solution) | Mouse | Reduces amyloid aggregates and improves memory | Alzheimer's disease | [232] |
| Caspase-1 inhibitor | 17 | -- | Caspase-1 inhibitor (5 μg/μL) administered via nose drops (2.5 μL/drop) over 20 min, for a total volume of 20 μL (solution) | Rat | Decreases hippocampal neuronal loss and improves neurocognitive action | Global cerebral ischemia | [233] |
| TNF-α siRNA | NA | Cationic nanoemulsion | 5 μL/nostril of siRNA nanoemulsion or saline solution, 1 min hold between doses | Rat | Site-specific downregulation of TNF-α cytokines | Prevention of neuroinflammation | [164] |

**Table 3.** *Cont.*

| Active | Mol wt. (kDa) | Carrier System | Formulation Type | Species | Observations | Potential Treatment/Application | Ref |
|---|---|---|---|---|---|---|---|
| Erythropoietin (EPO) | 30.4 | --- | 20 μL volumes of 0.6, 2.4, 6, and 12 U rhEPO/20 μL sterile saline delivered to each nostril | Mouse | Improves neurological- function, memory alterations, reduces infarct volume and improves neurologic function | Alzheimer's disease, cerebral ischemia, epilepsy | [234] |
| | | | EPO diluted in PBS (pH 7.0) at 0.15 Mm. Administration at 125 and 250 μg/kg | Mouse | Alleviated memory alterations, oxidative stress, neuroinflammation, apoptosis induction, and amyloid load | Cerebral ischemia, neuroinflammation, Alzheimer's disease | [235] |
| Exendin (9–39) | 4.186 | Pegylated Ex-4 | PEGEx-4 analogs in 100 mM PBS pH 7.4 | Rat | Reduces the insulin responses to enteral glucose | Congenital hyperinsulinism | [236] |
| Radio-labeled exendin (9–39) (I-Ex) | 3.4 | Cyclodextrin | 2 μL of phosphate buffer/normal saline with 500,000 cpm of I-Ex ± 5% β-cyclodextrin (CD) | Mouse | Improved brain uptake | CNS disorders | [187] |
| Full-length IgG | 150 | --- | Aβ25–35 + Glu-Ab: 300 μg/kg Glu-Ab water solution Aβ25–35 + γ-globulin: 300 μg/kg rabbit γ-globulin water solution | Rat | Anti-amnesic effect in an AD model; improved conditioned passive avoidance response following ischemia | Alzheimer's disease, ischemic injury | [237] |
| Galanin-like peptide (radioactively labeled) | 6.5 | α-cyclodextrin, dimethyl β-cyclodextrin | 2 μL of 250,000 cpm/μL I-GALP alone, with cyclodextrins (β-CD or α-CD), or with 1 μg/mouse unlabeled GALP solution | Mouse | Increased brain uptake | Eating regulation | [238] |
| H102 peptide (novel β-sheet breaker peptide) | NA | Liposomes egg phosphatidylcholine, DSPE–PEG, and cholesterol | H102 solution (2 mg/kg) with 1% chitosan, 0.1% BSA, and H102 liposomes (2 mg/kg) | Mouse | Improved spatial memory impairment and enhanced brain bioavailability | Alzheimer's disease | [239] |
| Human nerve growth factor | | 26.5 | 1 M phosphate-buffered saline (PBS, pH 7.4) | Rat | Improved memory and enhanced neurogenesis | Alzheimer's disease | [240] |

**Table 3.** *Cont.*

| Active | Mol wt. (kDa) | Carrier System | Formulation Type | Species | Observations | Potential Treatment/Application | Ref |
|---|---|---|---|---|---|---|---|
| Gly14-humanin (S14G-HN) | NA | Odorranalectin cubosomes | 1.0 mg/kg of cubosomes (10 µL per nostril) in 10 mmol PBS (pH 7.4) | Rat | Improved brain bioavailability and therapeutic activity | Alzheimer's disease | [241] |
| Insulin | 5.8 | Penetratin CPP | Exendin-4 solution (1 mg/mL) with L-penetratin (2 mM) ± insulin (8 IU/mL) | Mouse | Protection against neurodegeneration and improved brain bioavailability, partial neuroprotection | Alzheimer's disease, mild cognitive impairment | [135] |
| | | Penetratin CPP | L- or D-penetratin in pH 6.0 PBS with 0.001% methylcellulose, mixed with insulin to achieve 30 IU/mL and 2.0 mM solution | Mouse | Improved absorption of Insulin via nasal cavity | Alzheimer's disease, mild cognitive impairment | [177] |
| | | Liposome suspension | Suspension | Mouse | Enhanced permeation vs. insulin solution | ----- | [180] |
| | | Maltodextrin DE 3/22/ + Carbopol® 974P (90/10) DE 38 + (80/20) | Powder | Rabbit | Improved brain bioavailability | Alzheimer's disease | [242] |
| | | Starch + sodium glycodeoxycholate (GDC) 0.08 mg/kg starch microspheres + LPC 0.05 mg/kg | Powder | Sheep | Improved brain bioavailability | Alzheimer's disease | [243] |
| | | Maize starch + Carbopol® 974P (90/10), drum dried waxy maize starch. (DDWM)/Carbopol® 974P (90/10) or a spray-dried mixture of Amioca starch/Carbopol® 974P (25/75) | Powder | Rabbit | Improved brain bioavailability | ----- | [183] |

**Table 3.** *Cont.*

| Active | Mol wt. (kDa) | Carrier System | Formulation Type | Species | Observations | Potential Treatment/Application | Ref |
|---|---|---|---|---|---|---|---|
| | | Poly (N-vinyl pyrrolidone)-based nanogels | Gels | Mouse | High biocompatibility, no immunogenicity, rapid clearance within 24 h, enhanced delivery to all brain regions vs. free insulin | Alzheimer's disease | [179] |
| | | Polyacrylic acid | Gels | Mouse | Improved absorption of Insulin via nasal cavity | ------ | [181] |
| Insulin-like growth factor I | 7.650 | -- | 10 mM sodium succinate buffer containing 140 mM sodium chloride at pH 6.0 | Mouse | Enhances neurological function and prevents apoptosis, reduced infarct volume/brain oedema and enhanced neurologic function; in neonatal rats; prevented apoptosis after hypoxic-ischemic damage | Focal cerebral ischemic damage | [244] |
| | | | PBS solution containing 0.25% BSA | Mouse | Reduction in stroke volume and improved behavioral patterns | Alzheimer's disease, stroke | [188] |
| | | | PBS solution containing 0.25% BSA | Rat | Improved neurobehavioral performance, inhibition of apoptotic cell death | Cerebral hypoxia-ischemia | [189] |
| Interferon β1b | 18.5 | -- | Aqueous solution of human recombinant IFN-β and [$^{125}$I]-labeled human recombinant IFN-β at pH 4. | Adult cynomolgus monkey | Showed central distribution of the macromolecule along the olfactory and trigeminal pathway | Multiple sclerosis | [245] |
| | 19.86 | | $^{125}$I-IFNh-1b + rhIFNh-1b solution (1.53 mg/mL) | Rat | Produced tyrosine phosphorylation of IFN receptor in the CNS | Multiple sclerosis | [246] |
| Interleukin-1 receptor antagonist | 17 | N-trimethyl chitosan nanoparticles | Leu-Enk-loaded TMC nanoparticles (0.1 mg/mL in PBS pH 6.8) via a 50 μL Hamilton micro syringe | Rat | Protects neurons and improves neurological deficit | Cerebral ischemia | [151] |
| Leptin | 16 | Sodium taurodihydrofusidiate | 50 μL of 0.2, 0.1, and 0.03 mg/kg leptin solutions in 0.9% NaCl with 1% STDHF | Rat | Inhibits appetite | Obesity | [247] |

**Table 3.** *Cont.*

| Active | Mol wt. (kDa) | Carrier System | Formulation Type | Species | Observations | Potential Treatment/Application | Ref |
|---|---|---|---|---|---|---|---|
| mi R124 | 7.20 | PEG-PLGA nanoparticles | Emulsion | Rat | Relieved symptoms of cerebral ischemia-reperfusion damage, provides neuroprotection | Neurodegenerative diseases | [206] |
| miR132 | 14.084 | Fatty acid-modified octa-arginine CPP nanocomplexes | Suspension | Rat | Improved learning and memory | Alzheimer's disease | [207] |
| m-RNA | | Cationic liposomes | Solution | Rat | Improved brain bioavailability | Alzheimer's disease | [20] |
| NAP neuropeptide | 0.825 | Lactoferrin-conjugated PEG–PCLA | 20 µL nanoparticle solution containing 5 µg coumarin-6 | Rat | Improves neuroprotection and memory | Alzheimer's disease, schizophrenia, frontotemporal dementia Huntington's disease | [248] |
| Neuropeptide Substance P | 1.347 | Gelatine-cored nanostructured lipid carriers | Suspension | Rat | Demonstrated behavioral improvement and initiation of dopaminergic neuron recovery | Parkinson's disease | [249] |
| Neurotrophin-4 | 22.4 | -- | 70 µg of neurotrophic factor in 70 µL sterile PBS | Rat | Improves neuronal survival | Multiple sclerosis | [15] |
| Neurotoxin I | 6.9 | PLA nanoparticles | NT-I-NPs (45 mg lyophilized nanoparticles dissolved in 0.15 mL PBS with 1:1 polysorbate 80 | Rat | Enhanced brain bioavailability and facilitated brain transport of NT-I | Centrally active peptides | [250] |
| Neurotoxin 1 | 6.95 | PLA nanoparticles coated with polysorbate 80 | NT-P-NP (45 mg lyophilized nanoparticles in 0.15 mL PBS with 1:1 polysorbate 80, 17 mg NT/kg) and free NT solution | Mouse | Inhibits neurotransmission | Pain management | [251] |
| NR2B9c | 0.977 | WGA-functionalized PLA–PEG NPs | NR2B9c-NPs and WGA-NPs dispersed in physiological saline | Rat | Protects neurons against excitotoxicity, decreases ischemic brain injury and offers neurological function deficits | Ischemic stroke | [252] |

**Table 3.** *Cont.*

| Active | Mol wt. (kDa) | Carrier System | Formulation Type | Species | Observations | Potential Treatment/Application | Ref |
|---|---|---|---|---|---|---|---|
| Oxytocin | 1 | Oxytocin | Spray | Monkey, rabbit | Reduces anxiolytic effects social stress and enhances empathy. Increased trust; decreased stress-related cortisol; enhanced capacity to predict others' mental states; slowed amygdala response to fear in GAD; improved emotional identification in autism | Autism spectrum disorder, schizophrenia | [253] |
| | | | OXT dissolved at 40 mg/mL in purified water | Rat | Improved brain bioavailability | Autism | [254] |
| | | | Intranasal spray or nebulizer | Monkey | Influences social cognition and behavior, increased level of oxytocin in CSF | Autism spectrum disorder, schizophrenia | [255] |
| Orexin-A (hypocretin-1) | 3.5 | -- | Solution in PBS (spray) | Monkey | Reverses sleep deprivation | Narcolepsy | [256] |
| | | 1% and 5% phenylephrine | Mixture of unlabeled and $^{125}$I-labeled neuropeptide dissolved in PBS (solution) | Rat | Enhanced CNS targeting | Autoimmune disorders, Alzheimer's disease or meningitis | [257] |
| Ovalbumin | 45 | Cationic liposomes | Solution in PBS | Rat | Improves bioavailability | Immunity booster | [121,258] |
| Pituitary adenylate cyclase-activating peptide (PACAP) | 4.5 | --- | Aqueous solution with NaCl, citric acid monohydrate, disodium phosphate dehydrate, and benzalkonium chloride | Mouse | Enhances cognitive function Stimulated non-amyloidogenic processing and improved cognitive function. | Alzheimer's disease, cerebral ischemia | [259] |
| Phosphorothioate antisense oligonucleotides (PTO-ODNs) | 5 | Polycarbophilcysteine or unmodified PCP and reduced glutathione (GSH) | Emulsion | Porcine nasal mucosa (in vitro/in vivo) | Induced controlled release | CNS diseases | [202] |
| | | Thiolated polycarbophil and 0.5% glutathione | Solution | Human nasal epithelial cells, Porcine nasal mucosa | Enhanced controlled release, improved uptake | CNS diseases | [209] |

**Table 3.** *Cont.*

| Active | Mol wt. (kDa) | Carrier System | Formulation Type | Species | Observations | Potential Treatment/Application | Ref |
|---|---|---|---|---|---|---|---|
| Ribonucleic acid (tRNA) | 0.284 | Cell-permeating peptide nanocomplexes | Buffered solution | Mouse | Increases potentially therapeutic miRNA | Alzheimer's disease | [207] |
| [Ser(2)]exendin (1–9) +GLP 1 | NA | 10% β-cyclodextrin | Buffered solution | Mouse | Improved learning and memory, provides neuroprotection, lowers rates of kainic-induced apoptosis | Neurodegenerative and cognitive disorders | [186] |
| siRNA | 13–14 | MPEG-PCL-TAT nanomicelles | Alexa dextran solution | Mouse | MPEG-PCL TAT accelerated transport along the olfactory and trigeminal nerve pathways | Alzheimer's disease, Parkinson's disease and brain tumor | [199] |
| | 3.5–1350 | HA/DP7-C nanomicelles | Buffered solution | Rat | Inhibited tumor growth, reduced cytotoxicity | Glioblastoma therapy | [200] |
| | | Biodegradable PAMAM dendrimer | PBS solution | Rat | Target gene knockdown and neuroprotection, reduced infarct volumes and alleviated neurological and behavioral deficits | Postischemic brain disorders | [201] |
| BACE1 siRNA + Rapamycin | NA | PEGylated dendrigraft poly-L-lysines | Buffered solution | Rat | Improved cognition, promoted autophagy and improved nasal adsorption | Alzheimer's disease | [260] |
| i-NOS siRNA | NA | Gelatin NPs | PBS solution | Rat | Higher therapeutic potency compared to naked siRNA | Postischemic brain disorders | [261] |
| Thyrotropin-releasing hormone | 0.362 | D, L PLA NPs | Suspension | Rat | Recovers neuron and improves behavior | Epilepsy, seizures | [262] |
| Thyrotrophin-releasing hormone analogs | NA | PLA-co-glycolide NPs | Suspension | Rat | Improved target efficiency and reduced seizures | Epilepsy, seizures | [263] |
| TNF-α inhibitory single-chain antibody fragment | 26.3 | CPP (Pz-peptide) + penetration enhancer | Buffered solution | Mouse | Enhanced cognitive performance, reduced cerebral amyloid angiopathy and amyloid plaque pathology | Alzheimer's disease, Parkinson's disease, multiple sclerosis | [196] |

**Table 3.** *Cont.*

| Active | Mol wt. (kDa) | Carrier System | Formulation Type | Species | Observations | Potential Treatment/Application | Ref |
|---|---|---|---|---|---|---|---|
| Urocortin | <10 | Odorranalectin-conjugated PEG-PLGA NPs | OL-NPs dispersed in PBS Solution pH 7.4 | Rat | Improved bioavailability and therapeutic action | Parkinson's disease | [264] |
| Vascular endothelial growth factor | 38.2 | PEG-PLA NPs VEGF was radio-labeled with sodium $^{125}I$ using chloramines T method | 100 µL of VEGF solution | Rat | Develops behavior and enhances angiogenesis, decreased systemic side effects, increased neurotrophic and neuroprotective activity | Alzheimer's disease, CNS diseases | [265,266] |
| Vasoactive intestinal peptide | 16.6 | WGA-functionalized PEG-PLA NPs | 0.01 M HEPES buffer (pH 8.5) containing 0.1 mM $CaCl_2$ | Rat | Improved brain bioavailability and drug uptake | Alzheimer's disease | [267] |
| Plasmid DNA | 1950 ± 70 | Poloxamer 188 and 107 with polyethylene oxide and polycarbophil | 100 µL of plasmid DNA in 20 mL solution | Rat | Expression of encoded protein in brain and improved nasal adsorption | Alzheimer's disease | [208] |
| Progesterone | 0.314 | Viscous castor oil-based gels | Oleogel | Rat | Enhanced brain bioavailability, reduced anxiety and depression | Cognitive impairment, Alzheimer's disease, Parkinson's disease, and brain damage | [219–221] |
| Testosterone | 0.288 | | | | | | |
| Oestradiol | 0.272 | | | | | | |

## 6. Nasally Administered Biologics Currently on the Market and in Clinical Trials

Despite the success of N2B delivery at preclinical and sometimes clinical levels, screening of the drug base bank reveals a limited number of successfully marketed biologics, as shown in Table 4. A few decades ago, the majority of marketed medications were hormones, marking the first milestone in biologic nasal delivery. For example, the peptide buserelin (gonadotropin-releasing hormone (GnRh) analogue) is delivered nasally to treat hormone-dependent metastatic prostate cancer. It is quickly broken down completely in the digestive tract when taken orally and has a bioavailability of 2–3% when administered intranasally—at least in the current formulation. The IN bioavailability of buserelin is also substantially lower compared to subcutaneous injection (70%), but that is still effective against advanced prostate cancer and endometriosis [268]. Desmopressin, an antidiuretic hormone, is sold under the brand names Minirin™, Ddavp™, Noctiva™, Octostim spray™, and Stimate™ for the treatment of nocturnal enuresis and central cranial diabetes insipidus. The bioavailability of desmopressin following nasal administration is 10–20 times that of oral administration [269]. Glucagon is a peptide hormone that is administered intramuscularly to treat type 1 diabetes in youth. The bioavailability of glucagon nasal powder with the absorption enhancer dodecylphosphocholine was equivalent to that of an intramuscular glucagon injection [270]. Both intramuscular and IN (Baqsimi™) formulations of glucagon result in similar pharmacokinetic profile (reaching $C_{max}$ with 5 min). Nafarelin, commonly known as Synarel™, is a IN GnRH agonist spray that is used to treat endometriosis and early puberty [271]. It is also used to treat uterine fibroids, to control ovarian stimulation during IVF, and as part of transgender hormone therapy. IN salmon calcitonin (Miacalcin™ or Fortical™) is a peptide approved by the FDA for the treatment of osteoporosis in women over the age of 50 [272]. Table 4 lists intranasally administered biologics available on the market.

Table 5 lists the current status of clinical trials using biologics for the N2B delivery for several CNS disorders.

**Table 4.** Intranasally administered biologics available in the market.

| Drug | Drug Bank Accession No. | Biological Entity/Type | Condition/s | Brand Name | Marketed by | Market Approval Year | Ref. |
|---|---|---|---|---|---|---|---|
| Buserelin | DB06719 | Protein based | Prostate cancer, breast cancer, endometriosis, Uterine fibroids | Suprefact Intranasal solution 1 mg/mL (spray) | Hoechst Canada Inc. (Quebec, QC, Canada) | 1988 | [273] |
| | | | | Superfact Liq 1mg/mL (liquid) | Hoechst Roussel Canada Inc. (Montreal, QC, Canada) | 1993 | [172] |
| | | | | Superfact (solution) | Sanofi Aventis | 1998 | [274] |
| | | | | Suprecur (0.15 mg/spray) | Sanofi Aventis | 2001 | [273] |
| Desmopressin | DB00035 | Peptide drug | Nocturia, central cranial diabetes insipidus | Ddvap (0.01 mg/spray) | Ferring Pharmaceuticals Inc. (Saint-Prex, Switzerland) (discontinued) | 1978 | [274] |
| | | | | Ddvap (solution) | Sanofi Aventis | 1978 | [274] |
| | | | | Minirin (0.015 mg/spray) | Ferring Pharmaceuticals Inc. (discontinued) | 2000 | [274] |
| | | | | Noctiva (spray) | Avadel Speciality Pharmaceuticals LLC (Dublin, Ireland) (discontinued) | 2017 | [172] |
| | | | | Octostim Spray (1.5 mg/mL, spray) | Ferring Pharmaceuticals Inc. | 1998 | [273] |
| | | | | Stimate (1.5 mg/spray) | Ferring Pharmaceuticals Inc. (discontinued) | 2011 | [274] |
| Glucagon | DB00040 | Protein based | Severe hypoglycemia | Baqsimi (3 mg powder) | Eli Lilly & Co. Ltd. (Basingstoke, UK) | 2019 | [274] |
| Nafarelin | DB00666 | Synthetic agonist of gonadotrophin-releasing hormone | Central precocious, puberty, Endometriosis | Synarel (0.2 mg/ spray) | Pfizer Canada Ulc (Montreal, QC, Canada) | 1996 | [273,274] |
| | | | | Synarel (spray) | G.D. Searle LLC (Skokie, IL, USA) | 1990 | |
| | | | | Synarel (liquid) | Syntex Inc. (Houston, TX, USA) | 1991 | |
| Salmon calcitonin | DB00017 | Hormone | Paget's disease, osteoporosis | Fortical (200 IU/spray) | Upsher-Smith Laboratories (discontinued) | 2005 | [172,273,274] |
| | | | | Fortical (200 IU/spray) | Physicians Total Care, Inc. (Tulsa, OK, USA) | 2005 | |
| | | | | Miacalcin (200 IU/spray) | Novartis | 1995 | |
| Oxytocin | DB00107 | Peptide drug | Labour induction | Syntocinon (40 IU/mL, solution, spray) | Novartis | 1960 | [172,273] |

**Table 5.** Intranasally administered biologics under clinical investigation as enrolled at www.clinicaltrials.gov (accessed on 3 November 2023) [275].

| Drug | Study Title | Disease | Status | Year | Identifier |
|---|---|---|---|---|---|
| Insulin (Humulin R® U-100) | Study of nasal insulin to fight forgetfulness | Alzheimer's disease | Phase II and III completed | December 2018 | NCT01767909 |
| Insulin | Intranasal Insulin and Post-Stroke Cognition: A Pilot Study | Stroke | Phase II completed | March 2020 | NCT02810392 |
| Insulin analogue | Efficacy and Safety of Human Insulin Versus Analogue Insulin in Hospitalized Acute Stroke Patients with Hyperglycaemia | Stroke, hyperglycemia | Phase IV completed | June 2020 | NCT04834362 |
| Insulin aspart | Intranasal Insulin and Memory in Early AD | Alzheimer's disease | Phase I and II completed | May 2012 | NCT00581867 |
| Insulin aspart | Nasal Insulin to Fight Forgetfulness—Short-Acting Insulin | Alzheimer's disease<br>Mild cognitive impairment | Phase II completed | April 2019 | NCT02462161 |
| Insulin (humulin R U-100) | SNIFF 120: Study of Nasal Insulin to Fight Forgetfulness (120 Days) | Alzheimer's disease<br>Mild cognitive impairment | Phase II completed | December 2011 | NCT00438568 |
| Insulin (humulin R U-100)<br>Empagliflozin | Nasal Insulin to Fight Forgetfulness—Combination of Intranasal Insulin and Empagliflozin Trial | Mild cognitive impairment<br>Cognitive impairment<br>Alzheimer's disease | Phase II recruiting | Started October 2021 | NCT05081219 |
| Insulin | Treatment of Parkinson's Disease and Multiple System Atrophy Using Intranasal insulin | Parkinson's disease | Phase II completed | September 2015 | NCT02064166 |
| Insulin detemir | Study of Nasal Insulin to Fight Forgetfulness—Long-acting Insulin Detemir—120 Days (SL120) | Alzheimer's disease | Phase II completed | March 2015 | NCT01595646 |
| Insulin detemir | To evaluate its defect in diseased patients | Alzheimer's disease | Phase II completed | December 2012 | NCT01547169 |
| Oxytocin (syntocinon) | Intranasal Oxytocin for the Treatment of children and Adolescents with ASD | Autism spectrum disorder (ASD) | Phase II Completed | March 2016 | NCT01908205 |
| Oxytocin | Oxytocin and Social Cognition in Frontotemporal Dementia | Dementia | Completed | November 2010 | NCT01002300 |
| Oxytocin | To study the effect of drugs on PDD | Depression<br>Premenstrual dysphoric disorder (PDD) | Completed | July 2016 | NCT02508103 |
| Oxytocin (syntocinon) | To evaluate the safety and efficacy of exogenous oxytocin on social cognition and behavior in patients with recent-onset schizophrenia | Schizophrenia<br>Psychotic disorders | Early phase I completed | August 2019 | NCT02567032 |
| Oxytocin | Target Engagement and Response to Oxytocin | Schizophrenia | Phase IV active, not recruiting | Started January 2018 | NCT03245437 |
| Oxytocin and vasopressin | Effects of IN oxytocin and vasopressin on social behavior and decision making | Social behavior | Completed | December 2022 | NCT04890470 |
| Vasopressin | Effect of intranasal vasopressin on cooperative behavior of patients | Schizophrenia | Completed | November 2018 | NCT04190004 |

**Table 5.** *Cont.*

| Drug | Study Title | Disease | Status | Year | Identifier |
|---|---|---|---|---|---|
| Vasopressin | Intranasal Vasopressin Treatment in Children With Autism | Autism<br>Autism spectrum disorder | Phase II and III Recruiting | February 2018 | NCT03204786 |
| Calcitonin | Long-term Safety Study of BHV-3500 (Zavegepant *) for the Acute Treatment of Migraine (* BHV-3500, formerly "vazegepant") | Acute treatment of migraine | Phase II and III completed | December 2021 | NCT04408794 |
| | A Study to Learn About Zavegepant as the Acute Treatment of Migraine in Asian Adults | Acute treatment of migraine | Not yet recruiting | Estimated November 2023 | NCT05989048 |
| Insulin + semaglutide | Combination of Intranasal Insulin with Oral Semaglutide to Improve Cognition and Cerebral Blood Flow: A Feasibility Study | Metabolic syndrome and mild cognitive impairment (MCI) | Phase II Recruiting | Estimated start December 2023. | NCT06072963 |
| Human fibroblast growth factor | Intranasal Human FGF-1 for Subjects with Parkinson's Disease | Parkinson's disease | Phase I, not yet recruiting | September 2022 | NCT05493462 |
| Foralumab | Phase 1b Multiple Ascending Dose Study of Foralumab in Primary and Secondary Progressive MS patients | Multiple sclerosis (MS) | Phase 1 (withdrawn) | Started October 2021 | NCT05029609 |
| Progesterone | To study the safety and efficacy of progesterone for the treatment of Acute Haemorrhagic Stroke | Brain injury, stroke | Phase IV (unknown status) | Started February 2020 | NCT04143880 |

## 7. General Comments and Concluding Remarks

N2B delivery is a non-invasive, convenient, and patient-friendly route of drug administration that has the potential to provide a fast onset of action with accurate drug targeting and reduced systemic side effects. Moreover, it can provide the added advantage of transporting the drug into the brain directly by avoiding the BBB. However, the clinical translation of IN formulations still has some way to go. N2B delivery has numerous limitations, including mucociliary clearance, enzymatic degradation, and possible drug/formulation-related mucosal toxicity and neurotoxicity, that limit its potential uptake by the pharmaceutical industry. There are formulation-specific problems (e.g., availability/suitability of excipients, stability, scale-up, etc.), which can make it less attractive in comparison to other well-established routes. Although options to address some of these issues are already available, concerns remain. For example, the application of the nanoparticles in IN formulations requires long-term biosafety data. Although most nanoparticles for IN delivery are formulated with well-studied natural or biocompatible (PLGA, PCL, etc.) polymers or lipids, the impact of other components in the formulation is frequently ignored. For instance, the long-term safety and impact of lectins on the nasal mucosa from formulations designed for chronic therapies are still understudied, which needs to be established for these bioligands to be accepted by scientists and industry. Similarly, the evidence available on the biocompatibility and toxicity of inorganic nanoparticles in IN formulations is at best controversial, which limits their application as viable carriers in N2B drug delivery. Moreover, the fate of nanoparticles, especially in long-term therapy, needs careful attention, as their accumulation in the brain or circulation in extracellular fluids would not be desirable.

Another significant challenge in N2B drug delivery originates from the limited understanding of the spatial distribution of drugs in the brain tissue upon application. Although direct routes involving neuronal pathways (e.g., olfactory and/or trigeminal nerve systems) and indirect absorption via vasculature and lymphatic systems are commonly proposed, the exact mechanisms of drug absorption are anything but fully established. A thorough understanding of these routes and whether one or various mechanisms contribute to drug transportation simultaneously needs to be established for the successful development of IN formulations. Another challenge in establishing IN delivery as a major platform is the availability of in vivo models. The use of rodents is widespread while studying IN delivery, but anatomical differences between human and rodent noses can make pre-clinical results difficult to translate. Although progress has been made in developing fluorescent probes, imaging techniques, and in vitro/in vivo models, a concerted effort is still required to gain further understanding of these mechanisms.

Mucociliary clearance is also a major challenge in the nasal administration of applied formulations. It is difficult to resolve this via traditional formulations such as sprays. Hence, formulators need to explore novel ways that can increase the residence time of the formulation within the nasal cavity. The application of bioadhesive hydrogels or oleogels can rectify this to a certain extent. In situ gel-forming formulations can allow easy application and enhance the retention of the formulation without needing highly specialized delivery devices. However, the suitability of excipients in the IN delivery once again needs to be established to increase the available options.

Also, in numerous instances, the drug reaching the CNS can be very small compared with the amount of drug applied in the nasal cavity. The major issue with N2B delivery is the difficulty in reaching the olfactory region and then limited absorption (for peptides and protein-based drugs) once it has reached there. The application of absorption enhancers and mucoadhesive polymers can help in addressing these challenges, but their long-term toxicity in chronic nasal therapy remains unexplored. It is important to establish this before new products are made available for the N2B delivery of drugs that are not readily absorbed across the nasal mucosa. Similarly, other strategies, including charge neutralisation, solubilisation with additives, and stealth approaches to evade immune clearance, also need to be investigated specifically for their application in N2B delivery systems.

The outlook for N2B drug delivery in the pharmaceutical landscape is marked by both challenges and promising advancements. While hurdles exist, ongoing studies are anticipated to address limitations and contribute to a better understanding of the mechanisms associated with this route of drug delivery. We believe that the focus of future efforts in this area will be on elucidating the mechanisms involved in drug delivery from the nasal cavity to the brain, with an emphasis on the importance of properly designed formulations. The choice of excipients, along with their acceptance by the pharmaceutical industry and regulatory authorities, would allow formulators to work in a wider space, which would help to tune current approaches and develop novel delivery platforms.

This review discussed the challenge of delivering pharmaceutical actives, especially molecules such as peptides and proteins, to the brain while circumventing the BBB. The N2B route can be highly promising where the application of nanocarriers, targeting ligands, and mucoadhesive agents can assist drug transport through the nasal mucosa and promote delivery to the brain. The current landscape of N2B drug delivery research reveals a substantial concentration of small-molecular-weight drugs, along with some peptides and proteins, at the preclinical stage. However, the translation of these promising preclinical findings to clinical applications has been notably limited, encompassing only a few specific types of drugs. The bottleneck appears to stem from challenges associated with finding appropriate excipients, moving laboratory-level formulations to large-scale production, the availability of suitable animal models, and ensuring drug uniformity and stability in formulations. There is no doubt that the ongoing development of formulation technology and our improved understanding of the excipients will yield the development of novel strategies for N2B drug delivery that can offer potential solutions to the longstanding challenges associated with delivering high-molecular-weight drugs to the brain. Nonetheless, N2B delivery, especially for biologics, is still underexplored, even using currently available approaches. Undoubtedly, an intensified approach to expanding and clinically applying available delivery strategies to a wider array of drugs is needed, considering the various advantages that this route offers. There are a number of small-to-large molecular-weight drugs currently in clinical trials, which is encouraging, and it provides an optimistic outlook for the N2B delivery of the pharmaceutical actives. It can be anticipated that the ongoing advancements in formulation technologies and excipient availability will pave the way for a more diversified and clinically impactful N2B drug delivery approach in the near future.

**Author Contributions:** Conceptualization, V.T. and C.M.; investigation, A.L.A. and E.J.P.; resources, V.T.; writing—original draft preparation, A.L.A. and E.J.P.; writing—review and editing, A.L.A., E.J.P., V.T. and C.M.; project administration, V.T. and C.M. All authors have read and agreed to the published version of the manuscript.

**Funding:** This research received no external funding.

**Data Availability Statement:** Not applicable.

**Conflicts of Interest:** The authors declare no conflicts of interest. Claudia Mattern affiliates to MetP Pharma AG, the company had no role in the design of the study; in the collection, analyses, or interpretation of data; in the writing of the manuscript; or in the decision to publish the results.

## References

1. Di Nunzio, J.C.; Williams, R.O. CNS disorders—Current treatment options and the prospects for Advanced Therapies. *Drug Dev. Ind. Pharm.* **2008**, *34*, 1141–1167. [CrossRef] [PubMed]
2. Kesselheim, A.S.; Hwang, T.J.; Franklin, J.M. Two decades of new drug development for Central Nervous System Disorders. *Nat. Rev. Drug Discov.* **2015**, *14*, 815–816. [CrossRef] [PubMed]
3. Crawford, L.; Rosch, J.; Putnam, D. Concepts, technologies, and practices for drug delivery past the blood–brain barrier to the Central Nervous System. *J. Control. Release* **2016**, *240*, 251–266. [CrossRef] [PubMed]
4. Pardridge, W.M. Why is the global CNS pharmaceutical market so under-penetrated? *Drug Discov. Today* **2002**, *7*, 5–7. [CrossRef] [PubMed]

5. Chen, Y.; Liu, L. Modern methods for delivery of drugs across the blood–brain barrier. *Adv. Drug Deliv. Rev.* **2012**, *64*, 640–665. [CrossRef] [PubMed]
6. Alam, M.I.; Beg, S.; Samad, A.; Baboota, S.; Kohli, K.; Ali, J.; Ahuja, A.; Akbar, M. Strategy for effective brain drug delivery. *Eur. J. Pharm. Sci.* **2010**, *40*, 385–403. [CrossRef] [PubMed]
7. Khafagy, E.-S.; Kamei, N.; Nielsen, E.J.B.; Nishio, R.; Takeda-Morishita, M. One-month subchronic toxicity study of cell-penetrating peptides for insulin nasal delivery in rats. *Eur. J. Pharm. Biopharm.* **2013**, *85 Pt A*, 736–743. [CrossRef]
8. Merenlender-Wagner, A.; Pikman, R.; Giladi, E.; Andrieux, A.; Gozes, I. Nap (davunetide) enhances cognitive behavior in the stop heterozygous mouse—A microtubule-deficient model of schizophrenia. *Peptides* **2010**, *31*, 1368–1373. [CrossRef] [PubMed]
9. Dufes, C.; Olivier, J.C.; Gaillard, F.; Gaillard, A.; Couet, W.; Muller, J.M. Brain delivery of vasoactive intestinal peptide (VIP) following nasal administration to rats. *Int. J. Pharm.* **2003**, *255*, 87–97. [CrossRef]
10. Pan, W.; Kastin, A.J. Urocortin and the brain. *Prog. Neurobiol.* **2008**, *84*, 148–156. [CrossRef]
11. Sayani, A.P.; Chun, I.K.; Chien, Y.W. Transmucosal delivery of leucine enkephalin: Stabilization in rabbit enzyme extracts and enhancement of permeation through mucosae. *J. Pharm. Sci.* **1993**, *82*, 1179–1185. [CrossRef] [PubMed]
12. Acharya, B.; Meka, R.R.; Venkatesha, S.H.; Lees, J.R.; Teesalu, T.; Moudgil, K.D. A novel CNS-homing peptide for targeting neuroinflammatory lesions in experimental autoimmune encephalomyelitis. *Mol. Cell. Probes* **2020**, *51*, 101530. [CrossRef] [PubMed]
13. Niikura, T.; Sidahmed, E.; Hirata-Fukae, C.; Aisen, P.S.; Matsuoka, Y. A humanin derivative reduces amyloid beta accumulation and ameliorates memory deficit in triple transgenic mice. *PLoS ONE* **2011**, *6*, e16259. [CrossRef] [PubMed]
14. Heinrichs, M.; von Dawans, B.; Domes, G. Oxytocin, vasopressin, and human social behaviour. *Front. Neuroendocrinol.* **2009**, *30*, 548–557. [CrossRef] [PubMed]
15. Alcalá-Barraza, S.R.; Lee, M.S.; Hanson, L.R.; McDonald, A.A.; Frey, W.H.; McLoon, L.K. Intranasal delivery of neurotrophic factors BDNF, CNTF, EPO, and NT-4 to the CNS. *J. Drug Target.* **2009**, *18*, 179–190. [CrossRef] [PubMed]
16. Malerba, F.; Paoletti, F.; Capsoni, S.; Cattaneo, A. Intranasal delivery of therapeutic proteins for neurological diseases. *Expert Opin. Drug Deliv.* **2011**, *8*, 1277–1296. [CrossRef]
17. Falcone, J.A.; Salameh, T.S.; Yi, X.; Cordy, B.J.; Mortell, W.G.; Kabanov, A.V.; Banks, W.A. Intranasal administration as a route for drug delivery to the brain: Evidence for a unique pathway for albumin. *J. Pharm. Exp. Ther.* **2014**, *351*, 54–60. [CrossRef] [PubMed]
18. Das, S.; Mishra, K.P.; Ganju, L.; Singh, S.B. Intranasally delivered small interfering RNA-mediated suppression of scavenger receptor mac-1 attenuates microglial phenotype switching and working memory impairment following hypoxia. *Neuropharmacology* **2018**, *137*, 240–255. [CrossRef]
19. Dhaliwal, H.K.; Fan, Y.; Kim, J.; Amiji, M.M. Intranasal delivery and transfection of mRNA therapeutics in the brain using cationic liposomes. *Mol. Pharm.* **2020**, *17*, 1996–2005. [CrossRef]
20. Harmon, B.T.; Aly, A.E.; Padegimas, L.; Sesenoglu-Laird, O.; Cooper, M.J.; Waszczak, B.L. Intranasal administration of plasmid DNA nanoparticles yields successful transfection and expression of a reporter protein in rat brain. *Gene Ther.* **2014**, *21*, 514–521. [CrossRef]
21. Alarcón-Arís, D.; Recasens, A.; Galofré, M.; Carballo-Carbajal, I.; Zacchi, N.; Ruiz-Bronchal, E.; Pavia-Collado, R.; Chica, R.; Ferrés-Coy, A.; Santos, M.; et al. Selective α-synuclein knockdown in monoamine neurons by intranasal oligonucleotide delivery: Potential therapy for parkinson's disease. *Mol. Ther.* **2018**, *26*, 550–567. [CrossRef] [PubMed]
22. Sanchez-Ramos, J.; Song, S.; Kong, X.; Foroutan, P.; Martinez, G.; Dominguez-Viqueria, W.; Mohapatra, S.; Mohapatra, S.; Haraszti, R.A.; Khvorova, A.; et al. Chitosan-Mangafodipir nanoparticles designed for intranasal delivery of siRNA and DNA to brain. *J. Drug Deliv. Sci. Technol.* **2018**, *43*, 453–460. [CrossRef] [PubMed]
23. Simão Carlos, M.I.; Zheng, K.; Garrett, N.; Arifin, N.; Workman, D.G.; Kubajewska, I.; Halwani, A.; Moger, J.; Zhang, Q.; Schätzlein, A.G.; et al. Limiting the level of tertiary amines on polyamines leads to biocompatible nucleic acid vectors. *Int. J. Pharm.* **2017**, *526*, 106–124. [CrossRef] [PubMed]
24. Han, I.K.; Kim, M.Y.; Byun, H.M.; Hwang, T.S.; Kim, J.M.; Hwang, K.W.; Park, T.G.; Jung, W.W.; Chun, T.; Jeong, G.J.; et al. Enhanced brain targeting efficiency of intranasally administered plasmid DNA: An alternative route for brain gene therapy. *J. Mol. Med.* **2007**, *85*, 75–83. [CrossRef] [PubMed]
25. Zheng, P. Neuroactive steroid regulation of neurotransmitter release in the CNS: Action, mechanism and possible significance. *Prog. Neurobiol.* **2009**, *89*, 134–152. [CrossRef] [PubMed]
26. Meena, C.L.; Thakur, A.; Nandekar, P.P.; Sangamwar, A.T.; Sharma, S.S.; Jain, R. Synthesis of CNS active thyrotropin-releasing hormone (TRH)-like peptides: Biological evaluation and effect on cognitive impairment induced by cerebral ischemia in mice. *Bioorg. Med. Chem.* **2015**, *23*, 5641–5653. [CrossRef] [PubMed]
27. Korczeniewska, O.A.; Tatineni, K.; Faheem, S.; Fresin, W.; Bonitto, J.; Khan, J.; Eliav, E.; Benoliel, R. Effects of intra-nasal melanocortin-4 receptor antagonist on trigeminal neuropathic pain in male and female rats. *Neurosci. Lett.* **2023**, *796*, 137054. [CrossRef] [PubMed]
28. Cattepoel, S.; Hanenberg, M.; Kulic, L.; Nitsch, R.M. Chronic intranasal treatment with an anti-aβ(30-42) scfv antibody ameliorates amyloid pathology in a transgenic mouse model of Alzheimer's disease. *PLoS ONE* **2011**, *6*, e18296. [CrossRef]
29. Cheng, C.; Chen, Y.H.; Lennox, K.A.; Behlke, M.A.; Davidson, B.L. In vivo SELEX for Identification of Brain-penetrating Aptamers. *Mol. Ther. Nucleic Acids* **2013**, *2*, e67. [CrossRef]

30. Correa, D.; Scheuber, M.I.; Shan, H.; Weinmann, O.W.; Baumgartner, Y.A.; Harten, A.; Wahl, A.S.; Skaar, K.L.; Schwab, M.E. Intranasal delivery of full-length anti-Nogo-A antibody: A potential alternative route for therapeutic antibodies to central nervous system targets. *Proc. Natl. Acad. Sci. USA* **2023**, *120*, e2200057120. [CrossRef]
31. Neuwelt, E.; Abbott, N.J.; Abrey, L.; Banks, W.A.; Blakley, B.; Davis, T.; Engelhardt, B.; Grammas, P.; Nedergaard, M.; Nutt, J.; et al. Strategies to advance translational research into Brain Barriers. *Lancet Neurol.* **2008**, *7*, 84–96. [CrossRef]
32. Sonvico, F.; Clementino, A.; Buttini, F.; Colombo, G.; Pescina, S.; Guterres, S.S.; Pohlmann, A.R.; Nicoli, S. Surface-Modified nanocarriers for nose-to-brain delivery: From bioadhesion to targeting. *Pharmaceutics* **2018**, *10*, 34. [CrossRef]
33. Santaguida, S.; Janigro, D.; Hossain, M.; Oby, E.; Rapp, E.; Cucullo, L. Side by side comparison between dynamic versus static models of blood–brain barrier in vitro: A permeability study. *Brain Res.* **2006**, *1109*, 1–13. [CrossRef]
34. Hawkins, B.T.; Egleton, R.D. Pathophysiology of the blood-brain barrier: Animal models and methods. *Curr. Top. Dev. Biol.* **2007**, *80*, 277–309.
35. Kusuhara, H.; Sugiyama, Y. Efflux transport systems for drugs at the blood-brain barrier and blood-cerebrospinal fluid barrier (Part 1). *Drug Discov. Today* **2001**, *6*, 150–156. [CrossRef] [PubMed]
36. Masserini, M. Nanoparticles for brain drug delivery. *ISRN Biochem.* **2012**, *2013*, 238428. [CrossRef] [PubMed]
37. Mikitsh, J.L.; Chacko, A.M. Pathways for small molecule delivery to the central nervous system across the blood-brain barrier. *Pers. Med. Chem.* **2014**, *6*, 11–24. [CrossRef] [PubMed]
38. Vecchio, G.D.; Tscheik, C.; Tenz, K.; Helms, H.C.; Winkler, L.; Blasig, R.; Blasig, I.E. Sodium caprate transiently opens claudin-5-containing barriers at tight junctions of epithelial and endothelial cells. *Mol. Pharm.* **2012**, *9*, 2523–2533. [CrossRef] [PubMed]
39. Hall, W.A.; Doolittle, N.D.; Daman, M.; Bruns, P.K.; Muldoon, L.; Fortin, D.; Neuwelt, E.A. Osmotic blood-brain barrier disruption chemotherapy for diffuse pontine gliomas. *J. Neuro-Oncol.* **2006**, *77*, 279–284. [CrossRef] [PubMed]
40. Hülper, P.; Veszelka, S.; Walter, F.R.; Wolburg, H.; Fallier-Becker, P.; Piontek, J.; Blasig, I.E.; Lakomek, M.; Kulger, W.; Deli, M.A. Acute effects of short-chain alkylglycerols on blood-brain barrier properties of cultured brain endothelial cells. *Br. J. Pharmacol.* **2013**, *169*, 1561–1573. [CrossRef]
41. Cooper, I.; Last, D.; Guez, D.; Sharabi, S.; Goldman, S.E.; Lubitz, I.; Daniels, D.; Salomon, S.; Tamar, G.; Tamir, T.; et al. Combined local blood-brain barrier opening and systemic methotrexate for the treatment of brain tumours. *J. Cereb. Blood Flow Metab.* **2015**, *35*, 967–976. [CrossRef] [PubMed]
42. Prokai, L.; Prokai-Tatrai, K.; Bodor, N. Targeting drugs to the brain by redox chemical delivery systems. *Med. Res. Rev.* **2000**, *20*, 367–415. [CrossRef] [PubMed]
43. Girod, J.; Fenart, L.; Régina, A.; Dehouck, M.P.; Hong, G.; Scherrmann, J.M.; Cecchelli, R.; Roux, F. Transport of cationized anti-tetanus Fab'2 fragments across an In vitro blood-brain barrier model: Involvement of the transcytosis pathway. *J. Neurochem.* **1999**, *73*, 2002–2008. [PubMed]
44. Lu, C.T.; Zhao, Y.Z.; Wong, H.L.; Cai, J.; Peng, L.; Tian, X.Q. Current approaches to enhance CNS delivery of drugs across the brain barriers. *Int. J. Nanomed.* **2014**, *9*, 2241–2257. [CrossRef] [PubMed]
45. Bodor, N.; Buchwald, P. Recent advances in the brain targeting of neuropharmaceuticals by chemical delivery systems. *Adv. Drug Deliv. Rev.* **1999**, *36*, 229–254. [CrossRef] [PubMed]
46. Zhang, Y.; Pardridge, W.M. Conjugation of brain-derived neurotrophic factor to a blood-brain barrier drug targeting system enables neuroprotection in regional brain ischemia following intravenous injection of the neurotrophin. *Brain Res.* **2001**, *889*, 49–56. [CrossRef] [PubMed]
47. Tosi, G.; Constantino, L.; Rivasi, F.; Ruozi, B.; Leo, E.; Vergoni, A.V.; Tacchi, R.; Bertolini, A.; Vandelli, M.A.; Forni, F. Targeting the central nervous system: In vivo experiments with peptide-derivatized nanoparticles loaded with Loperamide and Rhodamine-123. *J. Control. Release* **2007**, *122*, 1–9. [CrossRef] [PubMed]
48. Venishetty, V.K.; Samala, R.; Komuravelli, R.; Kuncha, M.; Sistla, R.; Diwan, P.V. β-Hydroxybutyric acid grafted solid lipid nanoparticles: A novel strategy to improve drug delivery to brain. *Nanomed. Nanotechnol. Biol. Med.* **2013**, *9*, 388–397. [CrossRef]
49. Temsamani, J.; Bonnafous, C.; Rousselle, C.; Fraisse, Y.; Clair, P.; Granier, L.A.; Rees, A.R.; Kaczorek, M.; Scherrmann, J.M. Improved brain uptake and pharmacological activity profile of morphine-6-glucuronide using a peptide vector-mediated strategy. *J. Pharm. Exp. Ther.* **2005**, *313*, 712–719. [CrossRef]
50. van Vliet, E.A.; Zibell, G.; Pekcec, A.; Schlichtiger, J.; Edelbroek, P.M.; Holtman, L.; Aronica, E.; Gorter, J.A.; Potschka, H. COX-2 inhibition controls P-glycoprotein expression and promotes brain delivery of phenytoin in chronic epileptic rats. *Neuropharmacology* **2010**, *58*, 404–412. [CrossRef]
51. Muzi, M.; Mankoff, D.A.; Link, J.M.; Shoner, S.; Collier, A.C.; Sasongko, L.; Unadkat, J.D. Imaging of cyclosporine inhibition of P-glycoprotein activity using 11C-verapamil in the brain: Studies of healthy humans. *J. Nucl. Med.* **2009**, *50*, 1267–1275. [CrossRef] [PubMed]
52. Batrakova, E.V.; Miller, D.W.; Li, S.; Alakhov, V.Y.; Kabanov, A.V.; Elmquist, W.F. Pluronic P85 enhances the delivery of digoxin to the brain: In Vitro and in Vivo studies. *J. Pharm. Exp. Ther.* **2001**, *296*, 551–557.
53. Jain, S.; Mishra, V.; Singh, P.; Dubey, P.K.; Saraf, D.K.; Vyas, S.P. RGD-anchored magnetic liposomes for monocytes/neutrophils-mediated brain targeting. *Pharmaceutics* **2003**, *261*, 43–55. [CrossRef] [PubMed]
54. Groothuis, D.R.; Benalcazar, H.; Allen, C.V.; Wise, R.M.; Dills, C.; Dobrescu, C.; Rothholtz, V.; Levy, R.M. Comparison of cytosine arabinoside delivery to rat brain by intravenous, intrathecal, intraventricular and intraparenchymal routes of administration. *Brain Res.* **2000**, *856*, 281–290. [CrossRef] [PubMed]

55. Murry, D.J.; Blaney, S.M. Clinical pharmacology of encapsulated sustained-release cytarabine. *Ann. Pharmacother.* **2000**, *34*, 1173–1178. [CrossRef] [PubMed]
56. Di Fausto, V.; Fiore, M.; Tirassa, P.; Lambiase, A.; Aloe, L. Eye drop NGF administration promotes the recovery of chemically injured cholinergic neurons of adult mouse forebrain. *Eur. J. Neurol.* **2007**, *26*, 2473–2480. [CrossRef] [PubMed]
57. Haque, S.; Md, S.; Fazil, M.; Kumar, M.; Sahni, J.K.; Ali, J.; Baboota, S. Venlafaxine loaded chitosan NPs for brain targeting: Pharmacokinetic and pharmacodynamic evaluation. *Carbohydr. Polym.* **2012**, *89*, 72–79. [CrossRef] [PubMed]
58. Constantino, H.R.; Illum, L.; Brandt, G.; Johnson, P.H.; Quay, S.C. Intranasal delivery: Physicochemical and therapeutic aspects. *Int. J. Pharm.* **2007**, *337*, 1–24. [CrossRef]
59. Jadhav, K.R.; Gambhire, M.N.; Shaikh, I.M.; Kadam, V.J.; Pisal, S.S. Nasal Drug Delivery System-Factors Affecting and Applications. *Curr. Drug Ther.* **2007**, *2*, 27–38. [CrossRef]
60. Samaridou, E.; Alonso, M.J. Nose-to-brain peptide delivery—The potential of nanotechnology. *Biol. Med. Chem.* **2018**, *26*, 2888–2905. [CrossRef]
61. Gänger, S.; Schindowski, K. Tailoring Formulations for Intranasal Nose-to-Brain Delivery: A Review on Architecture, Physico-Chemical Characteristics and Mucociliary Clearance of the Nasal Olfactory Mucosa. *Pharmaceutics* **2018**, *10*, 116. [CrossRef] [PubMed]
62. Gizurarson, S. The effect of cilia and the mucociliary clearance on successful drug delivery. *Biol. Pharm. Bull.* **2015**, *38*, 497–506. [CrossRef] [PubMed]
63. Bitter, C.; Suter-Zimmermann, K.; Surber, C. Nasal drug delivery in humans. *Curr. Probl. Dermatol.* **2011**, *40*, 20–35. [PubMed]
64. Erdő, F.; Bors, L.A.; Farkas, D.; Bajza, A.; Gizurarson, S. Evaluation of intranasal delivery route of drug administration for brain targeting. *Brain Res. Bull.* **2018**, *143*, 155–170. [CrossRef] [PubMed]
65. Bogdan, M.S.; Slavic, D.O.; Babovic, S.S.; Zvezdin, B.S.; Kolarov, V.P.; Kljajic, V.L. Olfactory Perception and Different Decongestive Response of the Nasal Mucosa During Menstrual Cycle. *Am. J. Rhinol.* **2021**, *35*, 693–699. [CrossRef] [PubMed]
66. Cingi, C.; Ozdoganoglu, T.; Songu, M. Nasal obstruction as a drug side effect. *Ther. Adv. Respir. Dis.* **2011**, *5*, 175–182. [CrossRef] [PubMed]
67. Crowe, T.P.; Greenlee, M.H.W.; Kanthasamy, A.G.; Hsu, W.H. Mechanism of intranasal drug delivery directly to the brain. *Life Sci.* **2018**, *195*, 44–52. [CrossRef] [PubMed]
68. Bourganis, V.; Kammona, O.; Alexopoulos, A.; Kiparissides, C. Recent advances in carrier mediated nose-to-brain delivery of pharmaceutics. *Eur. J. Pharm. Biopharm.* **2018**, *128*, 337–362. [CrossRef]
69. Pardeshi, C.; Belgamwar, V. Direct nose to brain drug delivery via integrated nerve pathways bypassing the blood–brain barrier: An excellent platform for brain targeting. *Expert Opin. Drug Deliv.* **2013**, *10*, 957–972. [CrossRef]
70. Turhan, B.; Kervancioglu, P.; Yalcin, E.D. The radiological evaluation of the nasal cavity, conchae and nasal septum volumes by stereological method: A retrospective cone-beam computed tomography study. *Adv. Clin. Exp. Med.* **2019**, *28*, 1021–1026. [CrossRef]
71. Beule, A.G. Physiology and pathophysiology of respiratory mucosa of the nose and the paranasal sinuses. *GMS Curr. Top. Otorhinolaryngol. Head Neck Surg.* **2010**, *9*, Doc07. [PubMed]
72. Washington, N.; Steele, R.J.; Jackson, S.J.; Bush, D.; Mason, J.; Gill, D.A.; Pitt, K.; Rawlins, D.A. Determination of baseline human nasal pH and the effect of intranasally administered buffers. *Int. J. Pharm.* **2000**, *198*, 139–146. [CrossRef] [PubMed]
73. Zanin, M.; Baviskar, P.; Webster, R.; Webby, R. The Interaction between Respiratory Pathogens and Mucus. *Cell Host Microbe* **2016**, *19*, 159–168. [CrossRef] [PubMed]
74. Dedrick, S.; Akbari, M.J.; Dyckman, S.K.; Zhao, N.; Liu, Y.Y.; Momeni, B. Impact of Temporal pH Fluctuations on the Coexistence of Nasal Bacteria in an in silico Community. *Front. Microbiol.* **2021**, *12*, 613109. [CrossRef] [PubMed]
75. Santacroce, L.; Charitos, I.A.; Ballini, A.; Inchingolo, A.F.; Luperto, P.; De Nitto, E.; Topi, S. The Human Respiratory System and its Microbiome at a Glimpse. *Biology* **2020**, *9*, 318. [CrossRef] [PubMed]
76. Kumpitsch, C.; Koskinen, K.; Schöpf, V.; Moissl-Eichinger, C. The microbiome of the upper respiratory tract in health and disease. *BMC Biol.* **2019**, *17*, 87. [CrossRef] [PubMed]
77. Do, T.Q.; Moshkani, S.; Castillo, P.; Anunta, S.; Pogosyan, A.; Cheung, A.; Marbois, B.; Faull, K.F.; Ernst, W.; Chiang, S.M.; et al. Lipids including cholesteryl linoleate and cholesteryl arachidonate contribute to the inherent antibacterial activity of human nasal fluid. *J. Immunol.* **2008**, *181*, 4177–4187. [CrossRef] [PubMed]
78. Lee, J.T.; Jansen, M.; Yilma, A.N.; Nguyen, A.; Desharnais, R.; Porter, E. Antimicrobial lipids: Novel innate defence molecules are elevated in sinus secretions of patients with chronic rhinosinusitis. *Am. J. Rhinol.* **2010**, *24*, 99–104. [CrossRef]
79. Dhamankar, V.S. Cytochrome P450-Mediated Drug Metabolizing Activity in the Nasal Mucosa. Doctor of Philosophy Thesis, University of Iowa, Iowa City, IA, USA, 2013.
80. Tengamnuay, P.; Shao, Z.Z.; Mitra, A.K. Systemic absorption of L- and D-phenylalanine across the rat nasal mucosa. *Life Sci.* **1991**, *48*, 1477–1481. [CrossRef]
81. Bhise, S.B.; Yadav, A.V.; Avachat, A.M.; Malayandi, R. Bioavailability of intranasal drug delivery system. *Asian J. Pharm.* **2008**, *4*, 201. [CrossRef]
82. Abbott, N.J.; Pizzo, M.E.; Preston, J.E.; Janigro, D.; Thorne, R.G. The role of brain barriers in fluid movement in the CNS: Is there a 'glymphatic' system? *Acta Neuropathol.* **2018**, *135*, 387–407. [CrossRef]

83. Polo-Castillo, L.E.; Villavicencio, M.; Ramírez-Lugo, L.; Illescas-Huerta, E.; Gil Moreno, M.; Ruiz-Huerta, L.; Gutierrez, R.; Sotres-Bayon, F.; Caballero-Ruiz, A. Reimplantable Microdrive for Long-Term Chronic Extracellular Recordings in Freely Moving Rats. *Front. Neurol.* **2019**, *13*, 128. [CrossRef] [PubMed]
84. Ariel, P. A beginner's guide to tissue clearing. *Int. J. Biochem. Cell Biol.* **2017**, *84*, 35–39. [CrossRef] [PubMed]
85. Branch, A.; Tward, D.; Vogelstein, J.; Wu, Z.; Gallagher, M. An optimized protocol for iDISCO+ rat brain clearing, imaging, and analysis. *STAR Protoc.* **2019**, *4*, 101968.
86. Molbay, M.; Kolabas, Z.I.; Todorov, M.I.; Ohn, T.; Ertürk, A. A guidebook for DISCO tissue clearing. *Mol. Syst. Biol.* **2021**, *17*, e9807. [CrossRef] [PubMed]
87. Martins, P.P.; Smyth, H.D.C.; Cui, Z. Strategies to facilitate or block nose-to-brain drug delivery. *Int. J. Pharm.* **2019**, *570*, 118635. [CrossRef] [PubMed]
88. Surber, C.; Elsner, P.; Farage, M.A. Topical Applications and the Mucosa. *Cur. Prob. Dermatol.* **2011**, *40*, 20–35.
89. Lofts, A.; Abu-Hijleh, F.; Rigg, N.; Mishra, R.K.; Hoare, T. Using the Intranasal Route to Administer Drugs to Treat Neurological and Psychiatric Illnesses: Rationale, Successes, and Future Needs. *CNS Drugs* **2022**, *36*, 739–770. [CrossRef] [PubMed]
90. Alexander, A.; Ajazuddin, M.; Swarna, M.; Sharma, M.; Tripathi, D. Polymers and Permeation Enhancers: Specialized Components of Mucoadhesives. *Stamford J. Pharm. Sci.* **2011**, *4*, 91–95. [CrossRef]
91. Alexander, A.; Agarwal, M.; Chougule, B.M.; Saraf, S.; Saraf, S. Nose-to-brain drug delivery. *Nanopharmaceuticals* **2020**, *1*, 175–200.
92. Guggi, D.; Bernkop-Schnürch, A. Improved paracellular uptake by the combination of different types of permeation enhancers. *Int. J. Pharm.* **2015**, *288*, 141–150. [CrossRef] [PubMed]
93. Bernkop-Schnurch, A. Thiomers: A new generation of mucoadhesive polymers. *Adv. Drug Deliv. Rev.* **2005**, *57*, 1569–1582. [CrossRef] [PubMed]
94. Meredith, M.E.; Salameh, T.S.; Banks, W.A. Intranasal delivery of proteins and peptides in the treatment of neurodegenerative diseases. *AAPS J.* **2015**, *17*, 780–787. [CrossRef] [PubMed]
95. Jiao, C.-Y.; Delaroche, D.; Burlina, F.; Alves, I.D.; Chassaing, G.; Sagan, S. Translocation and endocytosis for cell-penetrating peptide internalization. *J. Biol. Chem.* **2009**, *284*, 33957–33965. [CrossRef] [PubMed]
96. Bechara, C.; Sagan, S. Cell-penetrating peptides: 20 years later, where do we stand? *FEBS Lett.* **2013**, *587*, 1693–1702. [CrossRef] [PubMed]
97. Ziegler, A. Thermodynamic studies and binding mechanisms of cell-penetrating peptides with lipids and glycosaminoglycans. *Adv. Drug Deliv. Rev.* **2008**, *60*, 580–597. [CrossRef] [PubMed]
98. Elmquist, A.; Langel, U. In vitro uptake and stability study of pVEC and its all-D analog. *J. Biol. Chem.* **2003**, *384*, 387–393. [CrossRef]
99. Konsoula, R.; Barile, F.A. Correlation of in vitro cytotoxicity with paracellular permeability in Caco-2 cells. In Vitro. *Toxicol* **2005**, *19*, 675–684. [CrossRef]
100. Matsuyama, T.; Morita, T.; Horikiri, Y.; Yamahara, H.; Yoshino, H. Enhancement of nasal absorption of large molecular weight compounds by combination of mucolytic agent and nonionic surfactant. *J. Control. Release* **2006**, *110*, 347–352. [CrossRef]
101. Chen, M.; Li, X.R.; Zhou, Y.X.; Yang, K.W.; Chen, X.W.; Deng, Q.; Ren, L. Improved absorption of salmon calcitonin by ultraflexible liposomes through intranasal delivery. *Peptides* **2009**, *30*, 1288–1295. [CrossRef]
102. Evans, C.M.; Koo, J.S. Airway mucus: The good, the bad, the sticky. *Pharmacol. Ther.* **2009**, *121*, 332–348. [CrossRef]
103. Rohrer, J.; Partenhauser, A.; Hauptstein, S.; Gallati, C.M.; Matuszczak, B.; Abdulkarim, M.; Gumbleton, M.; Bernkop-Schnürch, A. Mucus permeating thiolated self-emulsifying drug delivery systems. *Eur. J. Pharm. Biopharm.* **2016**, *98*, 90–97. [CrossRef]
104. Andrews, G.P.; Laverty, T.P.; Jones, D.S. Mucoadhesive polymeric platforms for controlled drug delivery. *Eur. J. Pharm. Biopharm.* **2009**, *71*, 505–518. [CrossRef] [PubMed]
105. Chaturvedi, M.; Kumar, M.; Pathak, K. A review on mucoadhesive polymer used in nasal drug delivery system. *J. Adv. Pharm. Technol. Res.* **2011**, *2*, 215–222. [CrossRef] [PubMed]
106. Awad, R.; Avital, A.; Sosnik, A. Polymeric nanocarriers for nose-to-brain drug delivery in neurodegenerative diseases and neurodevelopmental disorders. *Acta Pharm. Sin. B* **2023**, *13*, 1866–1886. [CrossRef] [PubMed]
107. Karavasili, C.; Fatouros, D.G. Smart materials: In situ gel-forming systems for nasal delivery. *Drug Discov. Today* **2016**, *21*, 157–166. [CrossRef] [PubMed]
108. Zahir-Jouzdani, F.; Wolf, J.D.; Atyabi, F.; Bernkop-Schnürch, A. In situ gelling and mucoadhesive polymers: Why do they need each other? *Expert Opin. Drug Deliv.* **2018**, *15*, 1007–1019. [CrossRef] [PubMed]
109. Gizurarson, S.; Bechaard, E. Study of Nasal Enzyme Activity towards Insulin. In Vitro. *Chem. Pharm. Bull.* **1991**, *39*, 2155–2157. [CrossRef]
110. Zhang, L.; Wang, S.; Zhang, M.; Sun, J. Nanocarriers for oral drug delivery. *J. Drug Target.* **2013**, *21*, 515–527. [CrossRef] [PubMed]
111. Na, D.H.; Youn, Y.S.; Park, E.J.; Lee, J.M.; Cho, O.R.; Lee, K.R.; Lee, S.D.; Yoo, S.D.; DeLuca, P.P.; Lee, K.C. Stability of PEGylated salmon calcitonin in nasal mucosa. *J. Pharm. Sci.* **2004**, *93*, 256–261. [CrossRef]
112. Veronese, F.; Mero, A. The Impact of PEGylation on Biological Therapies. *BioDrugs* **2018**, *22*, 315–329. [CrossRef]
113. Matanović, M.R.; Kristl, J.; Grabnar, P.A. Thermoresponsive polymers: Insights into decisive hydrogel characteristics, mechanisms of gelation, and promising biomedical applications. *Int. J. Pharm.* **2014**, *472*, 262–275. [CrossRef] [PubMed]
114. Pathak, R.; Prasad Dash, R.; Misra, M.; Nivsarkar, M. Role of mucoadhesive polymers in enhancing delivery of nimodipine microemulsion to brain via intranasal route. *Acta Pharm. Sin. B* **2014**, *4*, 151–160. [CrossRef] [PubMed]

115. Nigam, K.; Kaur, A.; Tyagi, A.; Nematullah, A.M.; Khan, F.; Gabrani, R.; Dang, S. Nose-to-brain delivery of lamotrigine-loaded PLGA nanoparticles. *Drug Deliv. Transl. Res.* **2019**, *9*, 879–890. [CrossRef] [PubMed]
116. Sharma, D.; Sharma, R.K.; Sharma, N.; Gabrani, R.; Sharma, S.K.; Ali, J.; Dang, S. Nose-To-Brain Delivery of PLGA-Diazepam Nanoparticles. *AAPS PharmSciTech* **2015**, *16*, 1108–1121. [CrossRef] [PubMed]
117. Sunena, S.K.; Singh, D.N. Nose to Brain Delivery of Galantamine Loaded Nanoparticles: In-vivo Pharmacodynamic and Biochemical Study in Mice. *Curr. Drug Deliv.* **2019**, *16*, 51–58. [CrossRef] [PubMed]
118. de Oliveira Junior, E.R.; Nascimento, T.L.; Salomão, M.A.; da Silva, A.C.G.; Valadares, M.C.; Lima, E.M. Increased Nose-to-Brain Delivery of Melatonin Mediated by Polycaprolactone Nanoparticles for the Treatment of Glioblastoma. *Pharm. Res.* **2019**, *36*, 131. [CrossRef] [PubMed]
119. Costa, C.P.; Moreira, J.N.; Sousa Lobo, J.M.; Silva, A.C. Intranasal delivery of nanostructured lipid carriers, solid lipid nanoparticles and nanoemulsions: A current overview of in vivo studies. *Acta Pharm. Sin B* **2021**, *11*, 925–940. [CrossRef] [PubMed]
120. Salade, L.; Wauthoz, N.; Vermeersch, M.; Amighi, K.; Goole, J. Chitosan-coated liposome dry-powder formulations loaded with ghrelin for nose-to-brain delivery. *Eur. J. Pharm. Biopharm.* **2018**, *129*, 257–266. [CrossRef]
121. Migliore, M.M.; Vyas, T.K.; Campbell, R.B.; Amiji, M.M.; Waszczak, B.L. Brain delivery of proteins by the intranasal route of administration: A comparison of cationic liposomes versus aqueous solution formulations. *J. Pharm. Sci.* **2010**, *99*, 1745–1761. [CrossRef]
122. Abdou, E.M.; Kandil, S.M.; El Miniawy, H.M. Brain targeting efficiency of antimigraine drug loaded mucoadhesive intranasal nanoemulsion. *Int. J. Pharm.* **2017**, *529*, 667–677. [CrossRef]
123. Boche, M.; Pokharkar, V. Quetiapine Nanoemulsion for Intranasal Drug Delivery: Evaluation of Brain-Targeting Efficiency. *AAPS PharmSciTech* **2017**, *18*, 686–696. [CrossRef] [PubMed]
124. Hady, M.A.; Sayed, O.M.; Akl, M.A. Brain uptake and accumulation of new levofloxacin-doxycycline combination through the use of solid lipid nanoparticles: Formulation; Optimization and in-vivo evaluation. *Colloids Surf. B* **2020**, *193*, 111076. [CrossRef] [PubMed]
125. Li, J.C.; Zhang, W.J.; Zhu, J.X.; Zhu, N.; Zhang, H.M.; Wang, X.; Zhang, J.; Wang, Q.Q. Preparation and brain delivery of nasal solid lipid nanoparticles of quetiapine fumarate in situ gel in rat model of schizophrenia. *Int. J. Clin. Exp. Med.* **2015**, *8*, 17590–17600. [PubMed]
126. Gartziandia, O.; Herrán, E.; Ruiz-Ortega, J.A.; Miguelez, C.; Igartua, M.; Lafuente, J.V.; Pedraz, J.L.; Ugedo, L.; Hernández, R.M. Intranasal Administration of Chitosan-Coated Nanostructured Lipid Carriers Loaded with GDNF Improves Behavioral and Histological Recovery in a Partial Lesion Model of Parkinson's Disease. *J. Biomed. Nanotechnol.* **2016**, *12*, 2220–2280. [CrossRef] [PubMed]
127. Pokharkar, V.; Patil-Gadhe, A.; Palla, P. Efavirenz loaded nanostructured lipid carrier engineered for brain targeting through intranasal route: In-vivo pharmacokinetic and toxicity study. *Biomed. Pharmacother.* **2017**, *94*, 150–164. [CrossRef]
128. Li, Y.; Li, J.; Zhang, X.; Ding, J.; Mao, S. Non-ionic surfactants as novel intranasal absorption enhancers: In vitro and in vivo characterization. *Drug Deliv.* **2016**, *23*, 2272–2279. [CrossRef]
129. Espinoza, L.C.; Silva-Abreu, M.; Clares, B.; Rodríguez-Lagunas, M.J.; Halbaut, L.; Cañas, M.-A.; Calpena, A.C. Formulation Strategies to Improve Nose-to-Brain Delivery of Donepezil. *Pharmaceutics* **2019**, *11*, 64. [CrossRef]
130. Perinelli, D.R.; Vllasaliu, D.; Bonacucina, G.; Come, B.; Pucciarelli, S.; Ricciutelli, M.; Cespi, M.; Itri, R.; Spinozzi, F.; Palmieri, G.F.; et al. Rhamnolipids as epithelial permeability enhancers for macromolecular therapeutics. *Eur. J. Pharm. Biopharm.* **2017**, *119*, 419–425. [CrossRef]
131. Lin, T.; Liu, E.; He, H.; Shin, M.C.; Moon, C.; Yang, V.C.; Huang, Y. Nose-to-brain delivery of macromolecules mediated by cell-penetrating peptides. *Acta Pharm. Sin. B* **2016**, *6*, 352–358. [CrossRef]
132. Kamei, N.; Takeda-Morishita, M. Brain delivery of insulin boosted by intranasal coadministration with cell-penetrating peptides. *J. Control. Release* **2015**, *197*, 105–110. [CrossRef]
133. Kanazawa, T.; Akiyama, F.; Kakizaki, S.; Takashima, Y.; Seta, Y. Delivery of siRNA to the brain using a combination of nose-to-brain delivery and cell-penetrating peptide-modified nano-micelles. *Biomaterials* **2013**, *34*, 9220–9226. [CrossRef] [PubMed]
134. Khafagy, E.-S.; Kamei, N.; Fujiwara, Y.; Okumura, H.; Yuasa, T.; Kato, M.; Arime, K.; Nonomura, A.; Ogino, H.; Hirano, S.; et al. Systemic and brain delivery of leptin via intranasal coadministration with cell-penetrating peptides and its therapeutic potential for obesity. *J. Control. Release* **2020**, *319*, 397–406. [CrossRef] [PubMed]
135. Kamei, N.; Okada, N.; Ikeda, T.; Choi, H.; Fujiwara, Y.; Okumura, H.; Takeda-Morishita, M. Effective nose-to-brain delivery of exendin-4 via coadministration with cell-penetrating peptides for improving progressive cognitive dysfunction. *Sci. Rep.* **2018**, *8*, 17641. [CrossRef] [PubMed]
136. Dalpiaz, A.; Fogagnolo, M.; Ferraro, L.; Beggiato, S.; Hanuskova, M.; Maretti, E.; Sacchetti, F.; Leo, E.; Pavan, B. Bile salt-coating modulates the macrophage uptake of nanocores constituted by a zidovudine prodrug and enhances its nose-to-brain delivery. *Eur. J. Pharm. Biopharm.* **2019**, *144*, 91–100. [CrossRef] [PubMed]
137. Md, S.; Khan, R.A.; Mustafa, G.; Chuttani, K.; Baboota, S.; Sahni, J.K.; Ali, J. Bromocriptine loaded chitosan nanoparticles intended for direct nose to brain delivery: Pharmacodynamic, pharmacokinetic and scintigraphy study in mice model. *Eur. J. Pharm. Biopharm.* **2013**, *48*, 393–405. [CrossRef] [PubMed]
138. Gavini, E.; Rassu, G.; Ferraro, L.; Generosi, A.; Rau, J.V.; Brunetti, A.; Giunchedi, P.; Dalpiaz, A. Influence of chitosan glutamate on the in vivo intranasal absorption of rokitamycin from microspheres. *J. Pharm. Sci.* **2011**, *100*, 1488–1502. [CrossRef] [PubMed]

139. Gavini, E.; Rassu, G.; Ferraro, L.; Beggiato, S.; Alhalaweh, A.; Velaga, S.; Marchetti, N.; Bandiera, P.; Giunchedi, P.; Dalpiaz, A. Influence of polymeric microcarriers on the in vivo intranasal uptake of an anti-migraine drug for brain targeting. *Eur. J. Pharm. Biopharm.* **2013**, *83*, 174–183. [CrossRef] [PubMed]
140. Li, Y.; He, J.; Lyu, X.; Yuan, Y.; Wang, G.; Zhao, B. Chitosan-based thermosensitive hydrogel for nasal delivery of exenatide: Effect of magnesium chloride. *Int. J. Pharm.* **2018**, *553*, 375–385. [CrossRef]
141. Kanazawa, T.; Kaneko, M.; Niide, T.; Akiyama, F.; Kakizaki, S.; Ibaraki, H.; Shiraishi, S.; Takashima, Y.; Suzuki, T.; Seta, Y. Enhancement of nose-to-brain delivery of hydrophilic macromolecules with stearate- or polyethylene glycol-modified arginine-rich peptide. *Int. J. Pharm.* **2017**, *530*, 195–200. [CrossRef]
142. Acharya, S.R.; Reddy, P.R.V. Brain targeted delivery of paclitaxel using endogenous ligand. *Asian J. Pharm. Sci.* **2016**, *11*, 427–438. [CrossRef]
143. Haque, S.; Md, S.; Sahni, J.K.; Ali, J.; Baboota, S. Development and evaluation of brain targeted intranasal alginate nanoparticles for treatment of depression. *J. Psych. Res.* **2014**, *48*, 1–12. [CrossRef] [PubMed]
144. Sawant, K.; Pandey, A.; Patel, S. Aripiprazole loaded poly(caprolactone) nanoparticles: Optimization and in vivo pharmacokinetics. *Mater. Sci. Eng. C-Mater.* **2016**, *66*, 230–243. [CrossRef] [PubMed]
145. Singh, S.K.; Hidau, M.K.; Gautam, S.; Gupta, K.; Singh, K.P.; Singh, S.K.; Singh, S. Glycol chitosan functionalized asenapine nanostructured lipid carriers for targeted brain delivery: Pharmacokinetic and teratogenic assessment. *Int. J. Biol. Macromol.* **2018**, *108*, 1092–1100. [CrossRef] [PubMed]
146. Rassu, G.; Soddu, E.; Posadino, A.M.; Pintus, G.; Sarmento, B.; Giunchedi, P.; Gavini, E. Nose-to-brain delivery of BACE1 siRNA loaded in solid lipid nanoparticles for Alzheimer's therapy. *Colloids Surf. B Biointerfaces* **2017**, *152*, 296–301. [CrossRef] [PubMed]
147. Salatin, S.; Barar, J.; Barzegar-Jalali, M.; Adibkia, K.; Jelvehgari, M. Thermosensitive in situ nanocomposite of rivastigmine hydrogen tartrate as an intranasal delivery system: Development, characterization, ex vivo permeation and cellular studies. *Colloids Surf. B Biointerfaces* **2017**, *159*, 629–638. [CrossRef] [PubMed]
148. Colombo, M.; Figueiró, F.; Dias, A.d.F.; Teixeira, H.F.; Battastini, A.M.O.; Koester, L.S. Kaempferol-loaded mucoadhesive nanoemulsion for intranasal administration reduces glioma growth in vitro. *Int. J. Pharm.* **2018**, *543*, 214–223. [CrossRef] [PubMed]
149. Tan, J.; Voo, Z.; Lim, S.; Venkataraman, S.; Ng, K.; Gao, S.; Hedrick, J.; Yang, Y. Effective encapsulation of apomorphine into biodegradable polymeric nanoparticles through a reversible chemical bond for delivery across the blood–brain barrier. *Nanomed. NBM* **2019**, *17*, 236–245. [CrossRef]
150. Zhang, C.; Chen, J.; Feng, C.; Shao, X.; Liu, Q.; Zhang, Q.; Pang, Z.; Jiang, X. Intranasal nanoparticles of basic fibroblast growth factor for brain delivery to treat Alzheimer's disease. *Int. J. Pharm.* **2014**, *461*, 192–202. [CrossRef]
151. Kumar, M.; Pandey, R.; Patra, K.; Jain, S.; Soni, M.; Dangi, J.; Madan, J. Evaluation of neuropeptide loaded trimethyl chitosan nanoparticles for nose to brain delivery. *Int. J. Biol. Macromol.* **2013**, *61*, 189–195. [CrossRef]
152. Ahmad, N.; Ahmad, R.; Ahmad, F.; Ahmad, W.; Alam, M.; Amir, M.; Ali, A. Poloxamer-chitosan-based Naringenin nanoformulation used in brain targeting for the treatment of cerebral ischemia. *Saudi J. Biol. Sci.* **2020**, *27*, 500–517. [CrossRef] [PubMed]
153. Joachim, E.; Kim, I.; Jin, Y.; Kim, K.; Lee, J.; Choi, H. Gelatin nanoparticles enhance the neuroprotective effects of intranasally administered osteopontin in rat ischemic stroke model. *Drug Deliv. Transl. Res.* **2014**, *4*, 395–399. [CrossRef] [PubMed]
154. Gartziandia, O.; Herran, E.; Pedraz, J.L.; Carro, E.; Igartua, M.; Hernandez, R.M. Chitosan coated nanostructured lipid carriers for brain delivery of proteins by intranasal administration. *Colloids Surf. B Biointerfaces* **2015**, *134*, 304–313. [CrossRef] [PubMed]
155. Tenenbaum, L.; Chtarto, A.; Lehtonen, E.; Velu, T.; Brotchi, J.; Levivier, M. Recombinant AAV-mediated gene delivery to the central nervous system. *J. Gene Med.* **2004**, *6*, S212–S222. [CrossRef] [PubMed]
156. Zhao, Y.Z.; Li, X.; Lu, C.T.; Lin, M.; Chen, L.J.; Xiang, Q.; Zhang, M.; Jin, R.R.; Jiang, X.; Shen, X.T.; et al. Gelatin nanostructured lipid carriers-mediated intranasal delivery of basic fibroblast growth factor enhances functional recovery in hemiparkinsonian rats. *Nanomed. NBM* **2014**, *10*, 755–764. [CrossRef] [PubMed]
157. Yadav, S.; Gattacceca, F.; Panicucci, R.; Amiji, M.M. Comparative Biodistribution and Pharmacokinetic Analysis of Cyclosporine-A in the Brain upon Intranasal or Intravenous Administration in an Oil-in-Water Nanoemulsion Formulation. *Mol. Pharm.* **2015**, *12*, 1523–1533. [CrossRef] [PubMed]
158. Piazzini, V.; Landucci, E.; D'Ambrosio, M.; Fasiolo, L.T.; Cinci, L.; Colombo, G.; Pellegrini-Giampietro, D.E.; Bilia, A.R.; Luceri, C.; Bergonzi, M.C. Chitosan coated human serum albumin nanoparticles: A promising strategy for nose-to-brain drug delivery. *Int. J. Biol. Macromol.* **2019**, *129*, 267–280. [CrossRef] [PubMed]
159. Bshara, H.; Osman, R.; Mansour, S.; El-Shamy, A.E.-H.A. Chitosan and cyclodextrin in intranasal microemulsion for improved brain buspirone hydrochloride pharmacokinetics in rats. *Carbohydr. Polym.* **2014**, *99*, 297–305. [CrossRef]
160. Devkar, T.B.; Tekade, A.R.; Khandelwal, K.R. Surface engineered nanostructured lipid carriers for efficient nose to brain delivery of ondansetron HCl using Delonix regia gum as a natural mucoadhesive polymer. *Colloids Surf. B Biointerfaces* **2014**, *122*, 143–150. [CrossRef]
161. Upadhyay, P.; Trivedi, J.; Pundarikakshudu, K.; Sheth, N. Direct and enhanced delivery of nanoliposomes of anti-schizophrenic agent to the brain through nasal route. *Saudi Pharm J.* **2017**, *25*, 346–358. [CrossRef]
162. Li, W.; Zhou, Y.; Zhao, N.; Hao, B.; Wang, X.; Kong, P. Pharmacokinetic behavior and efficiency of acetylcholinesterase inhibition in rat brain after intranasal administration of galanthamine hydrobromide loaded flexible liposomes. *Environ. Toxicol. Pharmacol.* **2012**, *34*, 272–279. [CrossRef]

163. Hao, J.; Zhao, J.; Zhang, S.; Tong, T.; Zhuang, Q.; Jin, K.; Chen, W.; Tang, H. Fabrication of an ionic-sensitive in situ gel loaded with resveratrol nanosuspensions intended for direct nose-to-brain delivery. *Colloids Surf. B Biointerfaces* **2016**, *147*, 376–386. [CrossRef] [PubMed]
164. Yadav, S.; Gandham, S.K.; Panicucci, R.; Amiji, M.M. Intranasal brain delivery of cationic nanoemulsion-encapsulated TNFα siRNA in prevention of experimental neuroinflammation. *Nanomed. Nanotechnol. Biol. Med.* **2016**, *12*, 987–1002. [CrossRef] [PubMed]
165. Ahmed, S.; Gull, A.; Aqil, M.; Ansari, M.D.; Sultana, Y. Poloxamer-407 thickened lipid colloidal system of agomelatine for brain targeting: Characterization, brain pharmacokinetic study and behavioral study on Wistar rats. *Colloids Surf. B Biointerfaces* **2019**, *181*, 426–436. [CrossRef] [PubMed]
166. Praveen, A.; Aqil, M.; Sarim Imam, S.; Ahad, A.; Moolakadath, T.; Ahmad, F.J. Lamotrigine encapsulated intra-nasal nanoliposome formulation for epilepsy treatment: Formulation design, characterization and nasal toxicity study. *Colloids Surf. B Biointerfaces* **2019**, *174*, 553–562. [CrossRef] [PubMed]
167. Iqbal, R.; Ahmed, S.; Jain, G.K.; Vohora, D. Design and development of letrozole nanoemulsion: A comparative evaluation of brain targeted nanoemulsion with free letrozole against status epilepticus and neurodegeneration in mice. *Int. J. Pharm.* **2019**, *565*, 20–32. [CrossRef] [PubMed]
168. Gonçalves, J.; Bicker, J.; Gouveia, F.; Liberal, J.; Oliveira, R.C.; Alves, G.; Falcão, A.; Fortuna, A. Nose-to-brain delivery of levetiracetam after intranasal administration to mice. *Int. J. Pharm.* **2019**, *564*, 29–339. [CrossRef] [PubMed]
169. Shelke, S.; Shahi, S.; Jalalpure, S.; Dhamecha, D.; Shengule, S. Formulation and evaluation of thermoreversible mucoadhesive in-situ gel for intranasal delivery of naratriptan hydrochloride. *J. Drug Deliv. Sci. Technol.* **2015**, *29*, 238–244.6. [CrossRef]
170. Shah, B.; Khunt, D.; Misra, M.; Padh, H. Non-invasive intranasal delivery of quetiapine fumarate loaded microemulsion for brain targeting: Formulation, physicochemical and pharmacokinetic consideration. *Eur. J. Pharm. Sci.* **2016**, *91*, 196–207. [CrossRef]
171. Fortuna, A.; Alves, G.; Serralheiro, A.; Sousa, J.; Falcão, A. Intranasal delivery of systemic-acting drugs: Small-molecules and biomacromolecules. *Eur. J. Pharm. Biopharm.* **2014**, *88*, 8–27. [CrossRef]
172. Agrawal, M.; Saraf, S.; Saraf, S.; Antimisiaris, S.G.; Hamano, N.; Li, S.-D.; Chougule, M.; Shoyele, S.A.; Gupta, U.; Ajazuddin; et al. Recent advancements in the field of nanotechnology for the delivery of anti-Alzheimer drug in the brain region. *Expert Opin. Drug Deliv.* **2018**, *15*, 589–617. [CrossRef] [PubMed]
173. Tiwari, S.K.; Chaturvedi, R.K. Peptide therapeutics in neurodegenerative disorders. *Curr. Med Chem.* **2014**, *21*, 2610–2631. [CrossRef] [PubMed]
174. Baig, M.H.; Ahmad, K.; Saeed, M.; Alharbi, A.M.; Barreto, G.E.; Ashraf, G.M.; Choi, I. Peptide based therapeutics and their use for the treatment of neurodegenerative and other diseases. *Biomed. Pharmacother.* **2018**, *103*, 574–581. [CrossRef] [PubMed]
175. Guidotti, G.; Brambilla, L.; Rossi, D. Peptides in clinical development for the treatment of brain tumors. *Curr. Opin. Pharmacol.* **2019**, *47*, 102–109. [CrossRef] [PubMed]
176. Sigurdsson, P.; Thorvaldsson, T.; Gizurarson, S.; Gunnarsson, E. Olfactory absorption of insulin to the brain. *Drug Deliv.* **1997**, *4*, 195–200. [CrossRef]
177. Kamei, N.; Tanaka, M.; Choi, H.; Okada, N.; Ikeda, T.; Itokazu, R.; Takeda-Morishita, M. Effect of an enhanced nose-to-brain delivery of insulin on mild and progressive memory loss in the senescence-accelerated mouse. *Mol. Pharm.* **2017**, *14*, 916–927. [CrossRef] [PubMed]
178. Khafagy, E.-S.; Morishita, M.; Isowa, K.; Imai, J.; Takayama, K. Effect of cell-penetrating peptides on the nasal absorption of insulin. *J. Control. Release* **2009**, *133*, 103–108. [CrossRef]
179. Picone, P.; Sabatino, M.A.; Ditta, L.A.; Amato, A.; Biagio, P.L.S.; Mulè, F.; Giacomazza, D.; Dispenza, C.; Di Carlo, M. Nose-to-brain delivery of insulin enhanced by a nanogel carrier. *J Control Release* **2018**, *270*, 23–36. [CrossRef]
180. Maitani, Y.; Asano, S.; Takahashi, S.; Nakagaki, M.; Nagai, T. Permeability of insulin entrapped in liposome through the nasal mucosa of rabbits. *Chem. Pharm. Bull.* **1992**, *40*, 1569–1572. [CrossRef]
181. Morimoto, K.; Morisaka, K.; Kamada, A. Enhancement of nasal absorption of insulin and calcitonin using polyacrylic acid gel. *J. Pharm. Pharmacol.* **1985**, *37*, 134–136. [CrossRef]
182. Zhou, M.; Donovan, M.D. Intranasal mucociliary of putative bioadhesive polymer gels. *Int. J. Pharm.* **1996**, *135*, 115–125. [CrossRef]
183. Pringels, E.; Callens, C.; Vervaet, C.; Dumont, F.; Slegers, G.; Foreman, P.; Remon, J. Influence of deposition and spray pattern of nasal powders on insulin bioavailability. *Int. J. Pharm.* **2006**, *310*, 1–7. [CrossRef]
184. Tsuneji, N.; Yuji, N.; Naoki, N.; Yoshiki, S.; Kunio, S. Powder dosage form of insulin for nasal administration. *J. Control. Release* **1984**, *1*, 15–22. [CrossRef]
185. Oechslein, C.R.; Fricker, G.; Kissel, T. Nasal delivery of octreotide: Absorption enhancement by particulate carrier systems. *Int. J. Pharm.* **1996**, *139*, 25–32. [CrossRef]
186. During, M.J.; Cao, L.; Zuzga, D.S.; Francis, J.S.; Fitzsimons, H.L.; Jiao, X.; Bland, R.J.; Klugmann, M.; Banks, W.A.; Drucker, D.J.; et al. Glucagon-like peptide-1 receptor is involved in learning and neuroprotection. *Nat. Med.* **2003**, *9*, 1173–1179. [CrossRef] [PubMed]
187. Banks, W.A.; During, M.J.; Niehoff, M.L. Brain uptake of the glucagon-like peptide1 antagonist exendin (9–39) after intranasal administration. *J. Pharmacol. Exp. Ther.* **2004**, *309*, 469–475. [CrossRef] [PubMed]

188. Thorne, R.; Pronk, G.; Padmanabhan, V.; Frey, W. Delivery of insulin-like growth factor-i to the rat brain and spinal cord along olfactory and trigeminal pathways following intranasal administration. *Neuroscience* **2004**, *127*, 481–496. [CrossRef]
189. Lin, S.; Fan, L.W.; Rhodes, P.G.; Cai, Z. Intranasal administration of IGF-1 attenuates hypoxic–ischemic brain injury in neonatal rats. *Exp. Neurol.* **2009**, *217*, 361–370. [CrossRef]
190. Zhao, Y.Z.; Lin, M.; Lin, Q.; Yang, W.; Yu, X.C.; Tian, F.R.; Mao, K.L.; Yang, J.J.; Lu, C.T.; Wong, H.L. Intranasal delivery of bFGF with nanoliposomes enhances in vivo neuroprotection and neural injury recovery in a rodent stroke model. *J. Control. Release* **2016**, *224*, 165–175. [CrossRef]
191. Nelson, A.L.; Dhimolea, E.; Reichert, J.M. Development trends for human monoclonal antibody therapeutics. *Nat. Rev. Drug Discov.* **2010**, *9*, 767–774. [CrossRef]
192. Elgundi, Z.; Reslan, M.; Cruz, E.; Sifniotis, V.; Kayser, V. The state of-play and future of antibody therapeutics. *Adv. Drug Deliv. Rev.* **2017**, *122*, 2–19. [CrossRef] [PubMed]
193. Cummings, J.; Aisen, P.; Lemere, C.; Atri, A.; Sabbagh, M.; Salloway, S. Aducanumab produced a clinically meaningful benefit in association with amyloid lowering. *Alzheimers Res. Ther.* **2021**, *13*, 10–12. [CrossRef] [PubMed]
194. FDA's Decision to Approve New Treatment for Alzheimer's Disease. Available online: https://www.fda.gov/drugs/our-perspective/fdas-decision-approve-new-treatment-alzheimers-disease (accessed on 9 June 2023).
195. Furrer, E.; Hulmann, V.; Urech, D.M. Intranasal delivery of ESBA105, a TNF-alphainhibitory scFv antibody fragment to the brain. *J. Neuroimmunol.* **2009**, *215*, 65–72. [CrossRef] [PubMed]
196. Chu, L.; Wanga, A.; Ni, L.; Yan, X.; Song, Y.; Zhao, M.; Sun, K.; Mu, H.; Liu, S.; Wu, Z.; et al. Nose-to-brain delivery of temozolomide-loaded PLGA nanoparticles functionalized with anti-EPHA3 for glioblastoma targeting. *Drug Deliv.* **2018**, *25*, 1634–1641. [CrossRef] [PubMed]
197. Musumeci, T.; Di Benedetto, G.; Carbone, C.; Bonaccorso, A.; Amato, G.; Faro, M.J.L.; Burgaletto, C.; Puglisi, G.; Bernardini, R.; Cantarella, G. Intranasal Administration of a TRAIL Neutralizing Monoclonal Antibody Adsorbed in PLGA Nanoparticles and NLC Nanosystems: An In Vivo Study on a Mouse Model of Alzheimer's Disease. *Biomedicines* **2022**, *10*, 985. [CrossRef] [PubMed]
198. Mehta, M.; Deeksha; Tewari, D.; Gupta, G.; Awasthi, R.; Singh, H.; Pandey, P.; Chellappan, D.K.; Wadhwa, R.; Collet, T.; et al. Oligonucleotide therapy: An emerging focus area for drug delivery in chronic inflammatory respiratory diseases. *Chem.-Biol. Interact.* **2019**, *308*, 206–215. [CrossRef] [PubMed]
199. Yang, Y.; Zhang, X.; Wu, S.; Zhang, R.; Zhou, B.; Zhang, X.; Tang, L.; Tian, Y.; Men, K.; Yang, L. Enhanced nose-to-brain delivery of siRNA using hyaluronan-enveloped nanomicelles for glioma therapy. *J. Control. Release* **2022**, *342*, 66–80. [CrossRef] [PubMed]
200. Kim, I.D.; Shin, J.H.; Kim, S.W.; Choi, S.; Ahn, J.; Han, P.L.; Park, J.S.; Lee, J.K. Intranasal delivery of HMGB1 siRNA confers target gene knockdown and robust neuroprotection in the postischemic brain. *Mol. Ther.* **2012**, *20*, 829–839. [CrossRef]
201. Watts, J.K.; Brown, R.H.; Khvorova, A. Nucleic acid therapeutics for neurological diseases. *Neurotherapeutics* **2019**, *16*, 245–247. [CrossRef]
202. Dagle, J.M.; Weeks, D.L.; Walder, J.A.; Lennox, K.A.; Sabel, J.L.; Johnson, M.J.; Moreira, B.G.; Fletcher, C.A.; Rose, S.D.; Behlke, M.A.; et al. Pathways of degradation and mechanism of action of antisense oligonucleotides in Xenopus laevis embryos. *Antisense Res. Dev.* **1991**, *1*, 11–20. [CrossRef]
203. Borgonetti, V.; Galeotti, N. Intranasal delivery of an antisense oligonucleotide to the RNA-binding protein HuR relieves nerve injury-induced neuropathic pain. *Pain* **2021**, *162*, 1500–1510. [CrossRef] [PubMed]
204. Borgonetti, V.; Sanna, M.D.; Lucarini, L.; Galeotti, N. Targeting the RNA-Binding Protein HuR Alleviates Neuroinflammation in Experimental Autoimmune Encephalomyelitis: Potential Therapy for Multiple Sclerosis. *Neurotherapeutics* **2021**, *18*, 412–429. [CrossRef] [PubMed]
205. Hao, R.; Sun, B.; Yang, L.; Ma, C.; Li, S. RVG29-modified microRNA-loaded nanoparticles improve ischemic brain injury by nasal delivery. *Drug Deliv.* **2020**, *27*, 772–781. [CrossRef] [PubMed]
206. Samaridou, E.; Walgrave, H.; Salta, E.; Álvarez, D.M.; Castro-López, V.; Loza, M.; Alonso, M.J. Nose-to-brain delivery of enveloped RNA-cell permeating peptide nanocomplexes for the treatment of neurodegenerative diseases. *Biomaterials* **2020**, *230*, 119657. [CrossRef] [PubMed]
207. Park, J.S.; Oh, Y.K.; Yoon, H.; Kim, J.M.; Kim, C.K. In situ gelling and mucoadhesive polymer vehicles for controlled intranasal delivery of plasmid DNA. *J. Biomat. Res.* **2002**, *59*, 144–151. [CrossRef] [PubMed]
208. Evers, M.M.; Toonen, L.J.; van Roon-Mom, W.M. Antisense oligonucleotides in therapy for neurodegenerative disorders. *Adv. Drug Deliv. Rev.* **2015**, *87*, 90–103. [CrossRef] [PubMed]
209. Vetter, A.; Bernkop-Schnürch, A. Nasal delivery of antisense oligonucleotides: In vitro evaluation of a thiomer/glutathione microparticulate delivery system. *J. Drug Target.* **2010**, *18*, 303–312. [CrossRef]
210. Vetter, A.; Martien, R.; Bernkop-Schnürch, A. Thiolated polycarbophil as an adjuvant for permeation enhancement in nasal delivery of antisense oligonucleotides. *J. Pharm. Sci.* **2010**, *99*, 1427–1439. [CrossRef]
211. Gyermek, L.; Genther, G.; Fleming, N. Some effects of progesterone and related steroids on the central nervous system. *Int. J. Neuropharm.* **1967**, *6*, 191–198. [CrossRef]
212. Baulieu, E.E.; Robel, P. Neurosteroids: A new brain function? *J. Steroid Biochem. Mol. Biol.* **1990**, *37*, 395–403. [CrossRef]
213. Eser, D.; Baghai, T.C.; Schuele, T.C.; Nothdurfter, C.; Ruppercht, R. Neuroactive steroids as endogenous modulators of anxiety. *Curr. Pharm. Des.* **2008**, *14*, 3225–3253. [CrossRef]

214. Schumacher, M.; Guennoun, R.; Stein, D.G.; De Nicola, A.F. Progesterone: Therapeutic opportunities for neuroprotection and myelin repair. *Pharmacol. Ther.* **2007**, *116*, 77–106. [CrossRef] [PubMed]
215. Ducharme, N.; Banks, W.A.; Morley, J.E.; Robinson, S.M.; Niehoff, M.L.; Mattern, C.; Farr, S.A. Brain distribution and behavioural effects of progesterone and pregnenolone after intranasal or intravenous administration. *Eur. J. Pharmacol.* **2010**, *641*, 128–134. [CrossRef] [PubMed]
216. de Souza Silva, M.A.; Topic, B.; Huston, J.P.; Mattern, C. Intranasal administration of progesterone increases dopaminergic activity in amygdala and neostriatum of male rats. *Neuroscience* **2008**, *157*, 196–203. [CrossRef] [PubMed]
217. van den Berg, M.P.; Verhoef, J.C.; Romeijn, S.G.; Merkus, F.W. Uptake of estradiol or progesterone into the CSF following intranasal and intravenous delivery in rats. *Eur. Pharm. Biopharm.* **2004**, *58*, 131–135. [CrossRef] [PubMed]
218. Hermens, W.A.; Deurloo, M.J.; Romeijn, S.G.; Verhoef, J.C.; Merus, F.W. Nasal absorption enhancement of 17-b-oestradiol by dimethyl-b-cyclodextrin in rabbits and rats. *Pharm. Res.* **1990**, *7*, 500–503. [CrossRef] [PubMed]
219. Wang, X.; He, H.; Leng, W.; Tang, X. Evaluation of brain-targeting for the nasal delivery of estradiol by the microdialysis method. *Int. J. Pharm.* **2006**, *317*, 40–46. [CrossRef] [PubMed]
220. Banks, W.A.; Morley, J.E.; Niehoff, M.L.; Mattern, C. Delivery of testosterone to the brain by intranasal administration: Comparison to intravenous testosterone. *J. Drug Target.* **2009**, *17*, 91–97. [CrossRef]
221. de Souza Silva, M.A.; Mattern, C.; Topic, B.; Buddenberg, T.E.; Huston, J.P. Dopaminergic and serotonergic activity in neostriatum and nucleus accumbens enhanced by intranasal administration of testosterone. *Eur. Neuropsychopharm.* **2009**, *19*, 53–63. [CrossRef]
222. Zhang, G.; Shi, G.; Tan, H.; Kang, Y.; Cui, H. Intranasal administration of testosterone increased immobile-sniffing, exploratory behavior, motor behavior and grooming behavior in rats. *Horm. Behav.* **2011**, *59*, 477–483. [CrossRef]
223. Zolkowska, D.; Wu, C.Y.; Rogawski, M.A. Intranasal Allopregnanolone Confers Rapid Seizure Protection: Evidence for Direct Nose-to-Brain Delivery. *Neurotherapeutics* **2019**, *18*, 544–555. [CrossRef]
224. Pietrowsky, R.; Struben, C.; Molle, M.; Fehm, H.L.; Born, J. Brain potential changes after intranasal vs. intravenous administration of vasopressin: Evidence for a direct nose–brain pathway for peptide effects in humans. *Biol. Psychiatry* **1996**, *39*, 332–340. [CrossRef]
225. Derad, I.; Sayk, F.; Lehnert, H.; Marshall, L.; Born, L.J.; Nitschke, M. Intranasal angiotensin II in humans reduces blood pressure when angiotensin II type 1 receptors are blocked. *Hypertension* **2014**, *63*, 762–767. [CrossRef] [PubMed]
226. Buchthal, B.; Weiss, U.; Bading, H. Post-injury Nose-to-Brain Delivery of Activin A and SerpinB2 Reduces Brain Damage in a Mouse Stroke Model. Molecular Therapeutics. *Sci. Rep.* **2018**, *26*, 28599.
227. Manickavasagam, D.; Lin, L.; Oyewumi, M.O. Nose-to-brain codelivery of repurposed simvastatin and BDNF synergistically attenuates LPS-induced neuroinflammation. *Nanomed. NBM* **2020**, *23*, 102107. [CrossRef] [PubMed]
228. Sun, B.L.; Shen, F.P.; Wu, Q.J.; Chi, S.M.; Yang, M.F.; Yuan, H.; Xie, F.M.; Zhang, Y.B.; Chen, J.; Zhang, F. Intranasal delivery of calcitonin gene-related peptide reduces cerebral vasospasm in rats. *Front. Biosci.* **2010**, *2*, 1502–1513. [CrossRef] [PubMed]
229. Morimoto, K.; Katsumata, H.; Yabuta, T.; Iwanaga, K.; Kakemi, M.; Tabata, Y.; Ikada, Y. Evaluation of gelatin microspheres for nasal and intramuscular administrations of salmon calcitonin. *Eur. J. Pharm. Sci.* **2001**, *13*, 179–185. [CrossRef] [PubMed]
230. du Plessis, L.H.; Lubbe, J.; Strauss, T.; Kotzé, A.F. Enhancement of nasal and intestinal calcitonin delivery by the novel Pheroid™ Fatty Acid based delivery system, and by N-trimethyl chitosan chloride. *Int. J. Pharm.* **2010**, *385*, 181–186. [CrossRef] [PubMed]
231. Pietrowsky, R.; Thiemann, A.; Kern, W.; Fehm, H.L.; Born, J. A nose–brain pathway for psychotropic peptides: Evidence from a brain evoked potential study with cholecystokinin. *Psychoneuroendocrinology* **1996**, *21*, 559–572. [CrossRef] [PubMed]
232. Shaw, P.; Zhang, X. Intranasal Delivery of a Cystatin C-peptide as Therapy for Alzheimer's Disease. *FASEB J.* **2013**, *27*, 533.1. [CrossRef]
233. Zhao, N.; Zhuo, X.; Lu, Y.; Dong, Y.; Ahmed, M.E.; Tucker, D.; Scott, E.L.; Zhang, Q. Intranasal Delivery of a Caspase-1 Inhibitor in the Treatment of Global Cerebral Ischemia. *Mol. Neurobiol.* **2017**, *54*, 4936–4952. [CrossRef]
234. Yu, Y.P.; Xu, Q.Q.; Zhang, Q.; Zhang, W.P.; Zhang, L.H.; Wei, E.Q. Intranasal recombinant human erythropoietin protects rats against focal cerebral ischemia. *Neurosci. Lett.* **2005**, *387*, 5–10. [CrossRef] [PubMed]
235. Rodríguez, C.Y.; Strehaiano, M.; Rodríguez, O.T.; García Rodríguez, R.J.C.; Maurice, T. An Intranasal Formulation of Erythropoietin (Neuro-EPO) Prevents Memory Deficits and Amyloid Toxicity in the APPSwe Transgenic Mouse Model of Alzheimer's Disease. *J. Alzheimer's Dis.* **2017**, *55*, 231–248. [CrossRef] [PubMed]
236. Kim, T.H.; Park, C.W.; Kim, H.Y.; Chi, M.H.; Lee, S.K.; Song, Y.M.; Jiang, H.H.; Lim, S.M.; Youn, Y.S.; Lee, K.C. Low molecular weight (1 kDa) polyethylene glycol conjugation markedly enhances the hypoglycemic effects of intranasally administered exendin-4 in type 2 diabetic db/db mice. *Biol. Pharm. Bull.* **2012**, *35*, 1076–1083. [CrossRef] [PubMed]
237. Gorbatov, V.Y.; Trekova, N.A.; Fomina, V.G.; Davydova, T.V. Antiamnestic effects of antibodies to glutamate in experimental Alzheimer's disease. *Bull. Exp. Biol. Med.* **2010**, *150*, 23–25. [CrossRef] [PubMed]
238. Nonaka, N.; Farr, S.A.; Kageyama, H.; Shioda, S.; Banks, W.A. Delivery of galanin-like peptide to the brain: Targeting with intranasal delivery and cyclodextrins. *J. Pharmacol. Exp. Ther.* **2008**, *325*, 513–519. [CrossRef] [PubMed]
239. Zheng, X.; Shao, X.; Zhang, C.; Tan, Y.; Liu, Q.; Wan, X.; Zhang, Q.; Xu, S.; Jiang, X. Intranasal H102 Peptide-Loaded Liposomes for Brain Delivery to Treat Alzheimer's Disease. *Pharm. Res.* **2015**, *32*, 3837–3849. [CrossRef] [PubMed]
240. Capsoni, S.; Marinelli, S.; Ceci, M.; Vignone, D.; Amato, G.; Malerba, F.; Paoletti, F.; Meli, G.; Viegi, A.; Pavone, F.; et al. Correction: Intranasal "painless" Human Nerve Growth Factors Slows Amyloid Neurodegeneration and Prevents Memory Deficits in App X PS1 Mice. *PLoS ONE* **2012**, *7*, e37555. [CrossRef]

241. Wu, H.; Li, J.; Zhang, Q.; Yan, X.; Guo, L.; Gao, X.; Qiu, M.; Jiang, X.; Lai, R.; Chen, H. A novel small Odorranalectin-bearing cubosomes: Preparation, brain delivery and pharmacodynamic study on amyloid-$\beta_{25-35}$-treated rats following intranasal administration. *Eur. J. Pharm. Biopharm.* **2012**, *80*, 368–378. [CrossRef]
242. Callens, C.; Remon, J.P. Evaluation of starch–maltodextrin–carbopol®974 P mixtures for the nasal delivery of insulin in Rabbits. *J. Control. Release* **2000**, *66*, 215–220. [CrossRef]
243. Illum, L.; Fisher, A.N.; Jabbal-Gill, I.; Davis, S.S. Bioadhesive starch microspheres and absorption enhancing agents act synergistically to enhance the nasal absorption of polypeptides. *Int. J. Pharm.* **2001**, *222*, 109–119. [CrossRef] [PubMed]
244. Liu, X.-F.; Fawcett, J.R.; Thorne, R.G.; De For, T.A.; Frey, W.H., 2nd. Intranasal administration of insulin-like growth factor-I bypasses the blood–brain barrier and protects against focal cerebral ischemic damage. *J. Neurol. Sci.* **2001**, *187*, 91–97. [CrossRef] [PubMed]
245. Thorne, R.G.; Hanson, L.R.; Ross, T.M.; Tung, D.; Frey, W.H., 2nd. Delivery of interferon-beta to the monkey nervous system following intranasal administration. *Neuroscience* **2008**, *152*, 785–797. [CrossRef] [PubMed]
246. Ross, T.M.; Martinez, P.M.; Renner, J.C.; Thorne, R.G.; Hanson, L.R.; Frey, W.H., 2nd. Intranasal administration of interferon beta bypasses the blood–brain barrier to target the central nervous system and cervical lymph nodes: A non-invasive treatment strategy for multiple sclerosis. *J. Neuroimmunol.* **2004**, *151*, 66–77. [CrossRef] [PubMed]
247. Fliedner, S.; Schulz, C.; Lehnert, H. Brain uptake of intranasally applied radioiodinated leptin in Wistar rats. *Endocrinology* **2006**, *147*, 2088–2094. [CrossRef] [PubMed]
248. Liu, Z.; Jiang, M.; Kang, T.; Miao, D.; Gu, G.; Song, Q.; Yao, Q.L.; Hu, Q.; Tu, Y.; Pang, Z.; et al. Lactoferrin-modified PEG-co-PCL nanoparticles for enhanced brain delivery of NAP peptide following intranasal administration. *Biomaterials* **2013**, *34*, 3870–3881. [CrossRef] [PubMed]
249. Zhao, Y.Z.; Jin, R.R.; Yang, W.; Xiang, Q.; Yu, W.Z.; Lin, Q.; Tian, F.R.; Mao, K.L.; Lv, C.Z.; Wang, Y.X.J.; et al. Using gelatin nanoparticle mediated intranasal delivery of neuropeptide substance P to enhance neuro-recovery in hemiparkinsonian rats. *PLoS ONE* **2016**, *11*, e0148848. [CrossRef] [PubMed]
250. Cheng, Q.; Feng, J.; Chen, J.; Zhu, X.; Li, F. Brain transport of neurotoxin-I with PLA nanoparticles through intranasal administration in rats: A microdialysis study. *Biopharm. Drug Dispos.* **2008**, *29*, 431–439. [CrossRef]
251. Ruan, Y.; Yao, L.; Zhang, B.; Zhang, S.; Guo, J. Antinociceptive properties of nasal delivery of Neurotoxin-loaded nanoparticles coated with polysorbate-80. *Peptides* **2012**, *32*, 1526–1529. [CrossRef]
252. Li, R.; Huang, Y.; Chen, L.; Zhou, H.; Zhang, M.; Chang, L.; Shen, H.; Zhou, M.; Su, P.; Zhu, D. Targeted delivery of intranasally administered nanoparticles-mediated neuroprotective peptide NR2B9c to brain and neuron for treatment of ischemic stroke. *Nanomed. NBM* **2019**, *18*, 380–390. [CrossRef]
253. Hess, L.; Votava, M.; Málek, J.; Kurzová, A.; Slíva, J. Sedative effects of intranasal oxytocin in rabbits and rhesus monkeys. *Physiol. Res.* **2016**, *65*, S473–S480. [CrossRef] [PubMed]
254. Tanaka, A.; Furubayashi, T.; Arai, M.; Inoue, D.; Kimura, S.; Kiriyama, A.; Kusamori, K.; Katsumi, H.; Yutani, R.; Sakane, T.; et al. Delivery of oxytocin to the brain for the treatment of autism spectrum disorder by nasal application. *Mol. Pharm.* **2018**, *15*, 1105–1111. [CrossRef] [PubMed]
255. Monte, O.D.; Noble, P.L.; Turchi, J.; Cummins, A.; Averbeck, B.B. CSF and blood oxytocin concentration changes following intranasal delivery in macaque. *PLoS ONE* **2014**, *9*, e103677.
256. Deadwyler, S.A.; Porrino, L.; Siegel, J.M.; Hampson, R.E. Systemic and nasal delivery of orexin- A (Hypocretin-1) reduces the effects of sleep deprivation on cognitive performance in nonhuman primates. *J. Neurosci.* **2007**, *27*, 14239–14247. [CrossRef] [PubMed]
257. Dhuria, S.V.; Hanson, L.R.; Frey, W.H. Novel vasoconstrictor formulation to enhance intranasal targeting of neuropeptide therapeutics to the central nervous system. *J. Pharmacol. Exp. Ther.* **2009**, *328*, 312–320. [CrossRef] [PubMed]
258. Gordon, L.B.; Knopf, P.M.; Cserr, H.F. Ovalbumin is more immunogenic when introduced into brain or cerebrospinal fluid than into extracerebral sites. *J. Neuroimmunol.* **1992**, *40*, 81–87. [CrossRef] [PubMed]
259. Rat, D.; Schmitt, U.; Tippmann, F.; Dewachter, I.; Theunis, C.; Wieczerzak, E.; Postina, R.; Leuven, F.; Fahrenholz, F.; Kojro, E.; et al. Neuropeptide pituitary adenylate cyclase-activating polypeptide (PACAP) slows down Alzheimer's disease-like pathology in amyloid precursor protein-transgenic mice. *FASEB J.* **2011**, *25*, 3208–3218. [CrossRef] [PubMed]
260. Yang, X.; Yang, W.; Xia, X.; Lei, T.; Yang, Z.; Jia, W.; Zhou, Y.; Cheng, G.; Gao, H. Intranasal Delivery of BACE1 siRNA and Rapamycin by Dual Targets Modified Nanoparticles for Alzheimer's Disease Therapy. *Small* **2022**, *18*, 2203182. [CrossRef]
261. Kim, I.D.; Sawicki, E.; Lee, H.K.; Lee, E.H.; Park, H.J.; Han, P.L.; Kim, K.K.; Choi, H.; Lee, J.K. Robust neuroprotective effects of intranasally delivered iNOS siRNA encapsulated in gelatin nanoparticles in the postischemic brain. *Nanomedicine* **2016**, *12*, 1219–1229. [CrossRef]
262. Veronesi, M.C.; Aldouby, Y.; Domb, A.J.; Kubek, M.J. Thyrotropin-releasing hormone d,l polylactide nanoparticles (TRH-NPs) protect against glutamate toxicity in vitro and kindling development in vivo. *Brain Res.* **2009**, *1303*, 151–160. [CrossRef]
263. Kaur, S.; Manhas, P.; Swami, A.; Bhandari, R.; Sharma, K.K.; Jain, R.; Kumar, R.; Pandey, S.K.; Kuhad, A.; Sharma, R.K.; et al. Bioengineered PLGA-chitosan nanoparticles for brain targeted intranasal delivery of antiepileptic TRH analogues. *Chem. Eng. J.* **2018**, *346*, 630–639. [CrossRef]

264. Wen, Z.; Yan, Z.; Hu, K.; Pang, Z.; Cheng, X.; Guo, L.; Zhang, Q.; Jiang, X.; Fang, L.; Lai, R. Odorranalectinconjugated nanoparticles: Preparation, brain delivery and pharmacodynamic study on Parkinson's disease following intranasal administration. *J. Control. Release* **2011**, *151*, 131–138. [CrossRef] [PubMed]
265. Yang, J.P.; Liu, H.J.; Wang, Z.L.; Cheng, S.M.; Cheng, X.; Xu, G.L.; Liu, X.F. The dose effectiveness of intranasal VEGF in treatment of experimental stroke. *Neurosci. Lett.* **2009**, *461*, 212–216. [CrossRef] [PubMed]
266. Yang, J.P.; Liu, H.J.; Cheng, S.M.; Wang, Z.L.; Cheng, X.; Yu, H.X.; Liu, X.F. Direct transport of VEGF from the nasal cavity to brain. *Neurosci. Lett.* **2009**, *449*, 108–111. [CrossRef] [PubMed]
267. Gao, X.; Wu, B.; Zhang, Q.; Chen, J.; Zhu, J.; Zhang, W.; Rong, Z.; Chen, H.; Jiang, X. Brain delivery of vasoactive intestinal peptide enhanced with the nanoparticles conjugated with wheat germ agglutinin following intranasal administration. *J. Control. Release* **2007**, *121*, 156–167. [CrossRef] [PubMed]
268. Brogden, R.N.; Buckley, M.M.; Ward, A.; Buserelin, A. A review of its pharmacodynamic and pharmacokinetic properties, and clinical profile. *Drugs* **1990**, *39*, 399–437. [CrossRef] [PubMed]
269. Thwala, L.N.; Préat, V.; Csaba, N.S. Emerging delivery platforms for mucosal administration of biopharmaceuticals: A critical update on nasal, pulmonary and oral routes. *Expert Opin. Drug Deliv.* **2017**, *14*, 23–36. [CrossRef] [PubMed]
270. Sherr, J.L.; Ruedy, K.J.; Foster, N.C.; Piché, C.A.; Dulude, H.; Rickels, M.R.; Tamborlane, W.V.; Bethin, K.E.; Di Meglio, L.A.; Fox, L.A.; et al. T1D Exchange Intranasal Glucagon Investigators, A Promising Alternative to Intramuscular Glucagon in Youth with Type 1 Diabetes. *Diabetes Care.* **2016**, *39*, 555–562. [CrossRef]
271. Chrisp, P.; Goa, K.L. Nafarelin: A review of its pharmacodynamic and pharmacokinetic properties, and clinical potential in sex hormone-related conditions. *Drugs* **1990**, *39*, 523–551. [CrossRef]
272. Kaneb, A.; Berardino, K.; Hanukaai, J.S.; Rooney, K.; Kaye, A.D. Calcitonin (FORTICAL, MIACALCIN) for the treatment of vertebral compression fractures. *Orthop. Rev.* **2021**, *13*, 24976. [CrossRef]
273. Rohrer, J.; Lupo, N.; Bernkop-Schnürch, A. Advanced formulations for intranasal delivery of biologics. *Int. J. Pharm.* **2018**, *553*, 8–20. [CrossRef]
274. U.S. Food and Drugs Administration. Center for Drug Evaluation and Research Drug Approvals and Databases. Available online: https://www.fda.gov/drugs/development-approval-process-drugs/drug-approvals-and-databasesInformation (accessed on 20 October 2023).
275. National Library of Medicine. Available online: https://www.clinicaltrials.gov (accessed on 3 November 2023).

*pharmaceutics*

MDPI

*Article*

# Self-Assembled Lecithin-Chitosan Nanoparticles Improved Rotigotine Nose-to-Brain Delivery and Brain Targeting Efficiency

**Paramita Saha [1], Prabhjeet Singh [1], Himanshu Kathuria [2], Deepak Chitkara [1] and Murali Monohar Pandey [1,*]**

[1] Industrial Research Laboratory, Department of Pharmacy, Birla Institute of Technology & Science, Pilani Rajasthan 333031, India
[2] Nusmetics Pte Ltd., E-Centre@Redhill, 3791 Jalan Bukit Merah, Singapore 159471, Singapore
* Correspondence: mmpphd@gmail.com or pandeymm@pilani.bits-pilani.ac.in

**Abstract:** Rotigotine (RTG) is a non-ergoline dopamine agonist and an approved drug for treating Parkinson's disease. However, its clinical use is limited due to various problems, viz. poor oral bioavailability (<1%), low aqueous solubility, and extensive first-pass metabolism. In this study, rotigotine-loaded lecithin-chitosan nanoparticles (RTG-LCNP) were formulated to enhance its nose-to-brain delivery. RTG-LCNP was prepared by self-assembly of chitosan and lecithin due to ionic interactions. The optimized RTG-LCNP had an average diameter of 108 nm with 14.43 ± 2.77% drug loading. RTG-LCNP exhibited spherical morphology and good storage stability. Intranasal RTG-LCNP improved the brain availability of RTG by 7.86 fold with a 3.84-fold increase in the peak brain drug concentration ($C_{max(brain)}$) compared to intranasal drug suspensions. Further, the intranasal RTG-LCNP significantly reduced the peak plasma drug concentration ($C_{max(plasma)}$) compared to intranasal RTG suspensions. The direct drug transport percentage (DTP (%)) of optimized RTG-LCNP was found to be 97.3%, which shows effective direct nose-to-brain drug uptake and good targeting efficiency. In conclusion, RTG-LCNP enhanced drug brain availability, showing the potential for clinical application.

**Keywords:** rotigotine; lecithin-chitosan hybrid nanoparticles; intranasal delivery; nose-to-brain uptake; brain distribution study

**Citation:** Saha, P.; Singh, P.; Kathuria, H.; Chitkara, D.; Pandey, M.M. Self-Assembled Lecithin-Chitosan Nanoparticles Improved Rotigotine Nose-to-Brain Delivery and Brain Targeting Efficiency. *Pharmaceutics* **2023**, *15*, 851. https://doi.org/10.3390/pharmaceutics15030851

Academic Editors: Nicolas Tournier, Toshihiko Tashima and Maria Camilla Bergonzi

Received: 11 December 2022
Revised: 11 February 2023
Accepted: 3 March 2023
Published: 5 March 2023



## 1. Introduction

Parkinson's disease (PD) is the second most prevalent neurodegenerative disorder, following Alzheimer's disease [1]. It significantly impairs patients' quality of life and productivity. Although PD is primarily a motor condition, research indicates that most patients (>90%) also experience non-motor symptoms. Frequently used drugs to treat PD provide only symptomatic relief. The efficacy of most anti-Parkinson drugs is limited due to their low systemic bioavailability and poor availability into the brain.

Rotigotine (RTG) is a dopamine agonist approved for treating PD [2]. It impacts both the motor and non-motor symptoms of PD. The benefits of RTG are superior to other standard dopamine agonists. RTG is available as 1–8 mg transdermal sustained-release patches applied for 24 h. RTG has low (<1%) oral bioavailability due to high hepatic first-pass metabolism [3]. The transdermal patch shows a systemic bioavailability of approximately 37% [4]. The bioavailability also varies depending on the site of application of the transdermal patch [3]. The availability of RTG in the brain is further hampered due to the blood–brain barrier (BBB). Therefore, developing a suitable delivery system for RTG that can be administered via an alternate route is required to avoid first-pass metabolism and efficiently increase the brain availability of the drug.

The BBB hinders the brain's availability of drugs, affecting their efficacy. Several delivery systems have been developed to overcome the BBB, such as cerebral implants and intracerebroventricular injections, which increase the brain availability of drugs. However, the invasive nature of these methods comes with a considerable risk [5,6]. Intranasal (i.n.) delivery is a non-invasive approach that avoids the BBB by increasing the direct nose-to-brain uptake of drugs. It also offers ease of administration, quick onset of action, and avoids first-pass metabolism and systemic toxicity. It has been reported that olfactory neural pathways and the trigeminal nerves are involved in the transport of drugs to the brain via the nasal cavity [7,8]. However, mucociliary clearance prevents drug retention in the nasal cavity, affecting the direct nose-to-brain delivery of drugs. Therefore, a suitable formulation approach is required to slow the mucociliary clearance process and increase the drug's permeability via the nasal epithelium following i.n. administration. Several nanocarriers have been investigated for RTG to increase the brain bioavailability of the drug [9–12]. Considering the advantages and disadvantages of previously reported polymeric and lipidic systems, a self-assembling system containing both polymer and lipid was found to be advantageous as compared to the previous approaches. Chitosan (CS)-lecithin nanoparticles of hydrophilic and lipophilic drugs are reported in the literature for oral, transdermal, and intranasal delivery [13–17]. These nanoparticles have been found to enhance the drugs' oral, systemic, and brain bioavailability.

CS is a biodegradable polysaccharide with a positive charge. It is a widely used pharmaceutical excipient because it is biocompatible and mucoadhesive. CS is available in various molecular weights, degrees of deacetylation and viscosities. CS-based i.n. formulations have shown improved nasal residence time and better mucoadhesion [18]. CS-nanocarriers are known to affect the tight junctions that help to enhance the transport of nanocarriers via an olfactory neuronal pathway [19]. CS-based nanocarriers with a size of ~100 nm renders increased rate and extent of drug uptake following i.n. administration via either paracellular or transcellular transport [20]. Several other reports also show that the surface and size properties of nanoparticles play a key role in the transport and uptake via the intranasal route, affecting drug brain availability [9,21]. Soy lecithin is a negatively charged phospholipid combination consisting mainly of phosphatidylcholines. It is a biocompatible, safe, and non-immunogenic excipient. The interaction between lecithin and the CS can produce nanoparticles by self-assembling utilizing ionic interactions.

In this study, RTG-loaded lecithin-CS nanoparticles (RTG-LCNP) were prepared and optimized for i.n. administration. This study hypothesized that RTG-LCNP could improve nasal mucoadhesion due to CS and improve RTG brain absorption. RTG-LCNP were characterized for size distribution, the zeta potential, microscopic morphology, drug crystallinity, and in vitro drug release. An ex vivo nasal study was performed to evaluate the RTG nasal permeability from RTG-LCNP. The nasal clearance time and in vivo study of the optimized LCNP were performed to assess the direct nose-to-brain delivery and brain targeting efficiency.

## 2. Materials and Methods

### *2.1. Materials*

Mylan Laboratories (Hyderabad, India) provided RTG as a gift sample. Glipizide, an internal standard (IS), was acquired from TCI Chemicals Pvt Ltd. (Chennai, India). Isoflurane USP was purchased from Abbott (Mumbai, India) for inhalation anesthesia. Medium-molecular-weight chitosan (75–85% deacetylated), acetic acid glacial was purchased from SISCO Research Laboratories (SRL) Pvt. Ltd. (Delhi, India). Lecithin (Lipoid S 100, soybean lecithin with phosphatidylcholine) and Poloxamer 407 were obtained as gift samples from Lipoid (GmBH, Germany) and BASF (Mumbai, India), respectively. Sodium chloride, potassium chloride, mannitol, and different buffer salts ($KH_2PO_4$, $K_2HPO_4$) were acquired from SD Fine Chemicals Pvt. Ltd. (Mumbai, India). HPLC grade acetonitrile (ACN) was purchased from Merck (Mumbai, India). Milli-Q water was taken from a Milli-Q® Reference water purification system (GmbH, Germany) and was used in all experimental procedures and analysis. Wistar rats were acquired from Central animal facility,

BITS Pilani, Pilani, India. All the statistical analysis were performed using GraphPad Prism 7.0 (GraphPad software Inc., San Diego, CA, USA).

### 2.2. Preparation of Rotigotine Nanoparticles

The LCNP was prepared by a solvent injection method [16,17]. An ethanolic solution of the drug and lecithin was prepared by dissolving 20 mg of RTG and lecithin in 1 mL of ethanol. CS and Poloxamer 407 were dissolved in aqueous acidic solution prepared with glacial acetic acid. The ethanolic solution was injected into the aqueous phase using a 22G needle attached to a polypropylene syringe. The injection was performed for 5 min under high-speed homogenization (Polytron PT 1300D, Kinematica, Lucerne, Switzerland) at 12,000 rpm. The organic solvent was evaporated from nano-dispersion using rotavapor (Buchi, Mumbai, India) for 10 min. After removal of organic solvent, RTG-LCNP was ultracentrifuged (Thermo Fisher, Waltham, MA, USA) at 45,000 rpm for 1 h at 4 °C to attain pellet of RTG-LCNP. The supernatant was decanted, and the LCNP was collected. Further, LCNP pellets were washed thrice with Milli-Q water to remove any traces of free drug from the surface of LCNP. For lyophilization, the finally collected pellet of RTG-LCNP was re-dispersed in mannitol solution (10% *w*/*v*), where mannitol acted as a cryoprotectant (Figure 1). The lyophilized RTG-LCNP was stored under refrigerated conditions (2–8 °C) till further use. A control RTG suspension was prepared by dispersing RTG in 0.2% *w*/*v* methyl cellulose (400 cps).

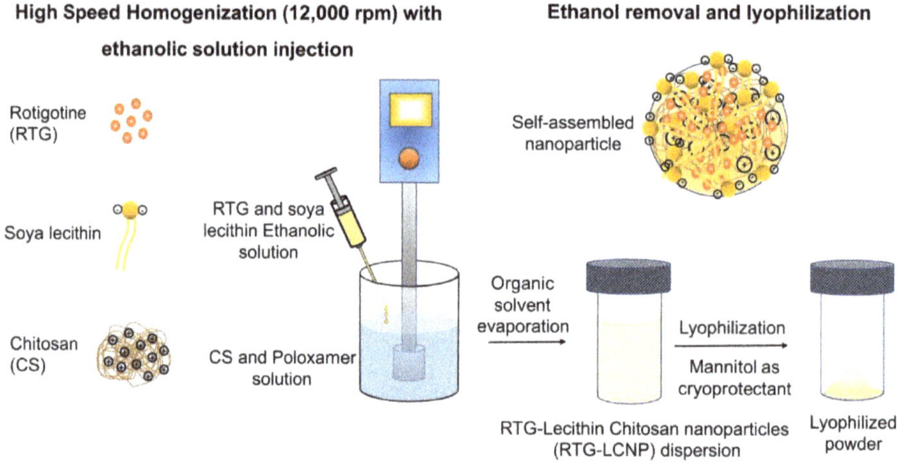


**Figure 1.** Schematic of RTG-LCNP preparation with soya lecithin, chitosan, and Poloxamer using high-speed homogenization. The soya lecithin and chitosan self-assembled due to ionic interaction upon ethanolic injection with homogenization, encapsulating RTG, and stabilized by Poloxamer.

The effect of several formulation parameters, viz. the ratio of drug:lecithin, the ratio of lecithin:CS, amount of Poloxamer 407, pH of CS solution on particle size, PDI, % entrapment efficiency (%EE), and % drug loading (%DL) were optimized to select the final LCNP batch. The final optimum composition of RTG-LCNP was 20 mg RTG, 60 mg lecithin, 2 mg chitosan, and 5 mg Poloxamer.

### 2.3. Size and Zeta Potential Measurements

The average particle size (d.nm) and PDI of RTG-LCNP were determined using the dynamic light scattering technique (Zetasizer nano ZS, Malvern Instruments, Malvern, UK). The zeta potential was measured using electrophoretic dynamic light scattering. The LCNP suspensions were diluted 10 fold with sodium acetate buffer (pH 5.5) and allowed to equilibrate for 2 min at 25 °C before each measurement. Three measurements were performed for every LCNP suspension, and the mean values were reported for the final particle size, PDI, and zeta potential.

### 2.4. Entrapment Efficiency and Drug Loading

The entrapment efficiency (%EE) was estimated from the unentrapped amount of RTG ($W_{Free\ drug}$). The free RTG was separated from LCNP suspension by ultracentrifuged at 45,000 rpm for 1 h. The supernatant was analyzed using the validated RP-HPLC analytical method to measure free RTG ($W_{free\ drug}$) [22]. %EE of LCNP was calculated using the following equation:

$$\%EE = \left( \frac{W_{Total\ drug} - W_{Free\ drug}}{W_{Total\ drug}} \right) \times 100 \quad (1)$$

where $W_{Total\ drug}$ is the total amount of RTG used in the preparation of RTG-LCNP, $W_{Free\ drug}$ is the unentrapped drug.

The drug loading (%DL) was estimated following the direct method. RTG-LCNP pellets were collected after ultracentrifugation (45,000 rpm for 1 h at 4 °C), washed, and dried under vacuum. The collected pellets were first weighed, dissolved in ACN to extract RTG, and diluted with the mobile phase. The quantity of RTG was determined using validated RP-HPLC analytical method [22]. Finally, %DL was calculated using the formula given in the equation below:

$$\%DL = \left( \frac{W_{RTG}}{W_{RTG-LCNP}} \right) \times 100 \quad (2)$$

where $W_{RTG}$ is the weight of RTG loaded in the LCNP and $W_{RTG\text{-}LCNP}$ is the total weight of NP.

### 2.5. Differential Scanning Calorimetry

Thermal analysis was carried out using differential scanning calorimetry (DSC) to analyze the physical state of RTG encapsulated in the optimized RTG-LCNP. Lyophilized RTG-LCNP was accurately weighed inside an aluminum pan and crimped. The samples were analyzed using DSC-60 Plus (Shimadzu, Nakagyo-ku, Kyoto, Japan) at a temperature range of 30–250 °C and heated at a rate of 5 °C/min in a nitrogen environment (50 mL/min). DSC analysis was also performed for pure RTG, CS, lecithin, and mannitol.

### 2.6. Field Emission Scanning Electron Microscopy

A field emission scanning electron microscope (FESEM) (FEI, Hillsboro, OR, USA) was used for the examination of surface morphology of the optimized LCNP. Briefly, 5 µL of optimized RTG-LCNP suspension was dropped onto a glass coverslip and left overnight to dry under the desiccator [23]. The sample containing glass coverslip was attached to the aluminum stab using double-sided carbon tape. Finally, the samples were sputter coated for 50 s by Q150TES sputter coater (Quorum Technologies, Laughton, East Sussex, UK). Gold-coated samples were analyzed using FESEM using a 15 kV high-voltage vacuum pump.

### 2.7. Transmission Electron Microscopy

The particle size and shape of RTG-LCNP and pure-RTG were evaluated using transmission electron microscopy (TEM) (JEOL Ltd., Akishima, Tokyo, Japan) at an accelerating voltage of 120 kV. The samples were prepared by drop cast on carbon grids. The formulation droplet was dropped on the carbon grid and casted on the grid for a few minutes. Then, the excess liquid was soaked using blotting paper before analysis. The cast grid was placed in TEM to take microscopic images for morphological analysis.

### 2.8. *Storage Stability of Nanoparticles*

The storage stability of the lyophilized RTG-LCNP was analyzed over 60 days in refrigerated conditions. RTG-LCNP were taken in airtight glass containers (15 mL) and stored at 2–8 °C. Samples (n = 3) were collected on 7 day, 30 day, and 60 day, redispersed in Milli-Q water by gentle manual shaking, and evaluated for the particle size (d.nm), PDI, zeta potential (mV), and %DL.

### 2.9. *In Vitro Drug Release*

RTG-LCNP drug release was performed using the dialysis bag method (Molecular weight cut-off of 12 kDa, Himedia, Mumbai, India). The dialysis bag was soaked in Milli-Q water for 2 h. An amount of 1 mg drug equivalent RTG-LCNP and RTG suspension were separately taken in a dialysis bag. Bags were sealed and immersed in the 50 mL phosphate buffer saline (PBS, pH 7.4). The system was maintained at 37 ± 2 °C with constant stirring at 100 rpm [24]. The 1 mL samples were withdrawn at predetermined intervals from 0.5 h to 24 h, and replenished with pre-heated fresh medium. The samples were diluted with mobile phase and analyzed using the validated RP-HPLC method [22]. The release profiles of RTG-LCNP were analyzed to understand the kinetics and release mechanism. The most common mathematical models, i.e., first-order, Higuchi, and Korsmeyer–Peppas were applied. The high correlation coefficient ($R^2$) was taken as the best fit. The 'n' value obtained in the Korsmeyer–Peppas model was used to assess the drug release mechanism. The similarity factor ($f_2$) was determined to compare RTG-LCNP and RTG suspension release profiles.

### 2.10. *Ex Vivo Nasal Drug Permeation*

Goat nasal mucosa was acquired from a local slaughterhouse. The Franz diffusion cell (Orchid Scientific, Nasik, India) with a diffusion area of 0.785 $cm^2$ was used. The mucosa was first hydrated in PBS (pH 6.4) for 15 min 5 mL of PBS (pH 6.4) as permeation media was filled in the receptor compartment. The nasal mucosa was facing toward the donor compartment. The diffusion cell was kept under magnetic stirring at 50 rpm and maintained at 33 ± 1 °C 1 mL of each formulation was placed in the donor compartment to study drug nasal permeation. The 500 μL samples were taken at various intervals, from 5 min to 360 min, and replenished with the pre-heated fresh media. All the samples were centrifuged (Eppendorf®, Hamburg, Germany) at 15,000 rpm for 15 min at 4 °C. Supernatants were collected, processed, and analyzed using validated RP-HPLC [22].

### 2.11. *In Vivo studies in Wistar Rats*

Male Wistar rats aged 9–10 weeks weighing 250–260 g were used. A 2 mg/Kg dose was administered for optimized RTG-LCNP and RTG suspension. Prior approval from the Institute's Animal Ethics Committee (IAEC) was obtained for all the in vivo animal studies (Protocol number- IAEC/RES/26/07/REV-1/30/19).

#### 2.11.1. Administration of Intranasal (i.n.) Formulation to Rats

Formulations were administered to the nasal cavity of rats using a 1.3 cm long soft cannula (Instech Laboratories, Plymouth, PA, USA) attached in front of microtip. Rats were anaesthetized inside an anesthetic chamber using isoflurane prior to dosing and during plasma collection. A volume of 75 μL of each formulation (dose of 2 mg/Kg) was administered in one of each nostrils [16], and animals were kept in supine position till recovery. The pharmacokinetics (PK) parameters of the brain and plasma of LCNP were compared with those of RTG suspension.

#### 2.11.2. Mucociliary Transport Time RTG-LCNP

After i.n. administration of formulations, the oropharyngeal cavity was swabbed using cotton buds at 5–90 min intervals. For 1 h after study initiation, animals were not fed the food. The samples were diluted 10 fold with the mobile phase and analyzed using a validated analytical method [22]. The time point when the drug was first detected in the oropharyngeal cavity was called mucociliary transport time.

2.11.3. Brain and Plasma PK Analysis

For the brain PK study, rats were divided into various groups with n = 4 in each group. The groups were divided based on time points of brain collection. The rats were sacrificed by cervical dislocation, and the whole brain was collected at predetermined intervals (0.5, 1, 2, 4, 6, and 8 h). At each time point, rats were sacrificed for brain PK studies. A separate group of rats (n = 4) was assigned for the plasma PK study. Blood samples were collected through retro-orbital plexus puncture at predetermined intervals (0, 0.08, 0.25, 0.5, 1, 2, 4, 6, and 8 h). Brain and plasma samples were processed and analyzed using a validated RP-HPLC bioanalytical method (Supplementary Materials S1). PK parameters (viz. $C_{max}$, $T_{max}$, $AUC_{0\rightarrow tlast}$, MRT, clearance) were determined by non-compartmental analysis (NCA) using Phoenix WinNonlin (Version 8.0) for both brain and plasma.

Drug targeting efficiency percentage (DTE (%)) and brain drug direct transport percentage (DTP (%)) were calculated to evaluate the brain targeting efficiency. DTE (%) signifies the total drug transported to the brain that contains direct nose-to-brain and indirect nose-to-brain via systemic circulation. DTP (%) demonstrates the drug fraction delivered directly to the brain through the nose. DTE (%) > 100 and a DTP (%) > 0, signify substantial direct nose-to-brain distribution of the drug. DTE (%) and DTP (%) were calculated using the following equations:

$$DTE\ (\%) = \frac{\left(AUC_{brain}/AUC_{plasma}\right)_{i.n.}}{\left(AUC_{brain}/AUC_{plasma}\right)_{i.v.}} \times 100 \quad (3)$$

where $AUC_{brain} = AUC_{0\rightarrow tlast}$ in brain, $AUC_{plasma} = AUC_{0\rightarrow tlast}$ in plasma

$$DTP(\%) = \frac{AUC_{brain\,i.n.} - B_x}{AUC_{brain\,i.n.}} \times 100 \quad (4)$$

where

$$B_x = \frac{AUC_{brain\,i.v.}}{AUC_{plasma\,i.v.}} \times AUC_{plasma\,i.n.}$$

where $AUC_{brain} = AUC_{0\rightarrow tlast}$ in brain, $AUC_{plasma} = AUC_{0\rightarrow tlast}$ in plasma. $B_x$ is the fraction of $AUC_{0\rightarrow last(brain)}$ from systemic circulation (via an indirect pathway) after i.n. administration of a given formulation.

### *2.12. Histopathology of Brain*

The brains were isolated from rats before i.n. administration (as control) and at 8 h after i.n. administration of drug suspension and RTG-LCNP. The isolated brains were washed in PBS (pH 7.4) to remove traces of blood and connective tissues. The cleaned brains were weighed and fixed in 10% *v/v* formalin solution. The brain tissues were embedded in paraffin wax, sectioned, and stained with hematoxylin and eosin. The histopathological slides were examined using an inverted light microscope (Carl Zeiss, Jena, Germany). Three rats from each group were used for this study.

## 3. Results and Discussion

### *3.1. Effect of Drug: Lecithin Ratio on Nanoparticle Size*

The amount of lecithin played an essential role in preparation of the nanoparticles. Lecithin concentration also directly affect %EE and %DL of nanoparticles. Firstly, drug:lecithin ratio was optimized for preparation of the formulation. The drug:lecithin ratio affected the particle size and PDI of the drug:lecithin dispersion (Table 1). Drug:lecithin ratio was varied between 1:1 to 1:6 (*w*/*w*) during the formulation optimization. The change in drug:lecithin ratio from 1:1 to 1:3 (*w*/*w*) resulted in significant ($p < 0.0001$, one-way ANOVA-Tukey test) decrease in the particle size. Further change in drug:lecithin ratio from 1:4 to 1:6 (*w/w*) caused an increased particle size and PDI significantly ($p < 0.0001$, one-way ANOVA-Tukey test). The ratio of 1:3 (*w*/*w*) had the lowest particle size and PDI. Hence, the drug:lecithin (1:3) ratio was considered the optimum for RTG-LCNP formulation. Both lower and higher lecithin concentrations resulted in increased particle size and PDI. The result might be attributed to the fact that an increase in lecithin amount results in aggregation of particles, whereas a decrease in lecithin amount fails to suitably stabilize the dispersion.

**Table 1.** Effect of drug:lecithin ratio on the particle size and PDI of RTG-LCNP.

| Formulation Code [a] | Drug:Lecithin Ratio (*w/w*) | Particle Size (nm) | PDI |
|---|---|---|---|
| LCNP 1 | 1:1 | 220 ± 1.33 | 0.451 ± 0.011 |
| LCNP 2 | 1:2 | 182 ± 2.34 | 0.412 ± 0.014 |
| LCNP 3 | 1:3 | 123 ± 2.12 | 0.292 ± 0.002 |
| LCNP 4 | 1:4 | 263 ± 1.22 | 0.409 ± 0.009 |
| LCNP 5 | 1:5 | 294 ± 1.56 | 0.495 ± 0.003 |
| LCNP 6 | 1:6 | 322 ± 2.86 | 0.309 ± 0.001 |

[a] LCNP 1 to LCNP 6 contain 20 mg of RTG

### *3.2. Effect of Lecithin:CS Ratio on the Particle Size and PDI*

Lecithin:CS ratio also affects the particle size and PDI of the LCNP. A proper complexation between lecithin and CS is a prerequisite for preparing self-assembled LCNP and resulting in the desired particle size. Lecithin:CS ratio was varied between 10 to 30, where the lecithin amount was kept constant at 60 mg. The increased lecithin:CS ratio resulted in a lower particle size (Table 2), whereas a lower lecithin:CS ratio resulted in a higher particle size. These results could be attributed to formation of larger aggregates at low lecithin:CS ratio [17]. Hence, the lecithin:CS ratio (30) was selected for further optimization of LCNP which demonstrated the lowest particle size.

**Table 2.** Effect of lecithin:CS ratio on the particle size and PDI of RTG-LCNP (n = 3).

| Formulation Code [a] | Lecithin:CS Ratio | Particle Size (nm) | PDI |
|---|---|---|---|
| LCNP 7 | 10 | 203.6 ± 1.22 | 0.430 ± 0.001 |
| LCNP 8 | 20 | 171.0 ± 2.31 | 0.394 ± 0.002 |
| LCNP 9 | 30 | 102.0 ± 1.22 | 0.312 ± 0.006 |

[a] LCNP 7 to LCNP 9 contain 20 mg of RTG.

### *3.3. Effect of the Amount of Poloxamer 407 on the Particle Size, PDI and %EE*

Poloxamer 407 can directly affect RTG-LCNP particle size, PDI, and %EE. The drug exhibited lower solubility in Poloxamer 407 than other stabilizers [9]. Thus, Poloxamer 407 was selected as a stabilizer. The amount of Poloxamer 407 was varied from 2.5 to 10 mg by keeping the previous two parameters constant (drug:lecithin ratio: 1:3 (*w*/*w*) and lecithin:CS ratio 30) (Table 3). Both low Poloxamer 407 amount (LCNP 10) and high Poloxamer amount (LCNP 12) showed a significantly ($p < 0.0001$) higher particle size of LCNP than LCNP 11. This can be attributed to insufficient Poloxamer (at low concentration) to stabilize the formulation. However, the high Poloxamer amount can result in higher steric hinderance, negatively affecting interaction of lecithin, chitosan and drug, rendering a high particle size. In addition, changes in drug solubility with poloxamer concentrations could also affect size parameters, whereas an increase in Poloxamer 407 amount negatively affected the %EE (Table 3). The high Poloxamer 407 increased the drug solubility, negatively impacting the %EE of RTG-LCNP. Hence, 5 mg of Poloxamer 407 was selected for the further optimization of %DL of the nanoparticles.

**Table 3.** Effect of the amount of Poloxamer 407 on the particle size, PDI, and %EE of RTG-LCNP (n = 3). One-way ANOVA with Tukey test was applied. *p*-value ≤ 0.05 was considered significant.

| Formulation Code [a] | Amount of Poloxamer 407 (mg) | Particle Size (nm) | PDI | %EE |
|---|---|---|---|---|
| LCNP 10 | 2.5 | 259.8 ± 5.17 | 0.309 ± 0.009 | 93.1 ± 3.61 |
| LCNP 11 | 5 | 110.3 ± 1.09 **** | 0.348 ± 0.012 | 87.6 ± 2.93 |
| LCNP 12 | 10 | 193.7 ± 4.05 **** | 0.421 ± 0.018 | 83.2 ± 1.90 |

[a] LCNP 10 to LCNP 12 contain 20 mg of RTG. '*' indicates levels of significance in comparison to LCNP 10. '****' indicates *p*-value ≤ 0.0001.

### 3.4. Effect of pH of CS Solution on the Particle Size and %DL

pH of CS solution is already reported to have a significant effect in the preparation of LCNP by ionic gelation method. CS gets solubilized in water due to the ionization of amine group. The positive charge causes the ionic interaction with the negatively charged lecithin [15]. CS solubility is decreased at pH > 6, because of poor ionization of the amine group [25]. Furthermore, in the case of i.n. delivery, the pH of the formulation is an important factor. Formulation pH different from the physiological pH (range) of the nasal cavity irritates the nasal cavity. Additionally, pH of CS solution might affect the solubility of RTG in the aqueous phase and finally effect the %DL. Hence, the pH of CS solution for optimization %DL was varied between pH 5 to 6. The effect of pH of CS solution on %DL of prepared RTG-LCNP is presented in Table 4.

**Table 4.** Effect of pH of CS solution on the particle size and %DL of RTG-LCNP.

| Formulation Code [a] | pH | Particle Size (nm) | %DL |
|---|---|---|---|
| LCNP 13 | 5.0 | 102.0 ± 0.0 | 6.33 ± 3.35 |
| LCNP 14 | 5.5 | 107.8 ± 2.0 | 10.72 ± 4.03 |
| LCNP 15 | 6.0 | 108.0 ± 4.0 | 14.43 ± 2.77 |

[a] LCNP 13 to LCNP 15 contain 20 mg of RTG, a lecithin CS ratio of 30 and Poloxamer 407 of 5 mg.

The result showed that with a decrease in pH of CS solution, the %DL was decreased when all the other formulation and process parameters were kept constant. This result might be attributed to the fact that the drug demonstrates a pH-dependent solubility. At lower pH of CS solution, the drug solubility increases, resulting in a lower %DL. RTG is soluble between pH 1 to 5, and with increasing pH, the solubility of the drug decreases. The change in pH (5 to 6) of the CS solution has no significant effect on the particle size of the prepared LCNP. Hence, LCNP 15 which showed a better %DL (14.43 ± 2.77) and a particle size of 108 ± 4 nm (Figure 2a) was selected as the optimal formulation. The %EE for LCNP 15 was 85.22 ± 1.83. The zeta potential of the optimized formulation was 14.9 ± 0.5 mV (Figure 2b).

### 3.5. Differential Scanning Calorimetry

DSC thermograms of pure RTG, lecithin, CS, mannitol (cryoprotectant), and lyophilized RTG-LCNP are presented in Figure 3a. The pure RTG showed a sharp endothermic melting peak at 97.87 °C [26], indicating that RTG is crystalline. Thermogram of CS shows no endothermic peak, whereas lecithin exhibits its characteristic sharp endothermic peak at 43.84 °C. Finally, the DSC thermogram of lyophilized RTG-LCNP exhibits a sharp endothermic peak at 166 °C which corresponds to the melting point of the cryoprotectant (mannitol) used for the lyophilization of LCNP [27]. The disappearance of RTG melting peak might be attributed to the entrapment of RTG in RTG-LCNP. The absence of peak might also be due to the conversion of RTG to its amorphous state within the LCNP.

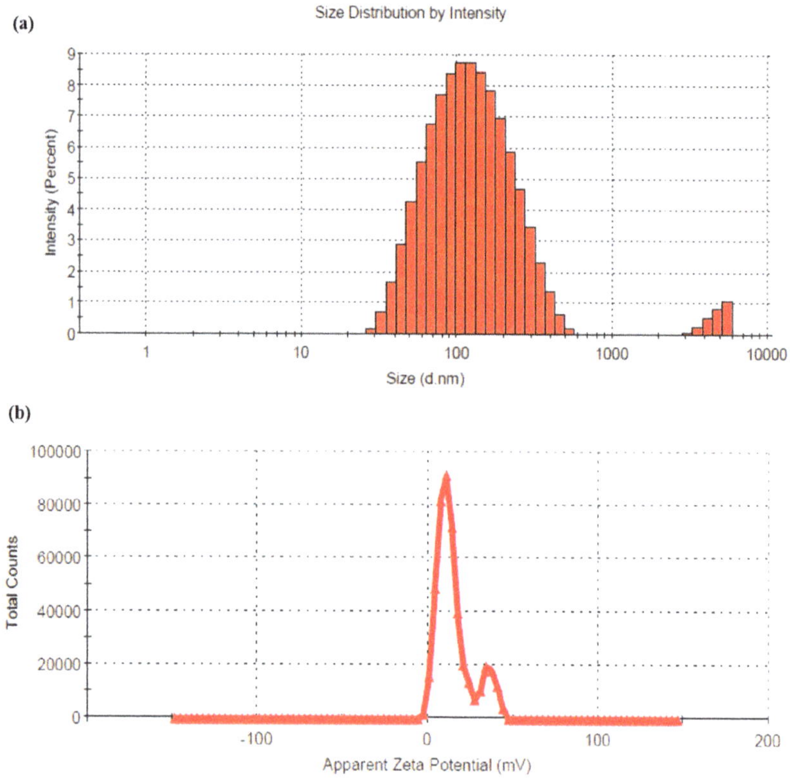


**Figure 2.** (**a**) Hydrodynamic diameter of optimized RTG-LCNP based on the % intensity; (**b**) zeta potential of optimized RTG-LCNP.

### *3.6. Field Emission Scanning Electron Microscopy*

The surface morphology of RTG-LCNP was characterized by FESEM. Figure 3b revealed almost spherical morphology of final RTG-LCNP. FESEM image revealed that the final RTG-LCNP were predominantly uniform in shape with smooth surfaces. The FESEM image also shows spherical particles of RTG-LCNP are of similar size as obtained by dynamic light scattering analysis. Figure 3c shows the FESEM images of crystalline RTG. Figure 3c revealed that the RTG crystal are orthorhombic in shape [28].

### *3.7. Tranmission Electron Microscopy*

TEM image of pure RTG revealed that the drug was crystalline with a sharp edge Figure 4a. In contrast, the morphology of LCNP showed a nearly spherical shape (Figure 4b). The core of the LCNP was surrounded by a compact outer layer which indicates the formation of a core-shell structure of the optimized LCNP [13,14].

### *3.8. Stability Study of RTG-LCNP*

The results obtained from the stability study of RTG-LCNP in refrigerated conditions are shown in Table 5. No significant variation was observed in any of the parameters such as the particle size (d.nm), PDI, zeta potential, and %DL between freshly prepared LCNP and stored LCNP over 60 days ($p > 0.05$).

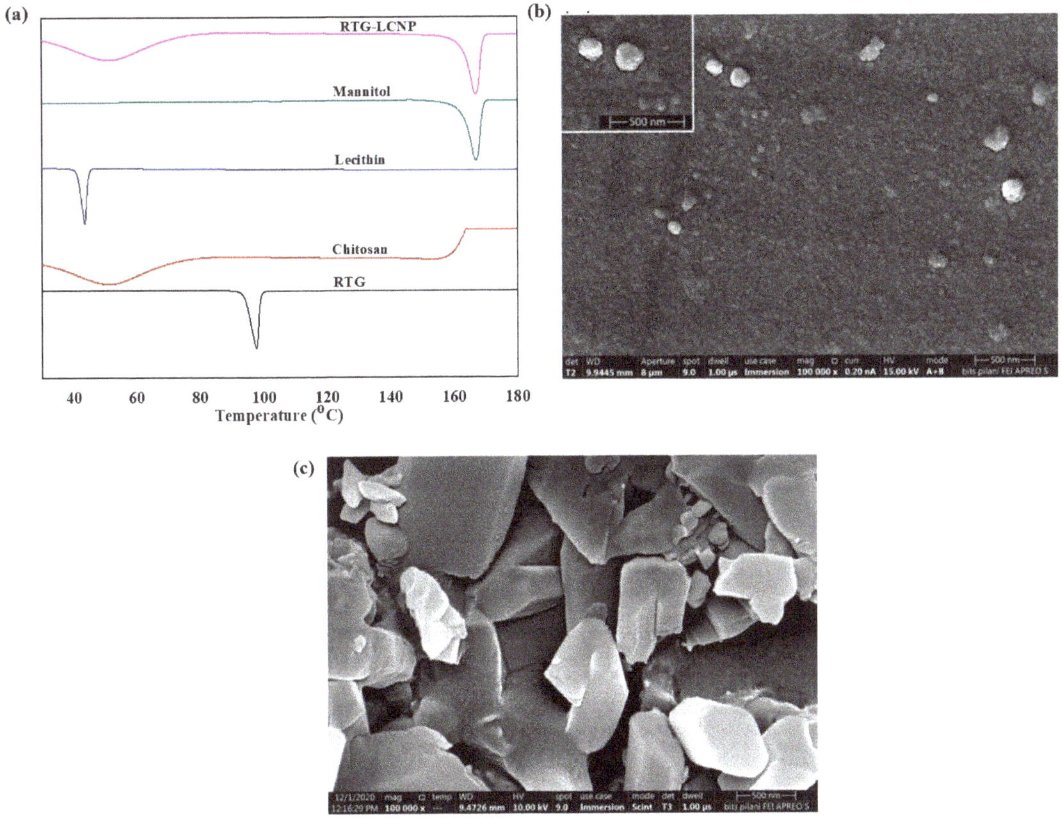


**Figure 3.** (**a**) DSC thermograms of RTG, Chitosan, Lecithin, Mannitol and lyophilized RTG-LCNP, (**b**) Surface morphology of the optimized RTG-LCNP by FESEM, (**c**) Surface morphology of pure crystalline RTG by FESEM.

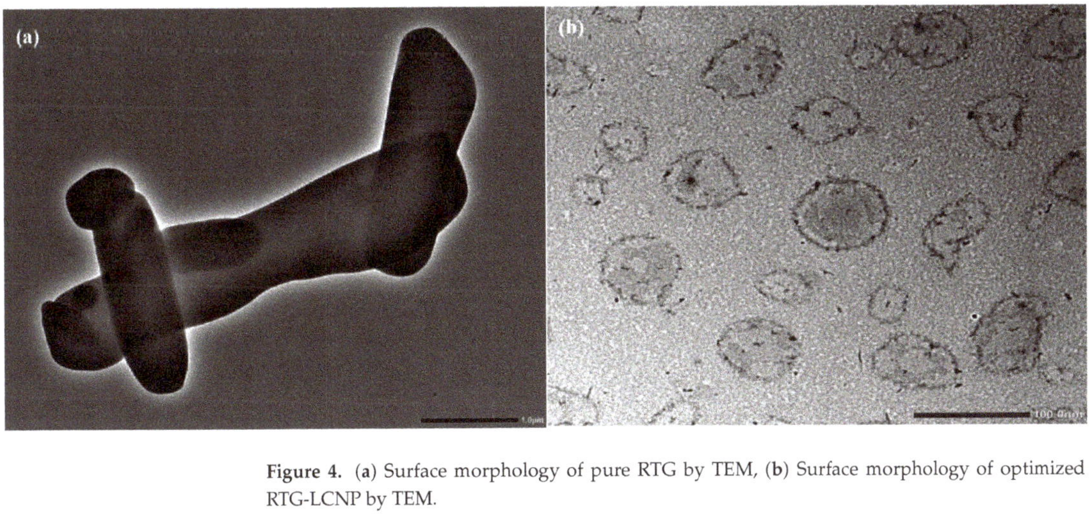


**Figure 4.** (**a**) Surface morphology of pure RTG by TEM, (**b**) Surface morphology of optimized RTG-LCNP by TEM.

**Table 5.** Stability data of lyophilized RTG-LCNP powder.

| Parameters | 0 Day | 7 Day | 30 Day | 60 Day |
|---|---|---|---|---|
| Particle size (d.nm) | 108.2 ± 4.40 | 105.1 ± 4.38 | 103.3 ± 1.56 | 119.8 ± 11.10 |
| PDI | 0.312 ± 0.001 | 0.310 ± 0.002 | 0.297 ± 0.022 | 0.371 ± 0.325 |
| Zeta potential (mV) | 14.9 ± 0.5 | 14.1 ± 0.3 | 13.8 ± 0.3 | 16.2 ± 0.3 |
| %DL | 14.43 ± 2.77 | 14.75 ± 0.12 | 15.01 ± 2.39 | 12.85 ± 4.03 |

### 3.9. *In Vitro Drug Release*

The in vitro release of pure RTG suspension and optimized RTG-LCNP were performed, and the profile is presented in Figure 5. From the drug suspension, almost 100% were released within 24 h. While from optimized LCNP, RTG released in a controlled pattern up to 24 h. Form RTG-LCNP percentage cumulative drug released (%CDR) was up to 32.44 ± 2.71% after 24 h. The drug release from RTG-LCNP showed best fit with the Korsmeyer–Peppas model with $R^2$ of 0.9296. The $R^2$ with first-order was 0.3526, and $R^2$ with the Higuchi model was 0.8289. The drug release mechanism from LCNP was best explained as non-Fickian diffusion type (n = 0.331) [29]. Similar results were also found in several literature reports. Alomrani et al. showed that lipophilic 5-fluorouracil-loaded chitosan-coated flexible liposomes exhibited Korsmeyer–Peppas model-dependent release profile [30]. Ilk et al. and Murthy et al. have reported that lecithin CS delivery system of lipophilic drugs demonstrated Korsmeyer–Peppas model-dependent release profile [17,31]. Additionally, a lower similarity factor ($f_2$ = 20) also demonstrated that the release profiles of RTG-LCNP and RTG are not similar to each other.

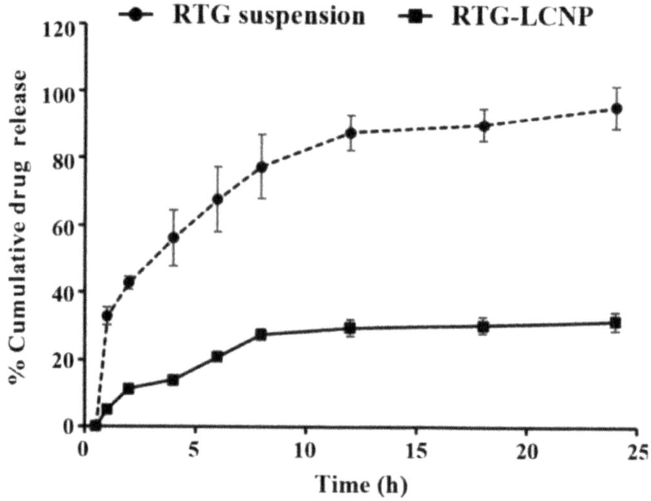


**Figure 5.** In vitro release profiles of RTG suspension and optimized RTG-LCNP (LCNP 15) in PBS (pH 7.4).

### 3.10. *Ex Vivo Nasal Permeation*

An ex vivo nasal permeation study was performed to observe the permeation behaviour of pure RTG suspension and RTG-LCNP. The mean cumulative ex vivo RTG permeated per unit area vs. time through the goat nasal mucosa is presented in Figure 6. The permeation profile revealed that RTG amount permeated (464.89 ± 58.22 μg/cm$^2$) from LCNP was significantly higher than that of the pure drug suspension ($p < 0.05$). Optimized RTG-LCNP showed a 9.66-fold increase in the amount permeated compared to the pure drug suspension. The result indicated that the LCNP formulation provides better permeability than pure drug. Better permeation of RTG from LCNP can be attributed to the presence of CS in the formulation. CS in the formulation might improve the ex vivo nasal permeation via paracellular transport by opening the tight junction of the biological membrane [14,32,33].

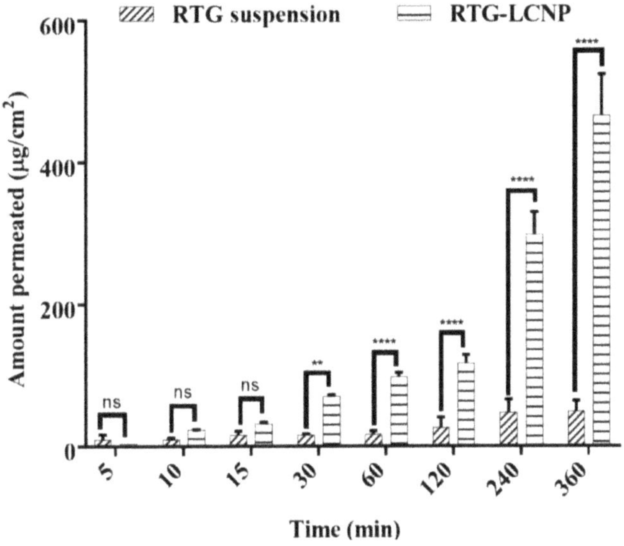


**Figure 6.** Ex vivo amount of drug permeated/unit area from optimized RTG-LCNP (LCNP 15) and drug suspension via goat nasal mucosa (n = 3, Mean ± SD). 'ns' indicates no significant difference, '**' indicates $p$-value $\leq$ 0.01 '****' indicates $p$-value $\leq$ 0.0001.

## 3.11. *In Vivo Studies*

### 3.11.1. Mucociliary Transport Time of Nanoparticles

Mucociliary transport time for pure RTG suspension and RTG-LCNP was 7.5 ± 3.53 min and 47.5 ± 3.53 min, respectively. RTG-LCNP demonstrated a higher ($p < 0.05$) mucociliary transport time than that RTG suspension (Figure 7). The increased mucociliary transport time of RTG-LCNP compared to the pure drug suspension indicates a higher residence time in the nasal cavity. The result might be attributed to the presence of mucoadhesive CS in the formulation. The high mucociliary transport time of RTG-LCNP indicated that the nanocarrier could resist the mucociliary clearance process and increased the retention time in the nasal cavity.

### 3.11.2. Plasma and Brain PK Analysis

The PK parameters of RTG-LCNP and the pure drug suspension are given in Table 6. Plasma $AUC_{0\rightarrow tlast}$ and $C_{max}$ for both formulations were not significantly different. The brain $AUC_{0\rightarrow tlast}$ for RTG-LCNP was approximately 8.77-fold higher than that of the brain $AUC_{0\rightarrow tlast}$ of the pure drug suspension. The brain $C_{max}$ of RTG-LCNP showed a 3.83-fold increment as compared to pure RTG suspension after i.n. administration. An unpair t-test comparison for brain $AUC_{0\rightarrow tlast}$ for both formulations showed a statistically significant ($p < 0.0001$) difference between the two formulations. The brain concentrations of RTG were compared between RTG-LCNP and pure RTG suspension using *t*-tests for all the time points. The drug concentrations from RTG-LCNP in the brain were significantly higher than RTG suspension at all respective time points at a 5% confidence interval (Figure 8a). To further evaluate the in vivo performance of LCNP formulation, DTP (%) and DTE (%)

were calculated as per Equation 3 and 4. Here, as a systemic route, the i.v. administration was used. The DTE (%) for RTG-LCNP was 3673.7, significantly higher than 100. This result implies that brain exposure of LCNP after i.n. administration is superior to that attained via the systemic route. This result finally indicates the nose-to-brain uptake efficacy of the prepared LCNP. The DTP (%) was 97.3 for RTG-LCNP, showing effective direct nose-to-brain uptake of RTG to the brain. The high and positive DTE (%) and DTP (%) of RTG-LCNP may be ascribed to the better retention of formulation at the site of administration than drug suspension. CS in LCNP formulation improved mucoadhesion in the nasal cavity [34]. The presence of CS might further help in reversibly opening tight junctions, facilitating drug uptake to the brain via the olfactory nerve pathway through paracellular transport [35]. Similar results were observed by few other researchers. Bhattamisra et al. showed a relatively high DTP (%) value (53.87 ± 10.14) when RTG was loaded in CS nanoparticles compared to RTG solution [12]. Md et al. reported that bromocriptine-loaded i.n. CS nanoparticles showed a high DTE (%) value (265.6 ± 37.3) compared to drug solution [36]. Wang et al. reported that RTG-loaded micellar thermosensitive gel improved DTP (%) in olfactory bulb, cerebrum, cerebellum, and striatum within a range of 49–70% [11]. These results confirm that the mucoadhesive properties of nanocarriers or a nanocarrier embedded in situ gel which has the ability to sustain the mucociliary clearance in the nasal cavity and also ability to open the tight junctions result in better brain bioavailability of the drugs via i.n. administration.

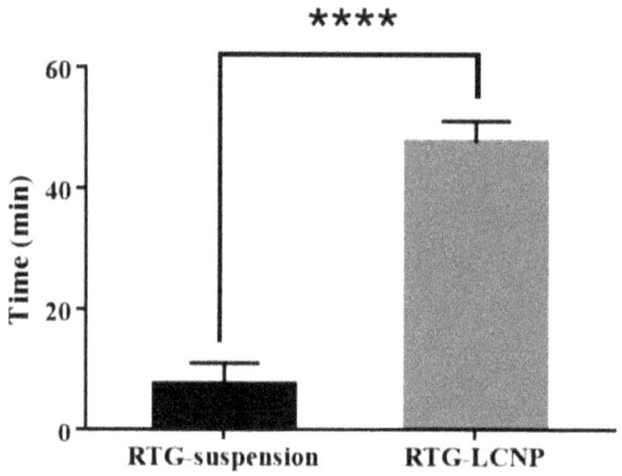


**Figure 7.** Mucociliary transport time of aqueous RTG suspension and RTG-LCNP (LCNP 15). Student's independent *t*-test with one-tail was applied. '****' shows *p*-value <0.05.

**Table 6.** Plasma and brain PK parameters for RTG-LCNP (LCNP 15) and RTG suspension after i.n. administration.

| PK Parameters | Brain | | Plasma | |
|---|---|---|---|---|
| | RTG-LCNP | RTG Suspension | RTG-LCNP | RTG Suspension |
| $AUC_{0\rightarrow tlast}$ (ng*h/g) [b], (ng*h/mL) [p] | 5507.57± 23.91 | 628.11 ± 12.21 | 1060.44 ± 29.95 | 779.01 ± 14.11 |
| $C_{max}$ (ng/g) [b], (ng/mL)[p] | 1013.47 ± 11.28 | 264.71 ± 21.12 | 230.87 ± 8.19 | 270.12 ± 18.50 |
| $T_{max}$ (h) | 2 ± 0.03 | 1 ± 0.01 | 1 ± 0.02 | 2 ± 0.01 |
| MRT (h) | 3.81 ± 0.38 | 1.82 ± 0.15 | 1.58 ± 0.05 | 3.15 ± 0.81 |
| Clearance (g/h) [b], (mL/h) [p] | 78.57 ± 12.19 | - | - | 312.65 ± 15.59 |

[b] unit for brain PK parameters; [p] unit for plasma PK parameters. RTG dose for both i.n. formulations: 2 mg/Kg; for plasma PK n = 4 animals were used, and n = 4 animal brains were used for brain PK at every time point. The brain and plasma data are represented as the mean ± SD.

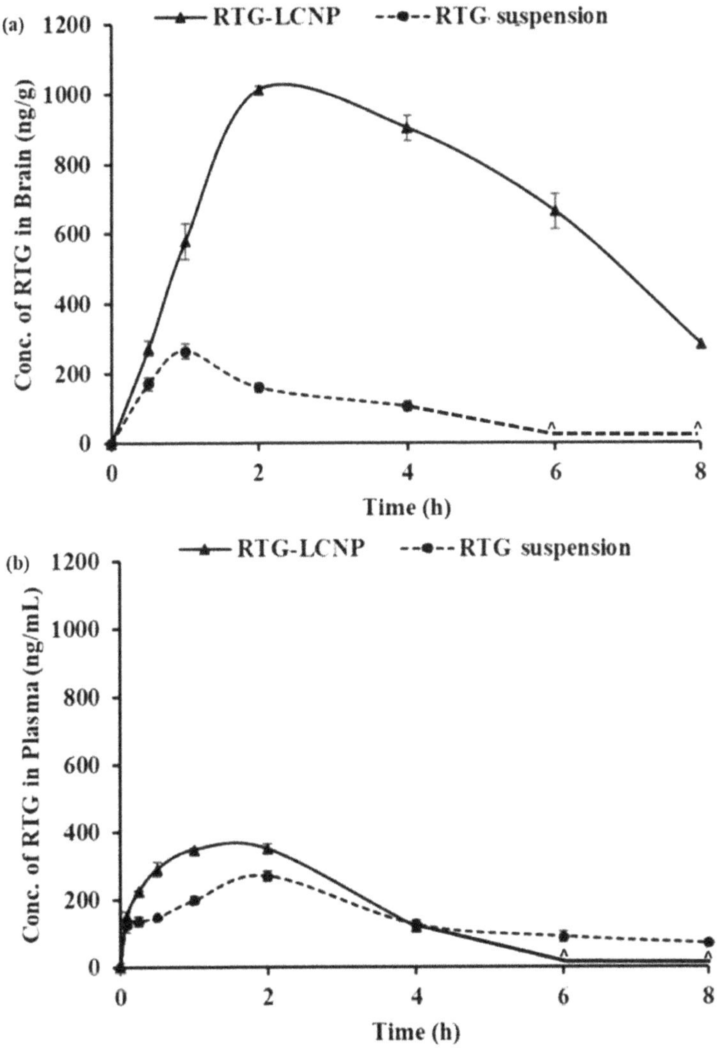


**Figure 8.** PK profiles of RTG attained after i.n. administration of RTG-LCNP (LCNP 15) and RTG suspension in (**a**): Brain and (**b**): Plasma. '^' in both the profiles denote that the concentration of RTG was not detected at those time points in brain matrices and plasma.

Plasma $AUC_{0\rightarrow tlast}$ from RTG-LCNP was significantly higher than drug suspension (Table 6). This result might be attributed to LCNP via an indirect pathway. RTG also reached the brain in higher amounts. CS present in the formulation might facilitate LCNP reaching the brain from systemic circulation by passing through the BBB [32,33]. The presence of CS in LCNP might also result in opening a tight junction of the nasal epithelium, which finally leads to better systemic exposure of drug from LCNP from the respiratory region compared to pure suspension. The high plasma drug concentration from LCNP might be another reason for high DTE (%).

### 3.12. *Histopathology of Brain*

At 0 h (control) and 8 h after receiving RTG-LCNP (treated), the morphology of the hippocampus region on brain slides was investigated for any toxicity (Figure 9) [37]. The morphology of the hippocampal area of LCNP the treated rat (Figure 9c,d) was similar to that of the control (Figure 9a,b). Figure 9d demonstrated that the in the hippocampal region, there were no indications of neuronal damage, such as cell body necrosis or shrinking. This suggested that RTG-LCNP did not cause any damage to the brain and was safe for clinical use.

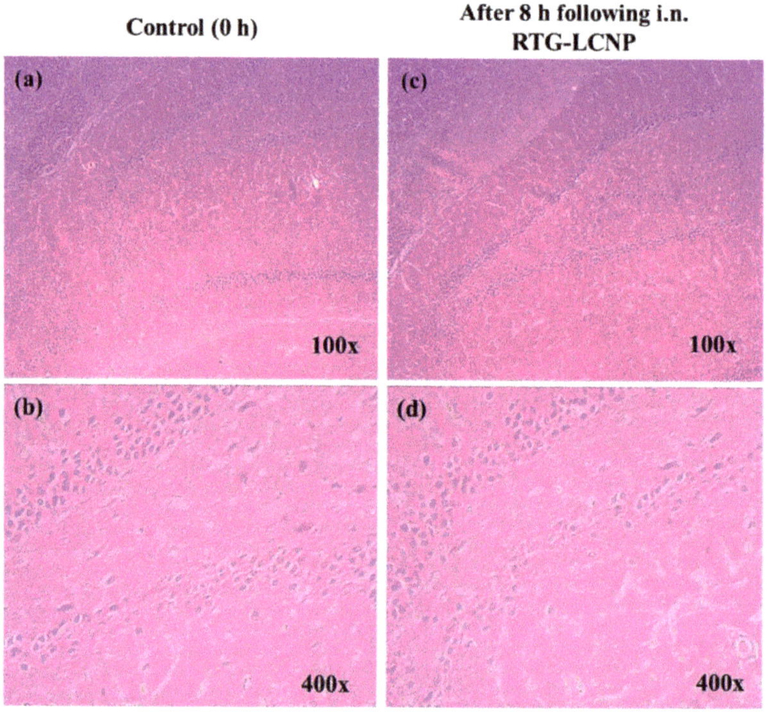


**Figure 9.** Histopathological evaluations of brain (hippocampal region) in different conditions: (**a**) Control animal at 100× magnification, (**b**) control animal at 400× magnification, (**c**) LCNP treated animal at 100× magnification, and (**d**) LCNP treated animal at 400× magnification.

## 4. Conclusions

Critical formulation variables of RTG-LCNP were optimized for an anticipated particle size, PDI, %EE, and %DL. The optimized RTG-LCNP was stable in refrigerated conditions for at least 2 months. The LCNP showed higher nasal permeation and mucociliary transport time than RTG suspension. RTG-LCNP improved PK parameters with high brain bioavailability and good targeting efficiency. Overall, RTG-LCNP can improve brain delivery following i.n. administration and has the potential for clinical application.

**Supplementary Materials:** The following supporting information can be downloaded at: https://www.mdpi.com/article/10.3390/pharmaceutics15030851/s1, S1: Processing of brain and plasma matrices.

**Author Contributions:** Conceptualization, M.M.P. and H.K.; methodology, P.S. (Paramita Saha); software, P.S. (Paramita Saha); validation, P.S. (Paramita Saha) and P.S.(Prabhjeet Singh); formal Analysis, P.S. (Paramita Saha); investigation, P.S. (Paramita Saha); resources, M.M.P. and D.C.; data curation, P.S. (Paramita Saha) and P.S.(Prabhjeet Singh); writing —original draft preparation, P.S. (Paramita Saha); writing—review and editing, M.M.P., H.K. and D.C.; visualization, P.S. (Paramita Saha), H.K., D.C.

and P.S. (Prabhjeet Singh); supervision, M.M.P.; project administration, M.M.P.; funding acquisition, M.M.P. All authors have read and agreed to the published version of the manuscript.

**Funding:** This research received no external funding.

**Institutional Review Board Statement:** The animal study protocol was approved by the Institute's Animal Ethics Committee of BITS Pilani (protocol number IAEC/RES/26/07/REV-1/30/19) for studies involving animals.

**Data Availability Statement:** Data can be provided on request.

**Acknowledgments:** We acknowledge BITS Pilani for the research fellowship to Paramita Saha and Prabhjeet S. We thank the Central analytical laboratory of BITS-Pilani, Pilani campus, for providing FESEM facility for analysis. We are grateful to Mylan Laboratories (Hyderabad, India) for providing rotigotine as a gift sample.

**Conflicts of Interest:** The authors declare no conflict of interest.

## References

1. Raza, C.; Anjum, R.; Shakeel, N.u.A. Parkinson's Disease: Mechanisms, Translational Models and Management Strategies. *Life Sci.* **2019**, *226*, 77–90. [CrossRef]
2. Saha, P.; Chitkara, D.; Pandey, M.M. (Re)Formulating Rotigotine: A Potential Molecule with Unmet Needs. *Ther. Deliv.* **2023**, *13*, 445–448. [CrossRef] [PubMed]
3. Elshoff, J.P.; Cawello, W.; Andreas, J.O.; Mathy, F.X.; Braun, M. An Update on Pharmacological, Pharmacokinetic Properties and Drug-Drug Interactions of Rotigotine Transdermal System in Parkinson's Disease and Restless Legs Syndrome. *Drugs* **2015**, *75*, 487–501. [CrossRef]
4. Elshoff, J.P.; Braun, M.; Andreas, J.O.; Middle, M.; Cawello, W. Steady-State Plasma Concentration Profile of Transdermal Rotigotine: An Integrated Analysis of Three, Open-Label, Randomized, Phase I Multiple Dose Studies. *Clin. Ther.* **2012**, *34*, 966–978. [CrossRef] [PubMed]
5. Nordling-David, M.M.; Yaffe, R.; Guez, D.; Meirow, H.; Last, D.; Grad, E.; Salomon, S.; Sharabi, S.; Levi-Kalisman, Y.; Golomb, G.; et al. Liposomal Temozolomide Drug Delivery Using Convection Enhanced Delivery. *J. Control. Release* **2017**, *261*, 138–146. [CrossRef] [PubMed]
6. Asadi, S.; Roohbakhsh, A.; Shamsizadeh, A.; Fereidoni, M.; Kordijaz, E.; Moghimi, A. The Effect of Intracerebroventricular Administration of Orexin Receptor Type 2 Antagonist on Pentylenetetrazol-Induced Kindled Seizures and Anxiety in Rats. *BMC Neurosci.* **2018**, *19*, 49. [CrossRef]
7. Dalvi, A.V.; Ravi, P.R.; Uppuluri, C.T.; Mahajan, R.R.; Katke, S.V.; Deshpande, V.S. Thermosensitive Nasal in Situ Gelling Systems of Rufinamide Formulated Using Modified Tamarind Seed Xyloglucan for Direct Nose-to-Brain Delivery: Design, Physical Characterization, and in Vivo Evaluation. *J. Pharm. Investig.* **2021**, *51*, 199–211. [CrossRef]
8. Dhaliwal, H.K.; Fan, Y.; Kim, J.; Amiji, M.M. Intranasal Delivery and Transfection of MRNA Therapeutics in the Brain Using Cationic Liposomes. *Mol. Pharm.* **2020**, *17*, 1996–2005. [CrossRef]
9. Saha, P.; Kathuria, H.; Pandey, M.M. Nose-to-Brain Delivery of Rotigotine Redispersible Nanosuspension: In Vitro and in Vivo Characterization. *J. Drug Deliv. Sci. Technol.* **2023**, *79*, 104049. [CrossRef]
10. Bi, C.C.; Wang, A.P.; Chu, Y.C.; Liu, S.; Mu, H.J.; Liu, W.H.; Wu, Z.M.; Sun, K.X.; Li, Y.X. Intranasal Delivery of Rotigotine to the Brain with Lactoferrin-Modified PEG-PLGA Nanoparticles for Parkinson's Disease Treatment. *Int. J. Nanomed.* **2016**, *11*, 6547–6559. [CrossRef] [PubMed]
11. Wang, F.; Yang, Z.; Liu, M.; Tao, Y.; Li, Z.; Wu, Z.; Gui, S. Facile Nose-to-Brain Delivery of Rotigotine-Loaded Polymer Micelles Thermosensitive Hydrogels: In Vitro Characterization and in Vivo Behavior Study. *Int. J. Pharm.* **2020**, *577*, 119046. [CrossRef] [PubMed]
12. Bhattamisra, S.K.; Shak, A.T.; Xi, L.W.; Safian, N.H.; Choudhury, H.; Lim, W.M.; Shahzad, N.; Alhakamy, N.A.; Anwer, M.K.; Radhakrishnan, A.K.; et al. Nose to Brain Delivery of Rotigotine Loaded Chitosan Nanoparticles in Human SH-SY5Y Neuroblastoma Cells and Animal Model of Parkinson's Disease. *Int. J. Pharm.* **2020**, *579*, 119148. [CrossRef]
13. Liu, L.; Zhou, C.; Xia, X.; Liu, Y. Self-Assembled Lecithin/Chitosan Nanoparticles for Oral Insulin Delivery: Preparation and Functional Evaluation. *Int. J. Nanomed.* **2016**, *11*, 761–769. [CrossRef] [PubMed]
14. Dong, W.; Ye, J.; Wang, W.; Yang, Y.; Wang, H.; Sun, T.; Gao, L.; Liu, Y. Self-Assembled Lecithin/Chitosan Nanoparticles Based on Phospholipid Complex: A Feasible Strategy to Improve Entrapment Efficiency and Transdermal Delivery of Poorly Lipophilic Drug. *Int. J. Nanomed.* **2020**, *15*, 5629. [CrossRef]
15. Hafner, A.; Lovrić, J.; Pepić, I.; Filipović-Grčić, J. Lecithin/Chitosan Nanoparticles for Transdermal Delivery of Melatonin. *J. Microencapsul.* **2011**, *28*, 807–815. [CrossRef] [PubMed]

16. Uppuluri, C.T.; Ravi, P.R.; Dalvi, A.V. Design and Evaluation of Thermo-Responsive Nasal in Situ Gelling System Dispersed with Piribedil Loaded Lecithin-Chitosan Hybrid Nanoparticles for Improved Brain Availability. *Neuropharmacology* **2021**, *201*, 108832. [CrossRef]
17. Murthy, A.; Ravi, P.R.; Kathuria, H.; Vats, R. Self-Assembled Lecithin-Chitosan Nanoparticles Improve the Oral Bioavailability and Alter the Pharmacokinetics of Raloxifene. *Int. J. Pharm.* **2020**, *588*, 119731. [CrossRef]
18. Dalvi, A.; Ravi, P.R.; Uppuluri, C.T. Rufinamide-Loaded Chitosan Nanoparticles in Xyloglucan-Based Thermoresponsive In Situ Gel for Direct Nose to Brain Delivery. *Front. Pharmacol.* **2021**, *12*, 1274. [CrossRef]
19. Mistry, A.; Glud, S.Z.; Kjems, J.; Randel, J.; Howard, K.A.; Stolnik, S.; Illum, L. Effect of Physicochemical Properties on Intranasal Nanoparticle Transit into Murine Olfactory Epithelium. *J. Drug Target.* **2009**, *17*, 543–552. [CrossRef] [PubMed]
20. Brooking, J.; Davis, S.S.; Illum, L. Transport of Nanoparticles Across the Rat Nasal Mucosa. *J. Drug Target.* **2001**, *9*, 267–279. [CrossRef] [PubMed]
21. Hinge, N.S.; Kathuria, H.; Pandey, M.M. Engineering of Structural and Functional Properties of Nanotherapeutics and Nanodiagnostics for Intranasal Brain Targeting in Alzheimer's. *Appl. Mater. Today* **2022**, *26*, 101303. [CrossRef]
22. Saha, P.; Pandey, M.M. DoE-Based Validation of a HPLC–UV Method for Quantification of Rotigotine Nanocrystals: Application to in Vitro Dissolution and Ex Vivo Nasal Permeation Studies. *Electrophoresis* **2022**, *43*, 590–600. [CrossRef] [PubMed]
23. Lujan, H.; Griffin, W.C.; Taube, J.H.; Sayes, C.M. Synthesis and Characterization of Nanometer-Sized Liposomes for Encapsulation and MicroRNA Transfer to Breast Cancer Cells. *Int. J. Nanomed.* **2019**, *14*, 5159–5173. [CrossRef] [PubMed]
24. Saka, R.; Chella, N.; Khan, W. Development of Imatinib Mesylate-Loaded Liposomes for Nose to Brain Delivery: In Vitro and in Vivo Evaluation. *AAPS PharmSciTech* **2021**, *22*, 192. [CrossRef]
25. Roy, J.C.; Salaün, F.; Giraud, S.; Ferri, A.; Roy, J.C.; Salaün, F.; Giraud, S.; Ferri, A. Solubility of Chitin: Solvents, Solution Behaviors and Their Related Mechanisms. In *Solubility of Polysaccharides*; IntechOpen: London, UK, 2017; pp. 20–60; ISBN 978-953-51-3650-7.
26. Wolff, H.-M.; Quere, L.; Riedner, J. Polymorphic Form of Rotigotine. 2008. Available online: https://patents.google.com/patent/EP2215072B1/en (accessed on 12 December 2022).
27. Paul, A.; Shi, L.; Bielawski, C.W. A Eutectic Mixture of Galactitol and Mannitol as a Phase Change Material for Latent Heat Storage. *Energy Convers. Manag.* **2015**, *103*, 139–146. [CrossRef]
28. Saha, P.; Pandey, M.M. Spectrochimica Acta Part A Molecular and Biomolecular Spectroscopy A New Fluorescence-Based Method for Rapid and Specific Quantification of Rotigotine in Chitosan Nanoparticles. *Spectrochim. Acta Part A Mol. Biomol. Spectrosc.* **2022**, *267*, 120555. [CrossRef] [PubMed]
29. Lisik, A. Witold Musial Conductomeric Evaluation of the Release Kinetics of Active Substances from Pharmaceutical Preparations Containing Iron Ions. *Materials* **2019**, *12*, 730. [CrossRef] [PubMed]
30. Alomrani, A.; Badran, M.; Harisa, G.I.; ALshehry, M.; Alshamsan, A.; Alkholief, M. The Use of Chitosan-Coated Flexible Liposomes as a Remarkable Carrier to Enhance the Antitumor Efficacy of 5-Fluorouracil against Colorectal Cancer. *Saudi Pharm. J.* **2019**, *27*, 603–611. [CrossRef] [PubMed]
31. Ilk, S.; Saglam, N.; Özgen, M. Kaempferol Loaded Lecithin/Chitosan Nanoparticles: Preparation, Characterization, and Their Potential Applications as a Sustainable Antifungal Agent. *Artif. Cells Nanomed. Biotechnol.* **2016**, *45*, 907–916. [CrossRef]
32. Şenyiğit, T.; Sonvico, F.; Rossi, A.; Tekmen, I.; Santi, P.; Colombo, P.; Nicoli, S.; Özer, Ö. In Vivo Assessment of Clobetasol Propionate-Loaded Lecithin-Chitosan Nanoparticles for Skin Delivery. *Int. J. Mol. Sci.* **2016**, *18*, 32. [CrossRef]
33. Şenyiğit, T.; Sonvico, F.; Barbieri, S.; Özer, Ö.; Santi, P.; Colombo, P. Lecithin/Chitosan Nanoparticles of Clobetasol-17-Propionate Capable of Accumulation in Pig Skin. *J. Control. Release* **2010**, *142*, 368–373. [CrossRef] [PubMed]
34. Jafarieh, O.; Md, S.; Ali, M.; Baboota, S.; Sahni, J.K.; Kumari, B.; Bhatnagar, A.; Ali, J. Design, Characterization, and Evaluation of Intranasal Delivery of Ropinirole-Loaded Mucoadhesive Nanoparticles for Brain Targeting. *Drug Dev. Ind. Pharm.* **2015**, *41*, 1674–1681. [CrossRef] [PubMed]
35. Shadab, M.D.; Khan, R.A.; Mustafa, G.; Chuttani, K.; Baboota, S.; Sahni, J.K.; Ali, J. Bromocriptine Loaded Chitosan Nanoparticles Intended for Direct Nose to Brain Delivery: Pharmacodynamic, Pharmacokinetic and Scintigraphy Study in Mice Model. *Eur. J. Pharm. Sci.* **2013**, *48*, 393–405. [CrossRef]
36. Md, S.; Haque, S.; Fazil, M.; Kumar, M.; Baboota, S.; Sahni, J.K.; Ali, J. Optimised Nanoformulation of Bromocriptine for Direct Nose-to-Brain Delivery: Biodistribution, Pharmacokinetic and Dopamine Estimation by Ultra-HPLC/Mass Spectrometry Method. *Expert Opin. Drug Deliv.* **2014**, *11*, 827–842. [CrossRef] [PubMed]
37. Sita, V.G.; Jadhav, D.; Vavia, P. Niosomes for Nose-to-Brain Delivery of Bromocriptine: Formulation Development, Efficacy Evaluation and Toxicity Profiling. *J. Drug Deliv. Sci. Technol.* **2020**, *58*, 101791. [CrossRef]

*pharmaceutics*

*Review*

# Mesenchymal Stem Cell (MSC)-Based Drug Delivery into the Brain across the Blood–Brain Barrier

**Toshihiko Tashima**

Tashima Laboratories of Arts and Sciences, 1239-5 Toriyama-cho, Kohoku-ku, Yokohama 222-0035, Japan; tashima_lab@yahoo.co.jp

**Abstract:** At present, stem cell-based therapies using induced pluripotent stem cells (iPSCs) or mesenchymal stem cells (MSCs) are being used to explore the potential for regenerative medicine in the treatment of various diseases, owing to their ability for multilineage differentiation. Interestingly, MSCs are employed not only in regenerative medicine, but also as carriers for drug delivery, homing to target sites in injured or damaged tissues including the brain by crossing the blood–brain barrier (BBB). In drug research and development, membrane impermeability is a serious problem. The development of central nervous system drugs for the treatment of neurodegenerative diseases, such as Alzheimer's disease and Parkinson's disease, remains difficult due to impermeability in capillary endothelial cells at the BBB, in addition to their complicated pathogenesis and pathology. Thus, intravenously or intraarterially administered MSC-mediated drug delivery in a non-invasive way is a solution to this transendothelial problem at the BBB. Substances delivered by MSCs are divided into artificially included materials in advance, such as low molecular weight compounds including doxorubicin, and expected protein expression products of genetic modification, such as interleukins. After internalizing into the brain through the fenestration between the capillary endothelial cells, MSCs release their cargos to the injured brain cells. In this review, I introduce the potential and advantages of drug delivery into the brain across the BBB using MSCs as a carrier that moves into the brain as if they acted of their own will.

**Keywords:** the blood–brain barrier; mesenchymal stem cell-based drug delivery; transmembrane drug delivery

**Citation:** Tashima, T. Mesenchymal Stem Cell (MSC)-Based Drug Delivery into the Brain across the Blood–Brain Barrier. *Pharmaceutics* **2024**, *16*, 289. https://doi.org/10.3390/pharmaceutics16020289

Academic Editor: Augusto Pessina

Received: 17 January 2024
Revised: 15 February 2024
Accepted: 16 February 2024
Published: 18 February 2024



## 1. Introduction

Stem cells offer a wide variety of possibilities for new medical treatments due to their ability to develop into many different cell types. Mesenchymal stem cells (MSCs), also known as mesenchymal stromal cells, have potential applications in therapeutic contexts due to their multilineage differentiation capacity and anti-inflammatory properties. Intriguingly, MSCs can serve as drug carriers, homing to specific target sites. In drug research and development, incorrect distribution and membrane impermeability pose serious challenges. Therefore, molecular target drugs, such as monoclonal antibody drugs, are being developed to address selectivity issues and are currently available for clinical use. Even molecular target drugs face challenges, including impermeability through passive diffusion due to size and hydrophilicity. Monoclonal antibodies, however, are utilized as a vector for monoclonal antibody-drug conjugates to traverse the blood–brain barrier (BBB) via receptor-mediated transcytosis in capillary endothelial cells through the transcellular route [1,2]. The BBB is primarily composed of (i) tight junctions between capillary endothelial cells facilitated by adhesion molecules like claudin, (ii) the hydrophobic lipid bilayer membrane of capillary endothelial cells, (iii) biological efflux transporters such as multiple drug resistance 1 (MDR1) (P-glycoprotein (P-gp)) on the apical membrane of capillary endothelial cells, and (iv) the support provided by pericytes and astrocytes. Furthermore, the development of drugs for the treatment of Parkinson's disease (PD) and Alzheimer's disease (AD) [3,4] in the central nervous system continues to face unmet medical needs, primarily due to impermeability caused by the BBB, in addition to their complicated pathogenesis and pathology. Therefore, utilizing MSCs for delivery could serve as a solution for highly selective and efficient delivery to disease sites, especially the injured or damaged brain. Indeed, drug delivery utilizing MSCs is currently under development. It is true that sone reviews focusing on the drug delivery using MSCs-derived exosomes are reported [5–7]. However, MSC-based drug delivery into the brain across the BBB can be considered a more dynamic strategy, particularly compared to isolated exosomes. Therefore, in this perspective review, I introduce the possibilities and approaches for drug delivery into the brain across the BBB using MSCs (Figure 1).

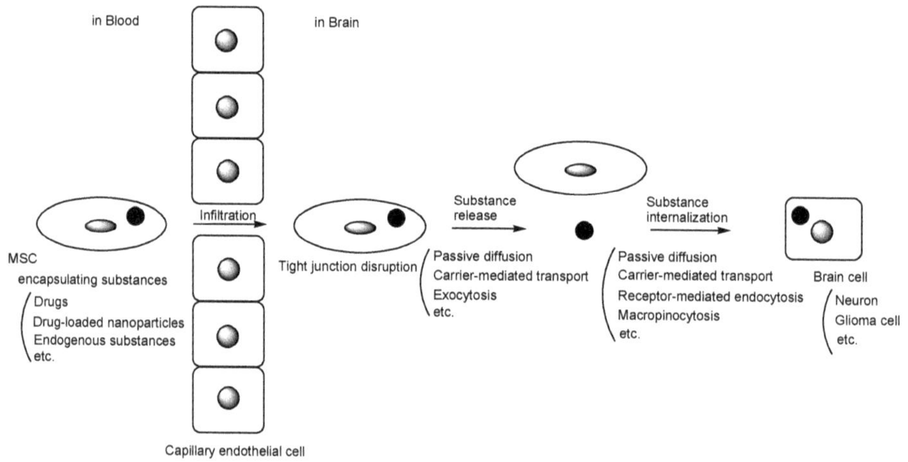


**Figure 1.** The pathway of mesenchymal stem cell (MSC)-based drug delivery into the brain across the blood–brain barrier. A black circle represents substances such as drugs, drug-loaded nanoparticles, or endogenous compounds. A gray circle or a gray ellipse represents a cell nucleus.

MSCs are pluripotent cells with self-renewal and differentiation potential. They can differentiate into mesodermal lineage cells, such as connective stromal cells, cartilage cells, fat cells, and bone cells; ectodermal lineage cells, such as epithelial cells and neurons; or endodermal lineage cells, such as muscle cells, gut epithelial cells, and lung cells (Figure 2) [8]. MSCs can be isolated from a variety of tissues. Intriguingly, MSCs sense signals from injured tissues or areas of disease and migrate to these locations to promote recovery. Moreover, MSCs play a vital role in regulating the cellular microenvironment, leading to immunomodulation, hematopoietic support, tissue repair, and tissue regeneration through interactions with various cells, including macrophages, neutrophils, cancer cells, hematopoietic stem cells, and others, mediated by cytokines [9]. Contrarily, MSC differentiation fates are influenced by the cellular microenvironment. It is known that MSCs secrete not only cytokines but also exosomes [10]. Therefore, the potential of MSCs is immeasurable.

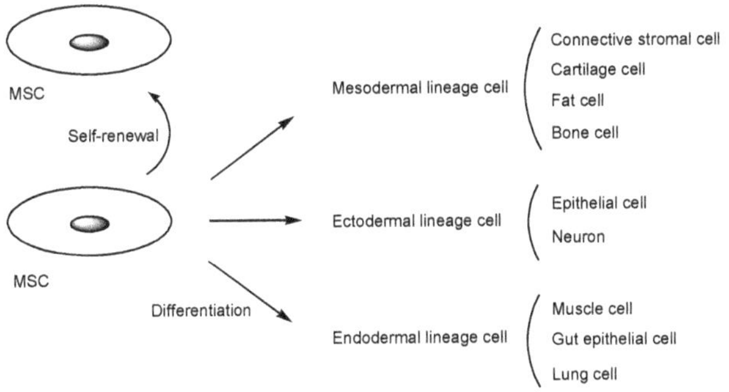


**Figure 2.** Schematic diagram illustrating mesenchymal stem cell (MSC) differentiation. A gray ellipse represents a cell nucleus.

## 2. Discussion

### 2.1. Human MSCs for Regenerative Medicine

Numerous clinical trials involving human MSCs for regenerative medicine are currently underway (Table 1). Some of these trials have already advanced to the pharmaceutical market. Representative cases are briefly introduced here [11], because the main theme of this perspective review is drug delivery. Other information can be obtained from references [12,13]. (i) Sutéramikku, autologous bone marrow-derived human MSCs (English name unknown, identified by the investigational drug code STR01 [14]), received conditional approval in 2018 in Japan for the improvement of neurological symptoms and functional impairment associated with spinal cord injury, marking a global milestone. Nevertheless, the approval, which was contingent on a study involving 13 patients in the active drug group, has generated controversy [15,16]. It is worth noting that the medications were administered promptly after undergoing the highest level of scrutiny mandated by modern scientific standards, laws, and regulations [17]. This medication is currently available clinically. Regulatory frameworks for new modalities should be established, aiming not only to offer patients the latest medical care, but also to prevent medical accidents. (ii) Temcell HS [18], allogeneic bone marrow-derived human MSCs, received approval for the treatment of acute graft-versus-host disease in Japan in 2015. (iii) Alofisel (darvadstrocel) [19], allogeneic bone marrow-derived human MSCs, received approval for the treatment of complex perianal fistula in adults with Crohn's disease in the European Union in 2017. (iv) SB623 (vandefitemcel) [20], allogeneic bone marrow-derived human MSCs, successfully completed a phase 2 clinical trial (STEMTRA trial) with positive results for traumatic brain injury. As a result, it was submitted for early approval with conditions in Japan in March 2022. (v) FF-31501, autologous bone marrow-derived human MSC, is currently undergoing a phase 3 clinical trial for meniscal injury in Japan, which commenced in February 2023. (vi) CYP-004, iPSC-derived human MSCs, have been undergoing a phase 3 clinical trial for osteoarthritis (ACTRN12620000870954) in Australia since November 2020. (vii) MutiStem (HLCM051), allogeneic bone marrow-derived human MSCs, underwent a phase 3 clinical trial for ischemic cerebral infarction (MASTERS-2 trial, NCT03545607) in the USA from July 2018 to June 2023. (viii) Rexlemestrocel-L, allogeneic bone marrow-derived human MSCs, underwent a phase 3 clinical trial for lower back pain (MSB-DR003 trial, NCT02412735) in the USA from March 2015 to June 2021. (ix) Remestemcel-L, an allogeneic bone marrow-derived human MSC product, underwent a phase 3 clinical trial for acute respiratory distress syndrome. This is an manufactured MSC product equivalent to Temcell HS. (x) gMSC1, allogeneic synovial membrane-derived human MSC, is currently undergoing a phase 3 clinical trial for knee cartilage damage since November 2017 in Japan.

**Table 1.** Numerous clinical trials utilizing human mesenchymal stem cells (MSCs) in regenerative medicine.

| # | Name | MSC Type | Diseases | Status | References |
|---|---|---|---|---|---|
| 1 | Sutéramikku | Autologous bone marrow-derived human MSCs | Spinal cord injury | Launched | [14–16] |
| 2 | Temcell HS | Allogeneic bone marrow-derived human MSCs | Acute graft-versus-host disease | Launched | [18] |
| 3 | Alofisel (darvadstrocel) | Allogeneic bone marrow-derived human MSCs | Complex perianal fistula in adults with Crohn's disease | Launched | [19] |
| 4 | SB623 (vandefitemcel) | Allogeneic bone marrow-derived human MSCs | Traumatic brain injury | Launched | [20] |
| 5 | FF-31501 | Autologous bone marrow-derived human MSCs | Meniscal injury | Phase 3 clinical trial | - |
| 6 | CYP-004 | iPSC-derived human MSCs | Osteoarthritis | Phase 3 clinical trial (AC-TRN12620000870954) | - |
| 7 | MutiStem (HLCM051) | Allogeneic bone marrow-derived human MSCs | Ischemic cerebral infarction | Phase 3 clinical trial (MASTERS-2 trial, NCT03545607), finished in2023 | - |
| 8 | Rexlemestrocel-L | Allogeneic bone marrow-derived human MSCs | Lower back pain | Phase 3 clinical trial (MSB-DR003 trial, NCT02412735), finished in 2021 | - |
| 9 | Remestemcel-L | Allogeneic bone marrow-derived human MSCs | Acute respiratory distress syndrome | Phase 3 clinical trial, finished | - |
| 10 | gMSC1 | Allogeneic synovial membrane-derived human MSCs | Knee cartilage damage | Phase 3 clinical trial | - |

The preparation of human MSCs and the clinical use of MSC-secretome are strictly subject to current good manufacturing practice (cGMP) standards [21]. MSCs from other donors might pose immunological challenges for allogeneic use, because they are not obtained from patient's own cells for autologous use. Thus, hypoimmunogenicity, low immunogenicity, immune tolerance should be necessary when allogeneic MSCs are used. Nonetheless, human MSCs are immunoprivileged because they possess very low levels of major histocompatibility complex (MHC) class I and no MHC class II, which are insufficient to induce activation of allogeneic lymphocytes [22].

Nevertheless, it is probable that human MSCs as carriers for drug delivery have not yet received clinical approval.

### 2.2. The Potential of MSC-Mediated Drug Delivery

It is known that the majority of intravenously administered rat MSCs are trapped in the lungs through the pulmonary first-pass effect. This is attributed to the cell size and the expression of adhesion molecules targeting receptors on the surface of pulmonary capillary endothelial cells, as observed in in vivo tests using rats [23]. This phenomenon might pose a relatively serious problem for MSC delivery, particularly into the brain. Moreover, when rat MSCs (with an average diameter of 23 μm) were bolused into the ipsilateral common iliac artery in rats, they spread out on the luminal side of the vessel and subsequently localized in a perivascular niche within 72 h [24]. In other words, the half-life of rat MSCs was roughly assumed to be around 36 h by approximating the attenuation curve as a straight line in this case. Generally, the diameter of human capillaries is approximately 5–20 μm [25]. Human red blood cells, with a disk diameter of 6.2–8.2 μm and a thickness of 2–2.5 μm at the thickest part [26], can pass through capillaries. There are various opinions regarding the size of MSCs. Nonetheless, the volume of rat MSCs could be roughly estimated at approximately 3000 $\mu m^3$, although there is variety in size [23]. Thus, their diameter is calculated to be approximately 18 μm when they are considered spherical. On the other hand, the average diameter of bone marrow-derived human MSCs cultured in low serum/serum-free media (SFM)/Xeno-free media (XFM) ranged from 16.02 to 19.20 μm [27]. MSCs can change their shape to a spindle-like shape. Therefore, while most MSCs might be small enough to pass through capillaries, it is thought that they move slowly in narrow regions and bind to the surface of capillary endothelial cells due to adhesion molecules interacting with cell surface receptors, and possibly due to wall fluid shear stress (FSS) (approximately 0.4 Pa) pushing them against the cell surface [28]. Anatomically, the surface area of human adult pulmonary capillaries is approximately 50–70 $m^2$ [29], whereas that of human adult brain capillaries is approximately 12–18 $m^2$ [30]. The pulmonary capillary mesh cannot be bypassed given its scale in the normal course. Systematically, all intravenously administered substances pass through pulmonary capillaries before reaching brain capillaries. It is preferable to administer MSCs through carotid artery injection or intranasal administration to avoid the pulmonary first-pass effect, based on the biological and physical systematic structures regulated by structuralism advocated by Dr. Lévi-Strauss [31,32]. Nose-to-brain routes through intranasal administration will be described at another time. Human MSCs, acting as both carriers and vectors, can store various pharmaceutical agents as cargo, such as drugs or nanoparticles containing drugs, within the cells or load them on the surface of the cells [33].

The suspension of human MSCs and various numbers of microcapsules was fixed in 2.5% glutaraldehyde and then centrifuged at 1500 g. The resulting precipitates were MSCs containing microcapsules. The cellular motility of MSCs was reduced as the number of loaded microcapsules increased. MSCs with microcapsules at a ratio of 1:10 demonstrated greater migration than those at 1:20 and 1:45, respectively, but still showed lower migration than the control group with no microcapsules. Morphologically, MSCs changed their shape from a spindle-like shape to an irregular shape, especially with microcapsules at a greater ratio of 1:20 [34]. Thus, it is suggested that MSCs should not be loaded with too many microcapsules to maintain migration ability and cell morphology.

### 2.3. *The Implementation of MSC Delivery into the Brain across the BBB*

#### 2.3.1. Glioma

Brain cancers are characterized by cancerous growth within the brain and are broadly categorized into various types, including glioma, metastatic brain tumors, medulloblastoma, malignant lymphoma, germ cell tumors, meningioma, hypophyseal adenoma, and neurilemmoma. Glioma [35] is the most common type of CNS neoplasm and originates from glial cells rather than metastasizing. Specifically, glioblastomas are highly malignant gliomas. Anti-brain cancer drugs face challenges in entering the brain due to the BBB, leading to unmet medical needs due to the lack of effective pharmaceutical agents. Therefore, an innovative drug delivery system should be established promptly.

MSCs can migrate to cancer foci due to cytokines secreted from the tumor microenvironment along a chemoattractant gradient [33]. On the other hand, metastasis from peripheral cancer tissues into the brain is gradually accomplished based on the 'seed and soil' theory proposed by Dr. Stephen Paget [36]. Exosomes released into the bloodstream from peripheral cancer cells fused with the membrane of capillary endothelial cells at the BBB, eventually disrupting the tight junctions. As a result, cancer cells migrated to the brain through the BBB disruption [37]. Therefore, MSCs could migrate to cancer foci in the brain across the BBB, similar to the BBB transmigration by cancer cells from peripheral cancer tissues in the metastasis process.

The BBB is significantly altered by brain cancer cells. During this process, brain cancer cells secrete vascular endothelial growth factors (VEGFs) that induce angiogenesis, cause the disappearance of astrocyte endfeet, and disrupt tight junctions to form fenestration. However, transport of substances between the bloodstream and the brain cancer stroma is regulated. This situation is referred to as the blood–tumor barrier. Anticancer drugs still face difficulty in entering the brain due to the blood–tumor barrier, even though there are fenestrations between the capillary endothelial cells. Hydrophilic nutrients and essential materials are delivered to the brain cancer stroma and cancer cells through the paracellular fenestration pathway and transcellular pinocytosis [38,39]. Thus, cytokines secreted from the tumor microenvironment in the brain might leak into the bloodstream through the fenestrations of the capillary endothelial cells at the BBB. It is believed that such cytokines might attract migrating cancer cells or MSCs into the brain.

It is true that low-molecular-weight anti-cancer agents are effective against glioma, but they cannot cross the BBB due to excretion by MDR1. Thus, MSC-mediated drug delivery into the brain across the BBB is one of the solutions. MSCs loaded with anti-cancer drugs might be a promising tool for delivery into brain cancer cells. MSCs might be relatively tolerant to commonly used anti-cancer agents such as doxorubicin or paclitaxel (PTX) (Figure 3), probably due to differences in cell division speed. In the case of MSC damage, the use of nanoparticles encapsulating anti-cancer drugs might transiently avoid such cell damage, particularly within 72 h until their localization in a perivascular niche. Some of the drugs might be released from the intracellular nanoparticles to the cytosol via passive diffusion or from the extracellular nanoparticles.

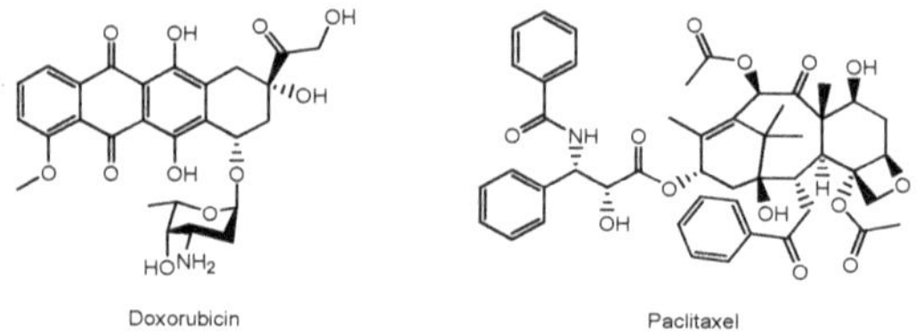


**Figure 3.** The structures of anti-cancer drugs.

(i) MSCs containing silica nanorattles encapsulating doxorubicin tracked down U251 glioma tumor cells more efficiently and enhanced tumor cell apoptosis in in vivo assays using rodents compared to doxorubicin alone or silica nanorattles encapsulating doxorubicin alone without using MSCs [40]. (ii) PTX-encapsulated hyaluronic acid-poly (D,L-lactide-co-glycolide) polymeric micelles (PTX/HA-PLGA micelles) (141.2 ± 0.5 nm in diameter) were efficiently internalized through receptor-mediated endocytosis, utilizing CD44 as a receptor in CD44 overexpressing MSCs. Both clathrin- and caveolae-mediated endocytosis pathways were involved in this internalization. MSCs exhibited tolerance to PTX due to the localization of PTX/HA-PLGA micelles in endosomes. MSCs containing PTX/HA-PLGA micelles demonstrated anti-glioma efficacy following contralateral injection in an in vivo assay using C6 glioma-bearing rats. PTX-encapsulated micelles were exocytosed into the brain and subsequently entered glioma cells via receptor-mediated endocytosis utilizing CD44. Finally, PTX was released from the micelles in endosomes and penetrated the cytosol through the endosomal membrane via passive diffusion [41].

Oncolytic viruses selectively infect cancer cells and eventually lyse them without infecting healthy cells [42]. In fact, glioma cells were destroyed by oncolytic viruses [43]. Teserpaturev (G47Δ, Delytact), a third generation (triple-mutated) recombinant oncolytic herpes simplex virus type 1, was conditionally approved for malignant glioma in June 2021 in Japan [44]. However, oncolytic viral agents were typically administered into the brain through stereotactic brain surgery. Oncolytic virotherapy for glioma tumors should be conducted in a non-invasive manner to reduce the burden on patients. Therefore, delivering oncolytic viruses into the brain using MSCs as a carrier and vector is a useful approach for glioma treatment. (iii) Human umbilical cord blood-derived MSCs loaded with a novel oncolytic adenovirus carrying interleukin (IL)-24 and/or endostatin demonstrated significantly greater antitumor effects in a xenograft model of glioma [45]. IL-24, a cytokine belonging to the IL-10 family, inhibited the growth of tumor cells and induced tumor-specific apoptosis [46]. Endostatin, a fragment of collagen XVIII, inhibits angiogenesis [47]. A synergistic anti-cancer effect was exhibited. (iv) Moreover, the oncolytic virus, CRAd.S.pK7, encapsulated within MSCs, entered and replicated in diffuse intrinsic pontine glioma using preclinical xenografted mouse models. Oncolytic virus-loaded MSCs, when combined with radiotherapy, exhibited prolonged survival compared to either therapy alone in mice bearing brainstem DIPG xenografts [48].

The modification of MSCs, such as overexpressing CXC chemokine receptor 4 (CXCR4) using a retroviral vector, is an improvement for homing to the tumor [49]. CXCR4 is a G-protein-coupled seven-transmembrane receptor on the cancer cell and is highly expressed in MSCs within the bone marrow, enabling MSCs to migrate to CXCR4 ligands at injured sites. Stromal cell-derived factor-1α (SDF-1α) (CXCL12) is a chemokine serving as a CXCR4 ligand that facilitates MSC tropism to tumors such as glioma. Additionally, the CXCR4/SDF-1α axis is highly relevant in cell recruitment during CNS injury [50]. Thus, strategies for actively homing MSCs to cancers might be feasible.

#### 2.3.2. Parkinson's Disease (PD)

PD [51] is a representative neurodegenerative disease caused by the loss of dopaminergic neurons in the nigrostriatal pathway due to the extracellular aggregation of α-synuclein, forming Lewy bodies. It manifests with symptoms such as motor dysfunction, including bradykinesia, tremor, and rigidity. Therefore, there is an expectation for innovative therapeutic agents. In general, nucleic acid-based drugs, such as antisense oligonucleotides, small interfering RNA (siRNA), and microRNA (miRNA), are enzymatically unstable in the serum due to nucleases. Endogenous miRNAs released from cells are protected within exosomes in the bloodstream. Similarly, MSCs can be used as carriers to protect delicate cargos such as RNAs. Nonetheless, MSC-derived exosomes or extracellular vesicles are likely to be sufficient for delivering miRNAs, such as miR-181a-2-3p, into the brain [52]. In PD treatment, MSCs are often used as regenerative medicine to differentiate into dopaminergic neurons [53]. However, genetically engineered MSCs are developed as an alternative approach for use as carriers. (i) Interestingly, MSCs encoding three critical genes for dopamine synthesis restored striatal dopamine levels and ameliorated motor function in PD rats [54]. (ii) MSCs primed with α-synuclein elicited neuroprotective effects by enhancing autophagy-mediated α-synuclein clearance. The expression of autophagy-regulating miRNAs, such as miR-376-3p, was increased in MSCs preliminarily primed with α-synuclein and subsequently packaged into exosomes derived from primed MSCs. Ultimately, MSCs primed with α-synuclein demonstrated more pronounced neuroprotective effects on dopaminergic neurons by inducing autophagy and lysosome activity in an in vivo assay using α-synuclein-overexpressing mice compared to naïve MSCs [55]. (iii) Matrix metalloproteinase-2 (MMP-2) derived from MSCs cleaved α-synuclein fibrils into smaller insoluble and oligomeric forms in the brain of a mouse PD model. The human MSCs used were not genetically manipulated. Conversely, MMP-2 knockdown MSCs through siRNA increased the intensity of α-synuclein aggregates in SH-SY5Y cells preincubated with α-synuclein, compared to normal MSCs [56]. Moreover, novel antisense oligonucleotides targeting mRNA coding for α-synuclein have been developed. Amido-bridged nucleic acid (AmNA)-modified antisense oligonucleotides targeting mRNA coding for α-synuclein demonstrated distribution to various brain areas in an in vivo assay through intrathecal administration using PD model mice, in the absence of any carrier or conjugation [57]. Is it possible to transport these antisense oligonucleotides more efficiently by using MSCs as a carrier to target the PD brain?

#### 2.3.3. Alzheimer's Disease (AD)

AD [58] is also a representative neurodegenerative disease caused by the loss of neurons due to the aggregation of amyloid β (Aβ), forming extracellular oligomers, protofibrils, and amyloid fibrils, and tau aggregation, forming intracellular neurofibrillary tangles (NFTs). It presents with symptoms such as memory loss, mild cognitive impairment, and dementia. Thus, innovative therapeutic agents are expected, although anti-Aβ antibodies have recently been launched in the pharmaceutical market. The anti-Aβ monoclonal antibody aducanumab [59] was approved by the Food and Drug Administration (FDA) in 2021. The anti-Aβ protofibril monoclonal antibody lecanemab [60] was approved by the FDA in 2023. Furthermore, the anti-Aβ monoclonal antibody donanemab [61] completed a phase 3 clinical trial with positive results for early AD in 2023 (NCT04437511). This strategy targeting Aβ is based on the amyloid hypothesis. However, there are several hypotheses regarding the onset and progression of AD due to the complex pathogenesis mechanism. It is implied that tau-derived NFTs are more closely correlated with AD pathogenesis than Aβ-derived senile plaques [3]. Although Aβ pathology and tau pathology initially proceeded independently, it is likely that Aβ pathology enhances the spreading of tau pathology at a certain point in the progression of AD symptoms [3]. In AD treatment, MSCs are often used as a regenerative medicine to differentiate into neurons or Schwann cell-like cells [62]. It has been suggested that neuroinflammation triggered by activated microglial cells plays a key role in the pathogenesis of AD [63]. Moreover, it is well-known that IL-10 deficiency exacerbates inflammation-induced tau pathology [64]. Thus, the use of IL-10 is considered effective for AD.

(i) Wharton's Jelly-derived MSCs improved spatial learning and alleviated memory decline after intravenous transplantation in the neuropathology and memory deficits in amyloid precursor protein (APP) and presenilin-1 (PS1) double-transgenic mice. Wharton's Jelly-derived MSCs increased the expression of IL-10, resulting in reduced microglial activation. The expressions of pro-inflammatory cytokines such as IL-1β and TNFα were decreased [65]. (ii) Furthermore, transplantation of MSCs via the tail vein improved spatial memory in the Morris water maze test using AD model mice (APdE9). Analysis based on electron paramagnetic resonance imaging revealed that oxidative stress was suppressed, evaluating the in vivo redox state of the brain. Intriguingly, the upregulation of CD14 expression in microglia by MSCs prompted the microglial uptake of Aβ via receptor-mediated endocytosis using the TLR4/CD14 complex and its clearance in the endo-lysosomal degradation pathway in vivo. MSCs altered the microglial phenotype from M1 to M2 by Th2 cytokines such as TGFβ and IL4 secreted from MSCs, eventually suppressing the production of proinflammatory cytokines in an in vitro assay using co-cultured mouse microglial cell line MG6 with MSCs [66]. (iii) Intracerebroventricularly injected bone marrow-derived MSCs improved cognitive impairment in APP/PS1 mice as an AD model by transferring exosomal miR-146a into astrocytes. The contents in exosomes secreted from MSCs into the cerebrospinal fluid (CSF) were internalized by astrocytes through fusion with the plasma membrane. The down-regulated expression of TRAF6 and NF-κB in astrocytes suppressed astrocyte inflammation and subsequently promoted synaptogenesis [67].

Therefore, MSCs demonstrated multifunctional remedial activity in AD pathology through the supply of IL-10, Th2 cytokines, miR-146a, and other substances. The use of MSCs as carriers for nanoparticles containing biologically active substances is not widely reported, although endogenous exosomes derived from MSCs can be considered natural nanoparticles.

#### 2.3.4. Stroke

Stroke [68] is strictly divided into cerebral infarction, cerebral hemorrhage, and subarachnoid hemorrhage. Cerebral infarction [69] occurs most frequently among them, causing necrosis of brain cells due to a lack of oxygen and nutrients resulting from blood vessel occlusion in the brain. Cerebral hemorrhage [70] involves the rupture of blood vessels in the brain, often forming an intracranial hematoma that may damage brain tissue. Subarachnoid hemorrhage [71] occurs in the subarachnoid space due to the rupture of blood vessels on the surface of the brain, often causing damage to brain tissue due to highly elevated intracranial pressure. Therefore, prognosis and recurrence prevention are crucial for affected individuals to lead a comfortable life. Stem cell therapy following a stroke is receiving considerable attention for its potential in improving neuroplasticity.

(i) Reactive oxygen species (ROS) play a role in brain injury following ischemic stroke [72]. To treat ischemic stroke, oxidative stress induced by ROS should be minimized. Mitochondrial Rho-GTPase 1 (Miro1) is a calcium-sensitive adaptor protein that facilitates the axonal transport of mitochondria in neurons. Intravenously injected Miro1-overexpressed multipotent MSCs significantly improved the recovery of neurological functions in rats modeled with middle cerebral artery occlusion-induced focal ischemia. The transfer of healthy mitochondria from Miro1-overexpressed multipotent MSCs to astrocytes exposed to ischemic damage, associated with elevated ROS levels, was performed. Consequently, the recipient astrocytes restored their bioenergetics. In fact, after 2 days of co-cultivation of (a) MSCs transfected with lentiviral constructs encoding red fluorescent protein fused with a mitochondrial localization signal and (b) astrocytes transfected with a similar construct encoding green fluorescent protein with a mitochondrial localization signal, red-fluorescing mitochondria derived from MSCs were observed alongside green-fluorescing mitochondria. Green-fluorescing mitochondria were not observed within MSCs. It is suggested that the mechanism of mitochondrial transport involved the passage through tunneling nanotubes [73]. (ii) Programmed cell death-ligand 1 (PD-L1) and AKT-modified umbilical cord-derived MSCs (UMSC-PD-L1-AKT), injected into a murine stroke model to overcome the hypoxic environment of the ischemic brain through intravenous and intracarotid routes, exhibited enhanced protection of neuroglial cells from ischemic injury based on the attenuation of systemic inflammation, compared to unmodified UMSCs. $CD8^+CD122^+IL\text{-}10^+$ regulatory T (Treg) cells were enhanced, while $CD11b^+CD80^+$ microglial/macrophages and $CD3^+CD8^+TNF\text{-}\alpha^+$ and $CD3^+CD8^+IFN\text{-}\alpha^+$ cytotoxic T cells were reduced. It is well-known that PD-L1 contributes to immune regulation. Akt activation is associated with pro-survival and anti-apoptotic effects. Akt is a serine/threonine protein kinase known as protein kinase B [74]. (iii) As an example of modified MSCs in a broad sense, three-dimensional (3D) spheroid-cultured MSCs, when intravenously injected, exhibited enhanced homing ability to the brain. Consequently, they decreased infarct volume and improved neurological function in rats that underwent middle cerebral artery occlusion and reperfusion, compared to 2D-cultured MSCs. The enhancement of the homing potential of MSCs is attributed to a reduced cell size that avoids lung entrapment and an increased expression of the chemokine receptor CXCR4. It is known that SDF-1$\alpha$ (CXCL12), a CXCR4 ligand, is produced by damaged neurons after cerebral ischemia. Furthermore, the anti-inflammatory properties of MSCs suppress a stimulated inflammatory response after ischemic stroke [75].

#### 2.3.5. Traumatic Brain Injury

Traumatic brain injury [76], often induced by an external force such as a violent blow, can result in cognitive dysfunction due to severe brain damage. (i) Indeed, in traumatic brain injury rats, genetically engineered MSCs overexpressing IL-10 significantly reduced the number of dead cells in the cortex and hippocampus three weeks after transplantation, compared to MSCs alone. It was suggested that IL-10 exhibited neuroprotective effects through its anti-inflammatory properties, suppressing the expression of various pro-inflammatory cytokines [77]. (ii) Brain-derived neurotrophic factor (BDNF) is involved in regulating the neurogenesis process through its binding to tropomyosin receptor kinase B (TrkB), which serves as a BDNF receptor on brain cells. Engineered MSCs overexpressing BDNF were intracerebroventricularly administered directly into the left lateral ventricle of the brain, ultimately improving the neurological and cognitive functions of traumatic brain injury rats in the Morris water maze test compared to a negative control. Thus, it was suggested that engineered MSCs secreted significantly more BDNF than naïve MSCs [78]. (iii) Fibroblast growth factor 21 (FGF21) is a type of secreted growth factor that acts as a metabolic regulator by binding to fibroblast growth factor receptors. MSCs overexpressing FGF21, administered through a hole drilled on the contralateral side of the injured hemisphere, enhanced neurogenesis in a mouse model of traumatic brain injury compared to a negative control. Thus, it was suggested that FGF21 released from MSCs induced neurogenesis [79].

### 2.3.6. Amyotrophic Lateral Sclerosis (ALS)

ALS [80] is a progressive neurodegenerative disease that causes muscle weakness due to the disorder of the motor neuron system. The causes of ALS are still unknown, although more than 30 causative gene mutations including Cu/Zn-superoxide dismutase (SOD1) have been discovered. Many clinical trials using MSCs are performed for the recovery of ALS [12]. These are not likely to be conducted as a carrier to aim the delivery or expression of specific compounds in the brain, although a type of effects including neuroinflammation or mitochondrial transfer are expected in addition to regenerative action [81]. Nonetheless, such accidental cargo might be improved. Tofersen, an oligonucleotide medicine targeting mRNA derived from SOD1 mutation, was clinically approved by the FDA in April, 2023 for the treatment of ALS associated with a mutation in the SOD1 gene [82]. Thus, MSC-mediated tofersen delivery into the brain can be a promising strategy due to enzymatic instability of oligonucleotide medicines and the impermeability across the BBB.

### 2.3.7. Multiple Sclerosis

Multiple sclerosis [83] is an immune-mediated inflammatory disease that affects the brain and spinal cord due to attacks mistaken by the body's immune system. The causes of multiple sclerosis are also still unknown, which are suggested to be a combination of genetic, immunologic, and environmental factors. Many clinical trials using MSCs are performed for the recovery of multiple sclerosis [12]. It turned out that MSCs were utilized to prevent circulating immune cells from crossing the BBB as disease-modifying therapies [84]. However, these processes are not considered as the drug delivers into the brain across the BBB using MSCs. Immunomodulatory strategies are thought to be effective on multiple sclerosis. (i) Ro-31-8425 is a cell-permeable, low-molecular weight ATP-competitive kinase inhibitor that inhibits human neutrophil superoxide generation (Figure 4) [85]. Systemically administered Ro-31-8425-loaded MSCs were more effective than MSCs alone or free Ro-31-8425 alone in the experimental autoimmune encephalomyelitis (EAE) mouse model of multiple sclerosis. Nonetheless, the serum level of Ro-31-8425 of Ro-31-8425-loaded MSCs was higher than Ro-31-8425 alone [86]. Accordingly, it was uncertain whether Ro-31-8425-loaded MSCs delivered their cargo into the brain across the BBB or not. Moreover, ocrelizumab, an anti-CD20 monoclonal antibody, was clinically approved by the FDA for the treatment of primary progressive multiple sclerosis (PPMS) disease progression in March 2017 [87]. Generally, monoclonal antibodies cannot cross the BBB via passive diffusion. Thus, MSC-mediated ocrelizumab delivery into the brain might enhance the activity.

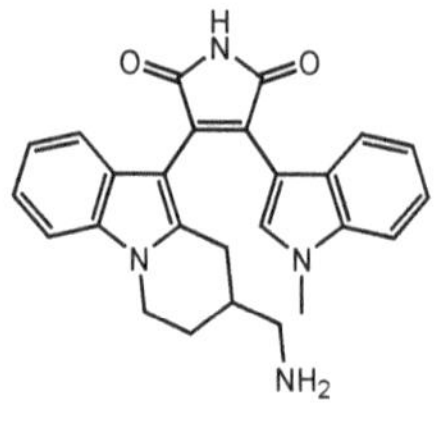


**Figure 4.** The structure of Ro-31-8425.

### 2.4. MSCs as a Carrier of Nanoparticles

It appears that the technology to use MSCs as carriers for nanoparticles containing biologically active substances has not been extensively developed, except in the field of brain tumors, such as doxorubicin- or PTX-encapsulated nanoparticles. The method of introducing nanoparticles onto the surface of MSCs (Figure 5) might be technologically easier than their internalization into MSCs, as demonstrated by neutrophils externally bound to functional microparticles entering the brain across the BBB for the treatment of glioblastoma [88]. Allogeneic sources are suitable for the preparation of modified MSCs to conduct sudden clinical use without any time difference. Furthermore, the surface modification on MSCs using nanoparticles is ideal for such sudden use due to easiness and high quality. Alternatively, internalizing cargo substances into exosomes produced by MSCs under the regulation of exosome biogenesis might be a solution, instead of using exosomes derived from isolated MSCs [5–7]. Otherwise, isolated MSCs-derived exosomes containing cargo substances might be reintroduced into the MSCs. The potential for MSC therapy will expand. Moreover, human artificial chromosomes are non-integrating chromosomal gene delivery vectors used for gene and cell therapies Duchene muscular dystrophy and for cancer therapy. Established MSCs with human artificial chromosomes might play an important role in MSC-based drug delivery [89], although human artificial chromosomes are a technology different from nanoparticles.

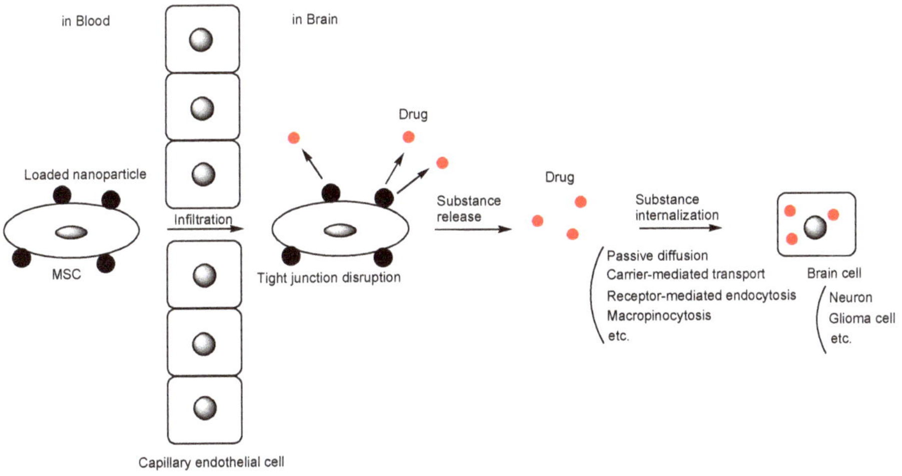


**Figure 5.** The pathway of nanoparticle loaded-mesenchymal stem cell (MSC)-based drug delivery into the brain across the blood–brain barrier. A black circle means nanoparticles containing drugs shown in a red circle. Released drugs from nanoparticles in the brain are internalized into brain cells.

## 3. Conclusions

Stem cells are gaining attention in the field of regenerative medicine, with MSCs being particularly noteworthy due to their easy obtainability from various tissues. Moreover, MSCs can serve as drug carriers that can home accurately and autonomously to target sites, including the brain, by traversing the BBB through transiently formed fenestrations between capillary endothelial cells. Cargos delivered by MSCs are divided into materials artificially included in advance, such as doxorubicin, and expected protein expression products of genetic modification, such as interleukins, including IL-10. Success has been observed in both cases, as mentioned above. Various types of materials are delivered to the target sites without serious off-target side effects (Table 2). Placing nanoparticles on the surface of MSCs is more realistic [88] than encapsulating them within MSCs, due to technical problems and material trajectory based on structuralism. Additionally, MSCs should be administered via carotid artery injection to avoid the pulmonary first-pass effect.

**Table 2.** The introduced applications of drug delivery into the brain using MSCs as a carrier.

| # | Formulation | Diseases | Cargo | Status | References |
|---|---|---|---|---|---|
| 1 | MSCs containing silica nanorattle encapsulating doxorubicin | Glioma | Doxorubicin | Basic research | [40] |
| 2 | PTX-encapsulated hyaluronic acid-poly (D,L-lactide-co-glycolide) polymeric micelles (PTX/HA-PLGA micelles) | Glioma | PTX | Basic research | [41] |
| 3 | Human umbilical cord blood MSCs loaded with the novel oncolytic adenovirus carrying interleukin (IL)-24 and/or endostatin | Glioma | IL-24 | Basic research | [45] |
| 4 | Oncolytic virus, CRAd.S.pK7, encapsulated within MSCs | Glioma | CRAd.S.pK7 | Basic research | [48] |
| 5 | MSCs encoding three critical genes for dopamine synthesis | Parkinson's disease | Dopamine | Basic research | [54] |
| 6 | MSC priming with α-synuclein | Parkinson's disease | miR 376-3p | Basic research | [55] |
| 7 | MSCs naturally possessing matrix metalloproteinase-2 (MMP-2) | Parkinson's disease | MMP-2 | Basic research | [56] |
| 8 | Transplantation of MSCs | Alzheimer's disease | IL-10 | Basic research | [65] |
| 9 | Bone marrow-derived MSCs | Alzheimer's disease | Th2 cytokines | Basic research | [66] |
| 10 | Bone marrow-derived MSCs | Alzheimer's disease | miR-146a | Basic research | [67] |
| 11 | Mitochondrial Rho-GTPase 1 (Miro1)-overexpressed multipotent MSCs | Stroke | Mitochondria | Basic research | [73] |
| 12 | Programmed cell death-ligand 1 (PD-L1) and AKT-modified umbilical cord-derived MSCs | Stroke | PD-L1 and AKT | Basic research | [74] |
| 13 | Three-dimensional (3D) spheroid cultured MSCs | Stroke | Unknown | Basic research | [75] |
| 14 | Genetically engineered MSCs overexpressing IL-10 | Traumatic brain injury | IL-10 | Basic research | [77] |
| 15 | Engineered MSCs overexpressing BDNF | Traumatic brain injury | BDNF | Basic research | [78] |
| 16 | MSCs overexpressing fibroblast growth factor 21 (FGF21) | Traumatic brain injury | FGF21 | Basic research | [79] |
| 17 | Ro-31-8425-loaded MSCs | Multiple sclerosis | Ro-31-8425 | Basic research | [85] |
| 18 | MSCs as a carrier of nanoparticles containing biologically active substances | CNS disease | Arbitrary substances | Under analysis in Tashima lab | - |

MSCs move to the injured sites as if acting of their own will, whereas compounds such as low-molecular-weight drugs, antibodies, nutrients, poisons, and waste materials move spontaneously and probabilistically to the target sites, completely based on the biological and physical machinery system regulated by structuralism. Nevertheless, it is true that MSC movement is subject to the biological and physical machinery system to some extent, but MSC therapy could have more immense possibilities, not only in the role of regenerative medicine, but also as a potent drug carrier than conventional medicine. Therefore, MSC therapy will rapidly evolve to deliver innovative medical care to patients in various roles.

**Funding:** This research received no external funding.

**Institutional Review Board Statement:** Not applicable.

**Informed Consent Statement:** Not applicable.

**Data Availability Statement:** Data available in a publicly accessible repository. The data presented in this study are openly available in References below. ClinicalTrials. govIdentifier can be found at https://clinicaltrials.gov/ (accessed on 1 January 2024).

**Acknowledgments:** This review is just my opinion based on or inferred from available published articles and public knowledge. Thus, the intellectual property rights are not infringed upon.

**Conflicts of Interest:** The author declares no conflict of interest.

## References

1. Alexander, P.; Thomson, H.A.; Luff, A.J.; Lotery, A.J. Retinal pigment epithelium transplantation: Concepts, challenges, and future prospects. *Eye* **2015**, *29*, 992–1002. [CrossRef]
2. Tashima, T. Smart Strategies for Therapeutic Agent Delivery into Brain across the Blood–Brain Barrier Using Receptor-Mediated Transcytosis. *Chem. Pharm. Bull.* **2020**, *68*, 316–325. [CrossRef]
3. Stimulus package. *Nat. Med.* **2018**, *24*, 247. [CrossRef]
4. Tashima, T. Delivery of Intravenously Administered Antibodies Targeting Alzheimer's Disease-Relevant Tau Species into the Brain Based on Receptor-Mediated Transcytosis. *Pharmaceutics* **2022**, *14*, 411. [CrossRef] [PubMed]
5. Ghasempour, E.; Hesami, S.; Movahed, E.; Keshel, S.H.; Doroudian, M. Mesenchymal stem cell-derived exosomes as a new therapeutic strategy in the brain tumors. *Stem Cell Res. Ther.* **2022**, *13*, 527. [CrossRef]
6. Yang, Z.; Li, Y.; Wang, Z. Recent Advances in the Application of Mesenchymal Stem Cell-Derived Exosomes for Cardiovascular and Neurodegenerative Disease Therapies. *Pharmaceutics* **2022**, *14*, 618. [CrossRef] [PubMed]
7. Rao, D.; Huang, D.; Sang, C.; Zhong, T.; Zhang, Z.; Tang, Z. Advances in Mesenchymal Stem Cell-Derived Exosomes as Drug Delivery Vehicles. *Front. Bioeng. Biotechnol.* **2022**, *9*, 797359. [CrossRef]
8. Uccelli, A.; Moretta, L.; Pistoia, V. Mesenchymal stem cells in health and disease. *Nat. Rev. Immunol.* **2008**, *8*, 726–736. [CrossRef] [PubMed]
9. Liu, J.; Gao, J.; Liang, Z.; Gao, C.; Niu, Q.; Wu, F.; Zhang, L. Mesenchymal stem cells and their microenvironment. *Stem Cell Res. Ther.* **2022**, *13*, 429. [CrossRef] [PubMed]
10. Wei, W.; Ao, Q.; Wang, X.; Cao, Y.; Liu, Y.; Zheng, S.G.; Tian, X. Mesenchymal Stem Cell–Derived Exosomes: A Promising Biological Tool in Nanomedicine. *Front. Pharmacol.* **2021**, *11*, 590470. [CrossRef] [PubMed]
11. Honda, T.; Yasui, M.; Shikamura, M.; Kubo, T.; Kawamata, S. What kind of impact does the Cell and Gene Therapy Product have on the medical and manufacturing industry? Part 3. *Pharm. Tech. Jpn.* **2023**, *39*, 2367–2374.
12. Fan, Y.; Goh, E.L.K.; Chan, J.K.Y. Neural Cells for Neurodegenerative Diseases in Clinical Trials. *Stem Cells Transl. Med.* **2023**, *12*, 510–526. [CrossRef] [PubMed]
13. Liu, X.; Robbins, S.; Wang, X.; Virk, S.; Schuck, K.; Deveza, L.A.; Oo, W.M.; Carmichael, K.; Antony, B.; Eckstein, F.; et al. Efficacy and cost-effectiveness of Stem Cell injections for symptomatic relief and strUctural improvement in people with Tibiofemoral knee OsteoaRthritis: Protocol for a randomised placebo-controlled trial (the SCUlpTOR trial). *BMJ Open* **2021**, *11*, e056382. [CrossRef] [PubMed]
14. Oka, S.; Yamaki, T.; Sasaki, M.; Ukai, R.; Takemura, M.; Yokoyama, T.; Kataoka-Sasaki, Y.; Onodera, R.; Ito, Y.M.; Kobayashi, S.; et al. Intravenous Infusion of Autoserum-Expanded Autologous Mesenchymal Stem Cells in Patients with Chronic Brain Injury: Protocol for a Phase 2 Trial. *JMIR Res. Protoc.* **2022**, *11*, e37898. [CrossRef] [PubMed]
15. Cyranoski, D. Japan's approval of stem-cell treatment for spinal-cord injury concerns scientists. *Nature* **2019**, *565*, 544–545. [CrossRef] [PubMed]
16. Japan should put the brakes on stem-cell sales. *Nature* **2019**, *565*, 535–536. [CrossRef]

17. Omae, K.; Yamamoto, K.; Teramukai, S.; Fukushima, M. The Principles of Regulatory Science in Regenerative Medicine Products. *Pharma. Med. Device Regul. Sci.* **2019**, *50*, 770–778. Available online: https://www.lhsi.jp/docs/05RS50-12_N-1.pdf (accessed on 1 January 2024).
18. Murata, M.; Teshima, T. Treatment of Steroid-Refractory Acute Graft-Versus-Host Disease Using Commercial Mesenchymal Stem Cell Products. *Front. Immunol.* **2021**, *12*, 724380. [CrossRef]
19. Scott, L.J. Darvadstrocel: A Review in Treatment-Refractory Complex Perianal Fistulas in Crohn's Disease. *BioDrugs* **2018**, *32*, 627–634. [CrossRef]
20. Tate, C.C.; Fonck, C.; McGrogan, M.; Case, C.C. Human mesenchymal stromal cells and their derivative, SB623 cells, rescue neural cells via trophic support following in vitro ischemia. *Cell Transplant.* **2010**, *19*, 973–984. [CrossRef]
21. Sanz-Nogués, C.; O'Brien, T. Current good manufacturing practice considerations for mesenchymal stromal cells as therapeutic agents. *Biomater. Biosyst.* **2021**, *2*, 100018. [CrossRef] [PubMed]
22. Schu, S.; Nosov, M.; O'Flynn, L.; Shaw, G.; Treacy, O.; Barry, F.; Murphy, M.; O'Brien, T.; Ritter, T. Immunogenicity of allogeneic mesenchymal stem cells. *J. Cell. Mol. Med.* **2012**, *16*, 2094–2103. [CrossRef]
23. Fischer, U.M.; Harting, M.T.; Jimenez, F.; Monzon-Posadas, W.O.; Xue, H.; Savitz, S.I.; Laine, G.A.; Cox, C.S., Jr. Pulmonary Passage is a Major Obstacle for Intravenous Stem Cell Delivery: The Pulmonary First-Pass Effect. *Stem Cells Dev.* **2009**, *18*, 683–692. [CrossRef]
24. Toma, C.; Wagner, W.R.; Bowry, S.; Schwartz, A.; Villanueva, F. Fate of Culture-Expanded Mesenchymal Stem Cells in the Microvasculature. *Circ. Res.* **2009**, *104*, 398–402. [CrossRef] [PubMed]
25. Kvernebo, K. Chapter 33—Microcirculation and Tissue Perfusion Assessment for Complex Cardiovascular Disease Care. In *Advances in Cardiovascular Technology. New Devices and Concepts*; Academic Press: Cambridge, MA, USA, 2022; pp. 501–513. [CrossRef]
26. Turgeon, M.L. *Clinical Hematology: Theory and Procedures*; Lippincott Williams & Wilkins: Philadelphia, PA, USA, 2004; p. 100. ISBN 9780781750073.
27. Bhat, S.; Viswanathan, P.; Chandanala, S.; Prasanna, S.J.; Seetharam, R.N. Expansion and characterization of bone marrow derived human mesenchymal stromal cells in serum-free conditions. *Sci. Rep.* **2021**, *11*, 3403. [CrossRef]
28. Tashima, T. Delivery of Drugs into Cancer Cells Using Antibody–Drug Conjugates Based on Receptor-Mediated Endocytosis and the Enhanced Permeability and Retention Effect. *Antibodies* **2022**, *11*, 78. [CrossRef] [PubMed]
29. Yang, J.; Pan, X.; Wang, L.; Yu, G. Alveolar cells under mechanical stressed niche: Critical contributors to pulmonary fibrosis. *Mol. Med.* **2020**, *26*, 95. [CrossRef]
30. Hartz, A.M.S.; Schulz, J.A.; Sokola, B.S.; Edelmann, S.E.; Shen, A.N.; Rempe, R.G.; Zhong, Y.; Seblani, N.E.; Bauer, B. Isolation of Cerebral Capillaries from Fresh Human Brain Tissue. *J. Vis. Exp.* **2018**, *139*, 57346. [CrossRef]
31. Laughlin, C.D.; D'Aquili, E.G. *Biogenetic Structuralism*; Columbia University Press: New York, NY, USA, 1974.
32. Leavy, S.A. Biogenetic Structuralism. *Yale J. Biol. Med.* **1976**, *49*, 420–421.
33. Zhang, T.; Lin, R.; Wu, H.; Jiang, X.; Gao, J. Mesenchymal stem cells: A living carrier for active tumor-targeted delivery. *Adv. Drug Deliv. Rev.* **2022**, *185*, 114300. [CrossRef]
34. Litvinova, L.S.; Shupletsova, V.V.; Khaziakhmatova, O.G.; Daminova, A.G.; Kudryavtseva, V.L.; Yurova, K.A.; Malashchenko, V.V.; Todosenko, N.M.; Popova, V.; Litvinov, R.I.; et al. Human Mesenchymal Stem Cells as a Carrier for a Cell-Mediated Drug Delivery. *Front. Bioeng. Biotechnol.* **2022**, *10*, 796111. [CrossRef]
35. Weller, M.; Wick, W.; Aldape, K.; Brada, M.; Berger, M.; Pfister, S.M.; Nishikawa, R.; Rosentha, M.; Wen, P.Y.; Stupp, R.; et al. Glioma. *Nat. Rev. Dis. Prim.* **2015**, *1*, 15017. [CrossRef]
36. Paget, S. The Distribution of Secondary Growths in Cancer of the Breast. *Lancet* **1889**, *133*, 571–573. [CrossRef]
37. Oliveira, F.D.; Castanho, M.A.R.B.; Neves, V. Exosomes and Brain Metastases: A Review on Their Role and Potential Applications. *Int. J. Mol. Sci.* **2021**, *22*, 10899. [CrossRef] [PubMed]
38. Mo, F.; Pellerino, A.; Soffietti, R.; Rudà, R. Blood–Brain Barrier in Brain Tumors: Biology and Clinical Relevance. *Int. J. Mol. Sci.* **2021**, *22*, 12654. [CrossRef] [PubMed]
39. Arvanitis, C.D.; Ferraro, G.B.; Jain, R.K. The blood–brain barrier and blood–tumour barrier in brain tumours and metastases. *Nat. Rev. Cancer* **2020**, *20*, 26–41. [CrossRef]
40. Li, L.; Guan, Y.; Liu, H.; Hao, N.; Liu, T.; Meng, X.; Fu, C.; Li, Y.; Qu, Q.; Zhang, Y.; et al. Silica nanorattle-doxorubicin-anchored mesenchymal stem cells for tumor-tropic therapy. *ACS Nano* **2011**, *5*, 7462–7470. [CrossRef]
41. Wang, X.-L.; Zhao, W.-Z.; Fan, J.-Z.; Jia, L.-C.; Lu, Y.-N.; Zeng, L.-H.; Lv, Y.-Y.; Sun, X.-Y. Tumor Tropic Delivery of Hyaluronic Acid-Poly (D,L-lactide-co-glycolide) Polymeric Micelles Using Mesenchymal Stem Cells for Glioma Therapy. *Molecules* **2022**, *27*, 2419. [CrossRef]
42. Muthukutty, P.; Yoo, S.Y. Oncolytic Virus Engineering and Utilizations: Cancer Immunotherapy Perspective. *Viruses* **2023**, *15*, 1645. [CrossRef]
43. Asija, S.; Chatterjee, A.; Goda, J.S.; Yadav, S.; Chekuri, G.; Purwar, R. Oncolytic immunovirotherapy for high-grade gliomas: A novel and an evolving therapeutic option. *Front. Immunol.* **2023**, *14*, 1118246. [CrossRef] [PubMed]
44. Frampton, J.E. Teserpaturev/G47Δ: First Approval. *BioDrugs* **2022**, *36*, 667–672. [CrossRef] [PubMed]

45. Zhang, J.; Chen, H.; Chen, C.; Liu, H.; He, Y.; Zhao, J.; Yang, P.; Mao, Q.; Xia, H. Systemic administration of mesenchymal stem cells loaded with a novel oncolytic adenovirus carrying IL-24/endostatin enhances glioma therapy. *Cancer Lett.* **2021**, *509*, 26–38. [CrossRef]
46. Zhu, W.; Wei, L.; Zhang, H.; Chen, J.; Qin, X. Oncolytic adenovirus armed with IL-24 Inhibits the growth of breast cancer in vitro and in vivo. *J. Exp. Clin. Cancer Res.* **2012**, *31*, 51. [CrossRef] [PubMed]
47. Pufe, T.; Petersen, W.J.; Miosge, N.; Goldring, M.B.; Mentlein, R.; Varoga, D.J.; Tillmann, B.N. Endostatin/collagen XVIII—An inhibitor of angiogenesis—is expressed in cartilage and fibrocartilage. *Matrix Biol.* **2004**, *23*, 267–276. [CrossRef] [PubMed]
48. Chastkofsky, M.I.; Pituch, K.C.; Katagi, H.; Zannikou, M.; Ilut, L.; Xiao, T.; Han, Y.; Sonabend, A.M.; Curiel, D.T.; Bonner, E.R.; et al. Mesenchymal Stem Cells Successfully Deliver Oncolytic Virotherapy to Diffuse Intrinsic Pontine Glioma. *Clin. Cancer Res.* **2021**, *27*, 1766–1777. [CrossRef] [PubMed]
49. Kalimuthu, S.; Oh, J.M.; Gangadaran, P.; Zhu, L.; Lee, H.W.; Rajendran, R.L.; Baek, S.H.; Jeon, Y.H.; Jeong, S.Y.; Lee, S.W.; et al. In Vivo Tracking of Chemokine Receptor CXCR4-Engineered Mesenchymal Stem Cell Migration by Optical Molecular Imaging. *Stem Cells Int.* **2017**, *2017*, 8085637. [CrossRef] [PubMed]
50. Al-Kharboosh, R.; ReFaey, K.; Lara-Velazquez, M.; Grewal, S.S.; Imitola, J.; Quiñones-Hinojosa, A. Inflammatory Mediators in Glioma Microenvironment Play a Dual Role in Gliomagenesis and Mesenchymal Stem Cell Homing: Implication for Cellular Therapy. Mayo Clin. Proc. Innov. *Mayo Clin. Proc. Innov. Qual. Outcomes* **2020**, *4*, 443–459. [CrossRef]
51. Bloem, B.R.; Okun, M.S.; Klein, C. Parkinson's disease. *Lancet* **2021**, *397*, 2284–2303. [CrossRef]
52. Ma, J.; Shi, X.; Li, M.; Chen, S.; Gu, Q.; Zheng, J.; Li, D.; Wu, S.; Yang, H.; Li, X. MicroRNA-181a–2–3p shuttled by mesenchymal stem cell-secreted extracellular vesicles inhibits oxidative stress in Parkinson's disease by inhibiting EGR1 and NOX4. *Cell Death Discov.* **2022**, *8*, 33. [CrossRef]
53. Heris, R.M.; Shirvaliloo, M.; Abbaspour-Aghdam, S.; Hazrati, A.; Shariati, A.; Youshanlouei, H.R.; Niaragh, F.J.; Valizadeh, H.; Ahmadi, M. The potential use of mesenchymal stem cells and their exosomes in Parkinson's disease treatment. *Stem Cell Res. Ther.* **2022**, *13*, 371. [CrossRef]
54. Li, J.; Li, N.; Wei, J.; Feng, C.; Chen, Y.; Chen, T.; Ai, Z.; Zhu, X.; Ji, W.; Li, T. Genetically engineered mesenchymal stem cells with dopamine synthesis for Parkinson's disease in animal models. *NPJ Park. Dis.* **2022**, *8*, 175. [CrossRef]
55. Shin, J.Y.; Kim, D.Y.; Lee, J.; Shin, Y.J.; Kim, Y.S.; Lee, P.H. Priming mesenchymal stem cells with α-synuclein enhances neuroprotective properties through induction of autophagy in Parkinsonian models. *Stem Cell Res. Ther.* **2022**, *13*, 483. [CrossRef]
56. Oh, S.H.; Kim, H.N.; Park, H.J.; Shin, J.Y.; Kim, D.Y.; Lee, P.H. The Cleavage Effect of Mesenchymal Stem Cell and Its Derived Matrix Metalloproteinase-2 on Extracellular α-Synuclein Aggregates in Parkinsonian Models. *Stem Cells Transl. Med.* **2017**, *6*, 949–961. [CrossRef]
57. Uehara, T.; Choong, C.J.; Nakamori, M.; Hayakawa, H.; Nishiyama, K.; Kasahara, Y.; Baba, K.; Nagata, T.; Yokota, T.; Tsuda, H.; et al. Amido-bridged nucleic acid (AmNA)-modified antisense oligonucleotides targeting α-synuclein as a novel therapy for Parkinson's disease. *Sci. Rep.* **2019**, *21*, 7567. [CrossRef] [PubMed]
58. Scheltens, P.; De Strooper, B.; Kivipelto, M.; Holstege, H.; Chételat, G.; Teunissen, C.E.; Cummings, J.; van der Flier, W.M. Alzheimer's disease. *Lancet* **2021**, *397*, 1577–1590. [CrossRef] [PubMed]
59. Pardridge, W.M. Blood-Brain Barrier and Delivery of Protein and Gene Therapeutics to Brain. *Front. Aging Neurosci.* **2020**, *11*, 373. [CrossRef] [PubMed]
60 van Dyck, C.H.; Swanson, C.J.; Aisen, P.; Bateman, R.J.; Chen, C.; Gee, M.; Kanekiyo, M.; Li, D.; Reyderman, L.; Cohen, S.; et al. Lecanemab in Early Alzheimer's Disease. *N. Engl. J. Med.* **2023**, *388*, 9–21. [CrossRef]
61. Rashad, A.; Rasool, A.; Shaheryar, M.; Sarfraz, A.; Sarfraz, Z.; Robles-Velasco, K.; Cherrez-Ojeda, I. Donanemab for Alzheimer's Disease: A Systematic Review of Clinical Trials. *Healthcare* **2023**, *11*, 32. [CrossRef] [PubMed]
62. Hernández, A.E.; García, E. Mesenchymal Stem Cell Therapy for Alzheimer's Disease. *Stem Cells Int.* **2021**, *2021*, 7834421. [CrossRef] [PubMed]
63. Sobue, A.; Komine, O.; Yamanaka, K. Neuroinflammation in Alzheimer's disease: Microglial signature and their relevance to disease. *Inflamm. Regen.* **2023**, *43*, 26. [CrossRef]
64. Weston, L.L.; Jiang, S.; Chisholm, D.; Jantzie, L.L.; Bhaskar, K. Interleukin-10 deficiency exacerbates inflammation-induced tau pathology. *J. Neuroinflamm.* **2021**, *18*, 161. [CrossRef]
65. Xie, Z.H.; Liu, Z.; Zhang, X.R.; Yang, H.; Wei, L.F.; Wang, Y.; Xu, S.L.; Sun, L.; Lai, C.; Bi, J.Z.; et al. Wharton's Jelly-derived mesenchymal stem cells alleviate memory deficits and reduce amyloid-β deposition in an APP/PS1 transgenic mouse model. *Clin. Exp. Med.* **2016**, *16*, 89–98. [CrossRef]
66. Yokokawa, K.; Iwahara, N.; Hisahara, S.; Emoto, M.C.; Saito, T.; Suzuki, H.; Manabe, T.; Matsumura, A.; Matsushita, T.; Suzuki, S.; et al. Transplantation of Mesenchymal Stem Cells Improves Amyloid-β Pathology by Modifying Microglial Function and Suppressing Oxidative Stress. *J. Alzheimers Dis.* **2019**, *72*, 867–884. [CrossRef]
67. Nakano, M.; Kubota, K.; Kobayashi, E.; Chikenji, T.S.; Saito, Y.; Konari, N.; Fujimiya, M. Bone marrow-derived mesenchymal stem cells improve cognitive impairment in an Alzheimer's disease model by increasing the expression of microRNA-146a in hippocampus. *Sci. Rep.* **2020**, *10*, 10772. [CrossRef]
68. Murphy, S.J.; Werring, D.J. Stroke: Causes and clinical features. *Medicine* **2020**, *48*, 561–566. [CrossRef]
69. Zhao, Y.; Zhang, X.; Chen, X.; Wei, Y. Neuronal injuries in cerebral infarction and ischemic stroke: From mechanisms to treatment (Review). *Int. J. Mol. Med.* **2022**, *49*, 15. [CrossRef] [PubMed]

70. Magid-Bernstein, J.; Girard, R.; Polster, S.; Srinath, A.; Romanos, S.; Awad, I.A.; Sansing, L.H. Cerebral Hemorrhage: Pathophysiology, Treatment, and Future Directions. *Circ. Res.* **2022**, *130*, 1204–1229. [CrossRef] [PubMed]
71. Neifert, S.N.; Chapman, E.K.; Martini, M.L.; Shuman, W.H.; Schupper, A.J.; Oermann, E.K.; Mocco, J.; Macdonald, R.L. Aneurysmal Subarachnoid Hemorrhage: The Last Decade. *Transl. Stroke Res.* **2021**, *12*, 428–446. [CrossRef] [PubMed]
72. Rodrigo, R.; Fernández-Gajardo, R.; Gutiérrez, R.; Matamala, J.M.; Carrasco, R.; Miranda-Merchak, A.; Feuerhake, W. Oxidative stress and pathophysiology of ischemic stroke: Novel therapeutic opportunities. *CNS Neurol. Disord. Drug Targets* **2013**, *12*, 698–714. [CrossRef]
73. Babenko, V.A.; Silachev, D.N.; Popkov, V.A.; Zorova, L.D.; Pevzner, I.B.; Plotnikov, E.Y.; Sukhikh, G.T.; Zorov, D.B. Miro1 Enhances Mitochondria Transfer from Multipotent Mesenchymal Stem Cells (MMSC) to Neural Cells and Improves the Efficacy of Cell Recovery. *Molecules* **2018**, *23*, 687. [CrossRef]
74. Lin, S.L.; Lee, W.; Liu, S.P.; Chang, Y.W.; Jeng, L.B.; Shyu, W.C. Novel Programmed Death Ligand 1-AKT-engineered Mesenchymal Stem Cells Promote Neuroplasticity to Target Stroke Therapy. *Mol. Neurobiol.* **2023**. [CrossRef]
75. Li, Y.; Dong, Y.; Ran, Y.; Zhang, Y.; Wu, B.; Xie, J.; Cao, Y.; Mo, M.; Li, S.; Deng, H.; et al. Three-dimensional cultured mesenchymal stem cells enhance repair of ischemic stroke through inhibition of microglia. *Stem Cell Res. Ther.* **2021**, *12*, 358. [CrossRef]
76. Ghajar, J. Traumatic brain injury. *Lancet* **2000**, *356*, 923–929. [CrossRef]
77. Maiti, P.; Peruzzaro, S.; Kolli, N.; Andrews, M.; Al-Gharaibeh, A.; Rossignol, J.; Dunbar, G.L. Transplantation of mesenchymal stem cells overexpressing interleukin-10 induces autophagy response and promotes neuroprotection in a rat model of TBI. *J. Cell. Mol. Med.* **2019**, *23*, 5211–5224. [CrossRef]
78. Choi, B.Y.; Hong, D.K.; Kang, B.S.; Lee, S.H.; Choi, S.; Kim, H.-J.; Lee, S.M.; Suh, S.W. Engineered Mesenchymal Stem Cells Over-Expressing BDNF Protect the Brain from Traumatic Brain Injury-Induced Neuronal Death, Neurological Deficits, and Cognitive Impairments. *Pharmaceuticals* **2023**, *16*, 436. [CrossRef] [PubMed]
79. Shahror, R.A.; Linares, G.R.; Wang, Y.; Hsueh, S.C.; Wu, C.C.; Chuang, D.M.; Chiang, Y.H.; Chen, K.Y. Transplantation of Mesenchymal Stem Cells Overexpressing Fibroblast Growth Factor 21 Facilitates Cognitive Recovery and Enhances Neurogenesis in a Mouse Model of Traumatic Brain Injury. *J. Neurotraum.* **2020**, *37*, 14–26. [CrossRef] [PubMed]
80. Feldman, E.L.; Goutman, S.A.; Petri, S.; Mazzini, L.; Savelieff, M.G.; Shaw, P.J.; Sobue, G. Amyotrophic lateral sclerosis. *Lancet* **2022**, *400*, 1363–1380. [CrossRef]
81. Morata-Tarifa, C.; Azkona, G.; Glass, J.; Mazzini, L.; Sanchez-Pernaute, R. Looking backward to move forward: A meta-analysis of stem cell therapy in amyotrophic lateral sclerosis. *NPJ Regen. Med.* **2021**, *6*, 20. [CrossRef]
82. Blair, H.A. Tofersen: First Approval. *Drugs* **2023**, *83*, 1039–1043. [CrossRef]
83. Dobson, R.; Giovannoni, G. Multiple sclerosis–a review. *Eur. J. Neurol.* **2019**, *26*, 27–40. [CrossRef] [PubMed]
84. Tabansky, I.; Messina, M.D.; Bangeranye, C.; Goldstein, J.; Blitz-Shabbir, K.M.; Machado, S.; Jeganathan, V.; Wright, P.; Najjar, S.; Cao, Y.; et al. Advancing drug delivery systems for the treatment of multiple sclerosis. *Immunol. Res.* **2015**, *63*, 58–69. [CrossRef] [PubMed]
85. Muid, R.E.; Dale, M.M.; Davis, P.D.; Elliott, L.H.; Hill, C.H.; Kumar, H.; Lawton, G.; Twomey, B.M.; Wadsworth, J.; Wilkinson, S.E.; et al. A novel conformationally restricted protein kinase C inhibitor, Ro 31-8425, inhibits human neutrophil superoxide generation by soluble, particulate and post-receptor stimuli. *FEBS Lett.* **1991**, *293*, 169–172. [CrossRef] [PubMed]
86. Levy, O.; Rothhammer, V.; Mascanfroni, I.; Tong, Z.; Kuai, R.; De Biasio, M.; Wang, Q.; Majid, T.; Perrault, C.; Yeste, A.; et al. A cell-based drug delivery platform for treating central nervous system inflammation. *J. Mol. Med.* **2021**, *99*, 663–671. [CrossRef] [PubMed]
87. Mulero, P.; Midaglia, L.; Montalban, X. Ocrelizumab: A new milestone in multiple sclerosis therapy. *Ther. Adv. Neurol. Disord.* **2018**, *11*, 1756286418773025. [CrossRef]
88. Fukuta, T. Development of functional microparticles capable of binding to neutrophils to overcome the blood-brain barrier for the treatment of ischemic stroke. *Pharm. Tech. Jpn.* **2023**, *39*, 81–83.
89. Uno, N.; Takata, S.; Komoto, S.; Miyamoto, H.; Nakayama, Y.; Osaki, M.; Mayuzumi, R.; Miyazaki, N.; Hando, C.; Abe, S.; et al. Panel of human cell lines with human/mouse artificial chromosomes. *Sci. Rep.* **2022**, *12*, 3009. [CrossRef]

*pharmaceutics* MDPI

*Article*

# Non-Invasive, Targeted Nanoparticle-Mediated Drug Delivery across a Novel Human BBB Model

**Shona Kaya, Bridgeen Callan and Susan Hawthorne ***

School of Pharmacy and Pharmaceutical Sciences, Ulster University, Coleraine BT52 1SA, N. Ireland, UK
* Correspondence: s.hawthorne@ulster.ac.uk

**Abstract:** The blood–brain barrier (BBB) is a highly sophisticated system with the ability to regulate compounds transporting through the barrier and reaching the central nervous system (CNS). The BBB protects the CNS from toxins and pathogens but can cause major issues when developing novel therapeutics to treat neurological disorders. PLGA nanoparticles have been developed to successfully encapsulate large hydrophilic compounds for drug delivery. Within this paper, we discuss the encapsulation of a model compound Fitc-dextran, a large molecular weight (70 kDa), hydrophilic compound, with over 60% encapsulation efficiency (EE) within a PLGA nanoparticle (NP). The NP surface was chemically modified with DAS peptide, a ligand that we designed which has an affinity for nicotinic receptors, specifically alpha 7 nicotinic receptors, found on the surface of brain endothelial cells. The attachment of DAS transports the NP across the BBB by receptor-mediated transcytosis (RMT). Assessment of the delivery efficacy of the DAS-conjugated Fitc-dextran-loaded PLGA NP was studied in vitro using our optimal triculture in vitro BBB model, which successfully replicates the in vivo BBB environment, producing high TEER ($\geq$230 $\Omega$/cm$^2$) and high expression of ZO1 protein. Utilising our optimal BBB model, we successfully transported fourteen times the concentration of DAS-Fitc-dextran-PLGA NP compared to non-conjugated Fitc-dextran-PLGA NP. Our novel in vitro model is a viable method of high-throughput screening of potential therapeutic delivery systems to the CNS, such as our receptor-targeted DAS ligand-conjugated NP, whereby only lead therapeutic compounds will progress to in vivo studies.

**Keywords:** in vitro model; blood–brain barrier (BBB); nanoparticles; drug delivery; targeted receptor-mediated transcytosis; ligand conjugation; nicotinic acetylcholine receptor

**Citation:** Kaya, S.; Callan, B.; Hawthorne, S. Non-Invasive, Targeted Nanoparticle-Mediated Drug Delivery across a Novel Human BBB Model. *Pharmaceutics* **2023**, *15*, 1382. https://doi.org/10.3390/pharmaceutics15051382

Academic Editors: Nicolas Tournier and Toshihiko Tashima

Received: 30 March 2023
Revised: 20 April 2023
Accepted: 28 April 2023
Published: 30 April 2023



## 1. Introduction

The central nervous system (CNS) is protected by a highly regulated physiological barrier known as the blood–brain barrier (BBB). The BBB consists of tightly regulated blood vessels formed by brain endothelial cells (BEC) and tight junction (TJ) proteins, forming part of the neurovascular unit (NVU), which also consists of pericytes, astrocytes, neurons and basement membrane (basal lamina) [1–4]. The endothelial cells that line the blood vessels of the BBB are unlike the endothelial cells that line blood vessels found within other organs of the body, as they are unfenestrated due to the presence of TJ proteins [2,3]. TJ proteins, such as occludin, claudin-5 and ZO-1, are expressed and regulated by cellular interaction and proximity between the endothelial cells and the other brain cell types that form part of the NVU and help prevent paracellular transport of toxins and pathogens. Even though TJ proteins are present within the BBB, the BBB facilitates the transportation of molecules that are essential for the maintenance of CNS homeostasis via diffusion (simple or facilitated), mediated or active transportation and the proximity of the circulating blood flow. However, due to the tightly regulated blood vessels of the BBB, paracellular diffusion is severely restricted and not a viable mode of transport for large hydrophilic molecules such as biologics (antibodies and proteins), causing issues with drug development, drug delivery and targeting of novel drugs for neurological conditions [1,2,4–9] Drugs that are lipid soluble and have a low molecular weight can transverse the BBB by transmembrane diffusion, which relies on the drug merging with the cell membrane by a non-saturable mechanism [1]. There can be issues however if the drug is highly lipid soluble, as some of the drug can remain in the cell, with only a small concentration of the drug reaching the CNS [1]. Transmembrane diffusion is not possible for therapeutics of high molecular weight and/or hydrophilic in nature; therefore, different mechanisms designed to transverse the BBB have been investigated. Currently, there are parenteral and non-parenteral routes of administration of drugs to treat neurological disorders, such as Parkinson's disease (PD), Alzheimer's disease (AD), dementia and stroke. Parenteral administrative routes for CNS delivery include intrathecal administration via intracerebroventricular (ICV) port, or intrathecal lumber (IT-L) injections or by convection-enhanced delivery (CED) such as polymeric implants [3,10]. Another method of administering a drug is peri-spinally using the cerebrospinal venous system (CSVS) [11]. Traditionally, these methods have a high success rate in terms of drug administration, but they are costly, requiring highly skilled clinicians and often hospitalisation for the patient as well as being uncomfortable and distressing for the patient. One such example of where invasive delivery prevents the full potential of a therapy is seen using etanercept.

Etanercept was first approved by the FDA in 1998 to treat rheumatoid arthritis. Etanercept is a potent anti-TNF (tumour necrosis factor) fusion protein and TNF inhibitor and was of interest for treating neuroinflammatory disorders such as stroke and Alzheimer's disease. However, to treat the neuroinflammatory disorders within the CNS, etanercept (a protein with a molecular weight of 150 kDa that cannot be delivered systemically), must be administered peri-spinally and transverse the dura mater utilising the CSVS [12–16]. Reports by Tobinick et al. (2014) have shown that after one dose of peri-spinal etanercept, patients with long-term acute brain injuries had improved aphasia and apraxia and the left hemiparesis is reduced [14]. A study carried out by Ralph et al. (2020) showed rapid and significant results for chronic post-stroke management by administration of peri-spinal etanercept, which shows that peri-spinal administration of large molecules such as etanercept is effective [15]. Even though etanercept has the potential to successfully treat neurological inflammation, the invasive delivery of the treatment can cause issues for long-term suffers of AD or PD, such as severe discomfort and distress; therefore, non-invasive administration would be a better mode for BBB drug delivery and expand upon its current use [3].

Chemical modifications of drugs to aid in their administration via non-invasive routes are currently utilised to modify small molecular weight drugs to become more lipophilic and increase their ability to permeate the BBB [3]. L-3,4-dihydroxyphenylalanine (L-DOPA) is a non-invasive form of treatment for neurological disorders, specifically PD, and is taken orally in tablet form. Unlike dopamine, L-DOPA, which is a precursor of dopamine, transverses the BBB by system L (LAT1), which is a form of amino acid transporter, and once across the BBB it undergoes a decarboxylation reaction to the active form, dopamine. L-DOPA has been used to treat the motor symptoms caused by PD for over 50 years [17–21].

One such mechanism that could be used to increase patient compliance, and reduce off-site targeting, toxicity and side effects, is the non-invasive method of drug delivery by an active transport mechanism known as receptor-mediated transcytosis (RMT). RMT transports molecules across the BBB into the CNS by targeting the receptors on the BEC; this is normally achieved either by preparing a complex between the drug of interest and the receptor-targeting entity, or by encapsulating the drug within a nanocarrier with the RMT-targeting ligand on the surface of the carrier [7,22–24]. Nanocarriers such as nanoparticles (NP) can be chemically modified by the conjugation of ligands to the surface of the loaded NP, which can then target the receptors on the BEC and facilitate the transportation of the novel drug across the BBB by RMT [25,26]. NP have the added benefit of protecting their internalised cargo, such as proteins and antibodies, from degradation by endogenous compounds. In addition, encapsulating compounds within the NP increases the accumulation of the therapeutic drug at the target site, increasing efficacy and requiring a reduction in drug dose, thereby reducing off-site targeting effects [22–24,27–29].

Ligand-conjugated NP have ligands attached which target receptors that are known to be found on the surface of BEC [26]; prior to any in vivo assessment, analysis of a variation in ligand-conjugated NP with different drug load concentrations and/or different ligand types or amounts needs to be analysed. Therefore, there is a requirement for the most cost-effective, time-efficient and ethical way to carry out this preliminary assessment by using in vitro BBB models where possible.

When developing new therapeutics, in vitro BBB models have been widely utilised to investigate drug targeting, drug permeability and drug toxicity. In vitro models can be constructed in various ways depending on cost, cell source (immortalised, primary or stem cells) and time frame, to mimic the in vivo physiology and architecture of the BBB. The in vitro models can be developed to maintain high integrity and low permeability by paracellular transport. There are different forms of in vitro models such as organoids/spheroids which are mainly developed using stem cells, microfluidic devices or transwell models which can be developed using primary, stem or immortalised cells [30–33]. However, both organoid/spheroids and micro-fluidic models are time-consuming, costly and complex, with microfluidic devices having limited scalability and prone to errors, whilst organoid/spheroid models have poor BEC coverage and poor vascularisation [30–33]. Transwell models are generally cost-effective, scalable, adaptable and easily produced, and have shown to be effective for high-throughput drug screening and are therefore a viable model to utilise when assessing the efficacy of novel compounds prior to lead compound in vivo analysis [34–36]. The inclusion of shear stress, cellular substrata and the co-localisation of astrocytes and pericytes produces an in vitro model which more accurately mimics the in vivo BBB architecture by enhancing TJ protein expression, increasing barrier integrity and thereby decreasing non-specific permeability. When developing drugs for the treatment of neurological disorders, the use of in vitro models such as transwell models is an important tool to enhance the development of targeted drug delivery systems (DDS) that have the ability to traverse the BBB via RMT, ensuring that novel neurological therapeutics can be delivered to the required site as efficiently and non-invasively as possible.

In this article, we demonstrate the development and optimisation of a novel, in vitro human-immortalised cell BBB model and also demonstrate that receptor-targeting PLGA NP are an ideal vehicle for transporting large, hydrophilic molecules across the BBB in vitro. We also demonstrate that the chemical modification of the surface of NP by a targeting ligand, aids in the transport of the loaded NP across the BBB via RMT. We have shown this by encapsulating Fitc-dextran, a large hydrophilic molecule (70,000 Da), within a PLGA NP and conjugating DAS peptide to the surface of the NP. DAS ($NH_2$-GCGGSGCLRVGGRrRrRr-COOH) is a ligand that we previously designed [37] which aids in the transportation of the loaded NP across the BBB by RMT, due to the DAS affinity for alpha 7 nicotinic acetylcholine receptors ($\alpha$-7 nAChR), which are found on the membranes of the BEC of the BBB.

## 2. Materials and Methods

### *2.1. Cell Culture*

#### 2.1.1. Materials

Cell Culture

Immortalised human brain microvascular endothelial cells (I-HBMEC) (Innoprot, Bizkaia, Spain) (P10361-1M), Immortalised human astrocytes (IA) (Innoprot, Bizkaia, Spain) (P10251-1M), CLTH/Immortalised Pericytes (IP) (Amsbio, Oxfordshire, U.K.) (CL05008-CLTH), D-MEM/F:12 (1:1) (CE) (Thermofisher, Cambridge, U.K.) (11320074), Insulin-trans-sel-G, 100× (Thermofisher, Cambridge, U.K.) (41400045), Penicillin streptomycin (PS) (Gibco, Paisley, U.K.) (15070-063), Fetal bovine serum (FBS) (Gibco, Paisley, U.K.) (A3160801), Hydrocortisone solution (50 um) (Merck, Dorset, U.K.) (H6909), Fibroblast growth factor-basic (BFGF) (Merck, Dorset, U.K.) (SRP3043), Heparin sodium salt (Merck, Dorset, U.K.) (H3149), Dulbecco's phosphate buffered saline, M (DPBS) (Merck, Dorset,

U.K.) (D8537), Accutase® solution (Merck, Dorset, U.K.) (A6964), Tissue culture flask, 75 $cm^2$ growth area (T75) (Sarstedt, Leicestershire, U.K.) (83.3911.002).

Transwell Model

Corning TW PC membrane 6.5 mm, 0.4 µm, TCT, S (Merck, Dorset, U.K.) (CLS3413-48EA), Tissue culture, 24-flat-well sterile plate (Sarstedt, Leicestershire, U.K.) (83.3922), Magnesium sulphate ($MgSO_4$) (Merck, Dorset, U.K.) (63136), Fibronectin bovine plasma (Merck, Dorset, U.K.) (F1141), Gelatin solution Bioreagent, Type B, 2% (Merck, Dorset, U.K.) (G1393).

2.1.2. Methods

Preparation of Cells for In Vitro EP + A transwell BBB Model

I-HBMEC, IP and IA were all seeded and grown in T75 flask with DMEM/F:12 medium supplemented with 10% FBS, 1% PS, 5 mL hydrocortisone solution, 2.5 mL Insulin-trans-sel-G, 100×, 30 µL BFGF, 15 mg of 100 KU Heparin sodium salt. Cells were aspirated and washed with DPBS, detached with Accutase and centrifuged using a Thermo Scientific Medifuge centrifuge, at 1000 rpm (I-HBMEC & IA) or 900 rpm (IP) for 5 min for formation of cell pellet.

Preparation of In Vitro Tri-Culture Transwell BBB Model

Day-2: The underside of the transwell polycarbonate inserts was precoated with 40 µL substratum (30 µg/mL fibronectin solution and 10 µg/mL gelatin solution). The precoated inserts were incubated for 4 h at 37 °C 5% $CO_2$. The underside of inserts was washed thrice with DPBS and inserts were inserted into wells on a 24-well plate that contained 200 µL DPBS to prevent underside of insert drying out. In apical layer of insert, 100 µL of substrata solution was pipetted and then incubated overnight at 37 °C 5% $CO_2$.

Day-1: Inserts and wells on 24-well plate were washed thrice with DPBS and allowed to airdry at RT. The IP and IA pellets were diluted to $8 \times 10^4$ cells/mL in complete medium containing 10 mM $MgSO_4$ ($Mg^{2+}$). Equal volumes of each $8 \times 10^4$ cells/mL IA and IP were combined to form $4 \times 10^4$ cells/mL IA/IP cell solution. Transwell inserts were inverted and 40 µL of the IA/IP cell solution was pipetted onto the pre-coated underside of inserts and incubated at RT for 40 min to allow cells to adhere. Then, 600 µL of the medium, was pipetted into wells on well plate and inserts were placed right side up into these wells, and 100 µL of the medium was pipetted into the apical layer of inserts and the plate was incubated overnight at 37 °C 5% $CO_2$.

Day 0: The I-HBMEC pellet was diluted to $6.25 \times 10^4$ cells/mL with medium. Apical layer of inserts was aspirated and 200 µL of the $6.25 \times 10^4$ cells/mL of I-HBMEC was pipetted into the apical layer of insert, and the medium in basolateral layer (well of well plate) was aspirated and replaced with fresh medium containing $Mg^2$+. Plate was incubated for 48 h at 37 °C 5% $CO_2$ with gentle shaking at 100 rpm on a Grant-bio Orbital shaker PSU-10i.

Day 1: Allowed cells to adhere to insert surfaces.

Days 2–5: Measured trans-endothelial electrical resistance (TEER) daily using WPI EVOM 2 voltohmmeter with WPI electrode set for EVOM and replaced medium in basolateral and apical layer of model with fresh medium then incubated at 37 °C 5% $CO_2$ at 100 rpm.

Day 6: Measured TEER, then tested compounds of interest on BBB model, replacing medium with serum-free medium (SFM) containing test compound in apical layer. In basolateral layer, the medium was replaced with 600 µL SFM. Plate was incubated at 37 °C 5% $CO_2$ at 100 rpm and samples were taken every half hour for 7 h and then at 24 h from basolateral layer. The medium removed from basolateral layer was replaced with an equivalent volume of SFM to maintain sink conditions (Figure 1).

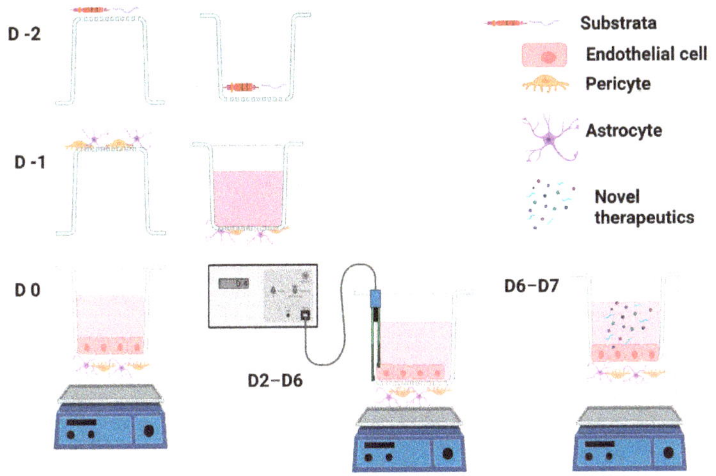


**Figure 1.** Image displays how the BBB model is developed over a 9-day period, including the application of shear stress by orbital shaker and TEER measurement using chopstick-style electrodes and a voltohmmeter (image created in BioRender).

### 2.2. *Evaluation of Barrier Integrity*

#### 2.2.1. Materials

MES hydrate (Merck, Dorset, U.K.) (M8250), N-(3-Dimethylaminopropyl)-N′-ethylcarbodiimide hydrochloride (EDC) (Merck, Dorset, U.K.) (E7750), N-Hydroxysuccinimide (NHS) (Merck, Dorset, U.K.) (130672), Fitc-CM-Dextran (Merck, Dorset, U.K.) (74817), DAS (GL Biochem Ltd., Shanghai, China), Dialysis tubing, benzoylated (Merck, Dorset, U.K.) (D7884).

#### 2.2.2. Methods: Preparation of DAS-Labelled Fitc-Dextran

A 25 mM MES buffer was prepared, and the pH was adjusted to pH 5–6. 30 mg/mL EDC, and 60 mg/mL NHS was added to the 5 mL 25 mM MES buffer and vortexed. Then, 10 mg/mL Fitc-CM-dextran was resuspended in 25 mM MES buffer and vortexed to aid dispersal. Then, 1 mL of EDC/NHS in 25 mM MES buffer was added to 1 mL of the 10 mg/mL Fitc-CM-dextran in 25 mM MES buffer, covered in foil and shaken at room temperature (RT) for 1 h to activate free carboxyl groups, and then 1.4 mg of DAS was added to 500 μL of $ddH_2O$ and vortexed to aid dissolution. The DAS solution was then added to the activated Fitc-dextran solution and incubated for 8 h at RT whilst shaking, to allow conjugation of DAS. This solution was dialysed overnight at RT, whilst shaking. This was then freeze-dried (Labconco, Freezone 4.5 Plus) for 48 h and stored at −20 °C until needed.

#### 2.2.3. Measurement of Barrier Permeability

On day 6 of BBB model, 1 mg/mL of Fitc-CM-dextran and 1 mg/mL of DAS-Fitc-dextran were resuspended in SFM, and 200 μL of each compound in SFM was added to the apical side of BBB model and incubated at 37 °C 5% $CO_2$ at 100 rpm. Then, 150 μL of samples was removed from the basolateral side of each in vitro model every 30 min for 7 h and at the 24 h timepoints, and the fluorescence of each sample was analysed utilising BMG LABTECH FLUOstar Omega platereader (exc. 485 nm, em. 520 nm). Amount removed from basolateral side of in vitro model was replaced with SFM to maintain sink conditions, maintaining the basolateral volume at 600 μL. Percentage of compound to permeate the BBB was calculated using Equation (1).

$$\%EE = \frac{\text{Mass of drug added} - \text{Mass of drug in supernatant}}{\text{Mass of drug added}} \times 100 \quad (1)$$

*2.3. Immunocytochemistry*

2.3.1. Materials

Anti-GFAP Alex fluor®488 (Invitrogen, Cambridge, U.K.) (53-9892-82), rabbit anti-α SMA (Abcam, Cambridge, U.K.) (ab5694), goat anti-rabbit TRITC (Abcam, Cambridge, U.K.) (ab6718), Poly-L-Lysine (Merck, Dorset, U.K.) (P4832), DPBS (Merck, Dorset, U.K.) (D8537), Methanol (Merck, Dorset, U.K.) (34860), Bovine serum albumin (BSA) (Merck, Dorset, U.K.) (A2153), DAPI readymade solution (Merck, Dorset, U.K.) (MBD0015), Slow fade™ Diamond antifade mounting medium (Invitrogen, Cambridge, U.K.) (S36967).

2.3.2. Methods

Briefly, 13 mm round glass coverslips pre-coated with poly-L-lysine were incubated overnight at 37 °C 5% $CO_2$. They were then washed with DPBS and seeded with 200 μL of $2 \times 10^5$ cells/mL of IA and IP and incubated for 48 h at 37 °C 5% $CO_2$. Media was aspirated and coverslips washed thrice with DPBS. Cells were fixated for 5 min with 100% methanol (−20 °C) and washed thrice with ice-cold DPBS. Coverslips were incubated cell faced down onto 100 μL drops of 1% BSA in DPBS for 1 h at RT. Coverslips were washed thrice with DPBS and incubated face down onto 50 μL drops of 1:5 dilution of rabbit anti-α SMA antibody in 1% BSA for 1.5 h in a humidified chamber. Coverslips were washed thrice with DPBS and incubated face down onto 1:10 dilution of anti-GFAP Alex fluor®488 antibody and 1:100 dilution of goat anti-rabbit TRITC antibody all in 1% BSA for 1.5 h in a dark humidified chamber, total volume of each drop being 50 μL. Coverslips were washed thrice with DPBS and incubated face down onto 50 μL drops of 300 nM DAPI in $ddH_2O$ solution for 2 min, in a dark chamber. Coverslips were washed thrice with DPBS and mounted onto slides using Slow fade™ Diamond antifade mounting medium, sealed and stored in dark at 4 °C until analysis. Analyses of the samples were completed by using Nikon Eclipse E400 microscope.

*2.4. Protein Expression*

2.4.1. Materials

Trizma® hydrochloride (Tris) (Merck, Dorset, U.K.) (10812846001), Sodium chloride (NaCl) (Merck, Dorset, U.K.) (71383), DPBS (Merck, Dorset, U.K.) (D8537), Sodium deoxycholate (Merck, Dorset, U.K.) (D6750), Triton 100 (Merck, Dorset, U.K.) (×100), Protease inhibitor cocktail (Merck, Dorset, U.K.) (P8340).

2.4.2. Methods

Protein lysis buffer was prepared using 10 mM tris, 150 mM NaCl, 0.5% sodium deoxycholate and 0.5% triton 100 to 20 mL $ddH_2O$ and stored at 4 °C. Media were aspirated from the cells and then rinsed with DPBS. Then, 500 μL of DPBS was added to cells, and surface was scraped using a cell scraper and sample was pipetted into a microcentrifuge tube. The sample was centrifuged for 3 min at 800 rpm using Hettich Zentrifugen MIKRO 120. Supernatant was aspirated and the pellet was resuspended in 250 μL of protein lysis buffer. The sample was placed on ice for 20 min and then centrifuged for 5 min at 3000 rpm. Supernatant was removed and pipetted into a fresh microcentrifuge tube and 25 μL protease inhibitor cocktail was added, and supernatant was stored at −20 °C until analysis.

#### 2.4.3. SDS-PAGE and Western Blotting

Materials

Trizma® base (Merck, Dorset, U.K.) (93350), Glycerol (Merck, Dorset, U.K.) (G5516), Sodium dodecyl-sulfate (SDS) (Merck, Dorset, U.K.) (11667289001), β-mercaptoethanol (Merck, Dorset, U.K.) (444203), Bromophenol blue (Merck, Dorset, U.K.) (114391), NUPAGE MOPS SDS running buffer (20×) (Thermofisher, Cambridge, U.K.) (NP0001), NUPAGE transfer buffer (20×) (Thermofisher, Cambridge, U.K.) (NP00061), NUPAGE nitrocellulose membrane filter paper sandwich (Thermofisher, Cambridge, U.K.) (LC2001), NUPAGE 10% Bis-Tris gel (1.0 MM 10 w) (Thermofisher, Cambridge, U.K.) (NP0301BOX), See Blue® Plus 2 Prestained standard (Invitrogen, Cambridge, U.K.) (LC5925), Bovine serum albumin (BSA) ( Merck, Dorset, U.K.) (A2153), ZO1 antibody (Abcam, Cambridge, U.K.) (ab276131), Actin antibody (Santa Cruz, Heidelberg, Germany) (40549), Anti-rabbit IgG (whole molecules)-Alkaline phosphatase antibody produced in goat (Merck, Dorset, U.K.) (A3687), BCIP/NBT solution (Merck, Dorset, U.K.) (B6404).

Methods

Reducing sample treatment buffer (×5) (RSTB) was prepared by combining 1.25 mL of stacking gel buffer (499 mM Trizma® base pH 6.8), 385 mM SDS, 4 mL glycerol, 2.5 mL β-mercaptoethanol, 1.25 mL $ddH_2O$ and a few grains of bromophenol blue and stored at −20 °C. Then, 20 μL of cell lysate samples was pipetted into a microcentrifuge tube and a 1:5 dilution of RSTB was added to each sample. The samples were then heated to 100 °C for 10 min and then electrophoresed on a NUPAGE 10% Bis-Tris gel (1.0 MM 10 w) using ×1 NUPAGE MOPS SDS running buffer. The proteins were transferred onto NUPAGE nitrocellulose membrane using ×1 NUPAGE transfer buffer.

The nitrocellulose membrane was blocked using 5% BSA in TBS for 2 h at RT. The nitrocellulose membrane was washed twice for 5 min in TBS, then 1:1000 dilution of anti-ZO1 antibody in 5% BSA in TBS and a 1:1000 dilution of anti-actin antibody in 5% BSA in TBS was added to the nitrocellulose membrane and incubated overnight, shaking at 4 °C. The nitrocellulose membrane was washed for 5 min twice in TBS and the incubated at RT for 2 h in 1:20,000 dilution of anti-rabbit IgG (whole molecules)-alkaline phosphatase antibody in 5% BSA in TBS solution and shaken. The wash step was repeated and BCIP/NBT substrate solution was added to the nitrocellulose membrane until purple bands appeared. Blot was scanned and analysed using Image J programme.

### 2.5. *Nanoparticles (NP)*

#### 2.5.1. Nanoparticle Formulation

Materials

Resomer® Rg 502H Poly(D,L-lactide-co-glycolide) (PLGA) (Merck, Dorset, U.K.) (719897), Poly(vinyl alcohol) (PVA) (Merck, Dorset, U.K.) (363081), Dichloromethane (DCM) (Merck, Dorset, U.K.) (66742) and Fluorescein isothiocyanate-dextran (Fitc-Dextran) (Merck, Dorset, U.K.) (46945).

Methods

Briefly, 4 mg of Fitc-Dextran was added to 500 μL $ddH_2O$ and added dropwise to PLGA solution (100 mg of PLGA dissolved in 4 mL DCM). The Fitc-dextran/PLGA solution was then sonicated for 60 s at 80% amplitude using Fisher scientific ultrasonic homogeniser CL-18 to form a w/o emulsion. The w/o emulsion was added dropwise to a 1.25% PVA solution (15 mL) and sonicated for 2 min at 80% amplitude to form a w/o/w emulsion. The w/o/w emulsion was placed onto a magnetic stirrer overnight in the dark at RT to allow DCM evaporation. The emulsion was centrifuged at 18,809× *g* at 4 °C for 30 min using Sigma® centrifuge 3–30 K. The supernatant was aspirated and stored at −20 °C for encapsulation efficiency analysis. The pellet was washed thrice with $ddH_2O$ and resuspended in 5 mL $ddH_2O$, and placed in −80 °C for 2 h. Once frozen, the NP were placed into Labconco Freezone 4.5 Plus freezedryer, for 48 h. NP were stored at −20 °C until sample sizing and PDI analysis.

2.5.2. Sizing and PDI

Materials

0.4 μM Minisart® syringe filter (Sartorius, Surrey, U.K.) (16555), Malvern disposable folded capillary cells DT51070 (Malvern, Worcestershire, U.K.).

Methods

Briefly, 1 mg of DAS-FD-NP or FD-NP were resuspended in 1 mL dd$H_2O$ to make a 1 mg/mL solution. The 1 mg/mL solution was vortexed and pipetted into folded capillary cells and analysed on the Malvern zetasizer Nano series at 10 °C with 5 series (15 runs each series) to obtain size and PDI of the NP.

2.5.3. Encapsulation Efficiency

Materials

Fluorescein isothiocyanate-dextran (Fitc-dextran) (Merck, Dorset, U.K.) (46945).

Methods

A calibration curve was produced using Fitc-dextran in dd$H_2O$ (exc. 485 nm, em. 520 nm, gain 750). The linear equation gained from the calibration curve was used to analyse the concentration of Fitc-Dextran within retained supernatant (Section 2.5.1. The encapsulation efficiency (EE) of Fitc-Dextran within the FD-NP was then determined by Equation (2).

$$\%EE = \frac{\text{Mass of drug added} - \text{Mass of drug in supernatant}}{\text{Mass of drug added}} \times 100 \quad (2)$$

2.5.4. Release Assay

Materials

3,3-dimethylglutaric acid (Merck, Dorset, U.K.) (D4379), Sodium hydroxide (NaOH) (Merck, Dorset, U.K.) (221465), Sodium chloride (NaCl) (Merck, Dorset, U.K.) (71383), DPBS (Merck, Dorset, U.K.) (D8537).

Methods

Briefly, 0.01 M DMGA buffer was prepared using 6 mM 3,3-dimethylglutaric acid, 3.9 mM NaOH, 150 mM $NaCl_2$ in 100 mL dd$H_2O$, pH 4.5. 1.5 mg of FD- NP was resuspended in either 1 mL DMGA buffer or 1 mL DPBS and incubated at 37 °C. At each hourly time point (for 7 h then 24 h), the samples were centrifuged at 5000 rpm for 5 min using Hettich Zentrifugen MIKRO 120. Then, 150 μL of each sample's supernatant was removed and replaced with 150 μL of fresh buffer and pellet redispersed in solution and incubated at 37 °C. The fluorescence of each sample was analysed (exc. 485 nm, em. 520 nm, 700 gain). The concentration of Fitc-Dextran released from NP was calculated using linear equation obtained from calibration curves and cumulative release results.

2.5.5. Conjugation Efficiency

Materials

DAS (GL Biochem Ltd., Shanghai, China), Phosphate buffered saline (PBS) (Dulbecco A) (Thermofisher, Cambridge, U.K.) (BR0014G), nd Pierce™ BCA protein assay kit (Thermofisher, Cambridge, U.K.) (23227).

Methods

DAS was conjugated to the surface of the FD-NP following the protocol published by Huey et al. (2019) [37].

2.5.6. Delivery across BBB Model

Materials

Mecamylamine (Merck, Dorset, U.K.) (M9020), hexamethonium chloride (Merck, Dorset, U.K.) (H2138), anti-Nicotinic acetylcholine receptor antibody alpha 7/CHRNA7 antibody (α-7 nAChR antibody) (Santa Cruz, Heidelberg, Germany) (sc-58607).

Methods

The in vitro BBB model was prepared as shown in Section 2.1.2. On day 6 of the in vitro BBB model, 100 μL of either 2 mM mecamylamine in SFM, 2 mM hexamethonium in SFM, or 1:100 dilution of α-7 nAChR antibody in SFM was added to the apical side of transwell inserts and incubated for 1 h at 37 °C 5% $CO_2$. Then, 0.4 mg/mL of Fitc-CM-dextran and 0.4 mg/mL of DAS-FD-NP were resuspended individually in SFM and 200 μL was added to the apical side of transwell insert containing antibodies or antagonist (which diluted NP concentration to 0.2 mg/mL). The models were incubated at 37 °C 5% $CO_2$ at 100 rpm until each hourly time point. Then, 150 μL samples were removed from the basolateral side of each in vitro model for 7 h and at the 24 h timepoints and the fluorescence of each sample was analysed (exc. 485 nm, em. 520 nm). The media removed from basolateral layer of the model were replaced with SFM to maintain sink conditions, maintaining the basolateral volume at 600 μL. Percentage of drug to permeate BBB was calculated using Equation (1) (Section 2.2.3).

## 3. Results

### 3.1. Determining Transwell Model Architecture

Figure 2 demonstrates the effect of substratum and shear stress on the integrity of a monolayer of I-HBMECs (cell concentration of 6.25 × $10^4$ cells/mL) using TEER measurement. The I-HBMEC concentration was determined from previous proliferation studies.

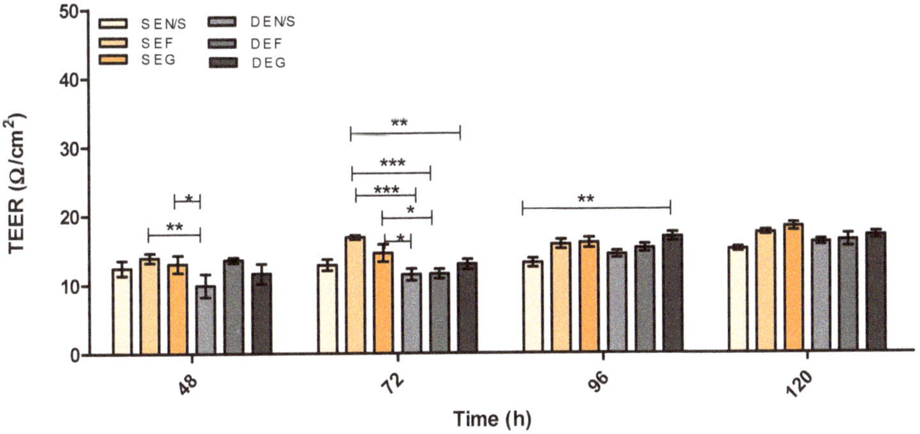


**Figure 2.** TEER ($\Omega/cm^2$) of static (S) versus dynamic (D) HMEC monolayer in vitro models utilising different substratum over 120 h. E = Endothelial cells, N/S = No substratum, F = Fibronectin and G = Gelatin. $n = 9 \pm$ SD, * = $p < 0.05$, ** = $p < 0.01$, *** = $p < 0.001$; statistical analysis was performed using two-way ANOVA Bonferroni post hoc tests.

Figures 3 and 4 demonstrate the integrity of the BBB model using the two optimal substrata from Figure 2, on their own or in combination, in both static and dynamic modes, using TEER measurement.

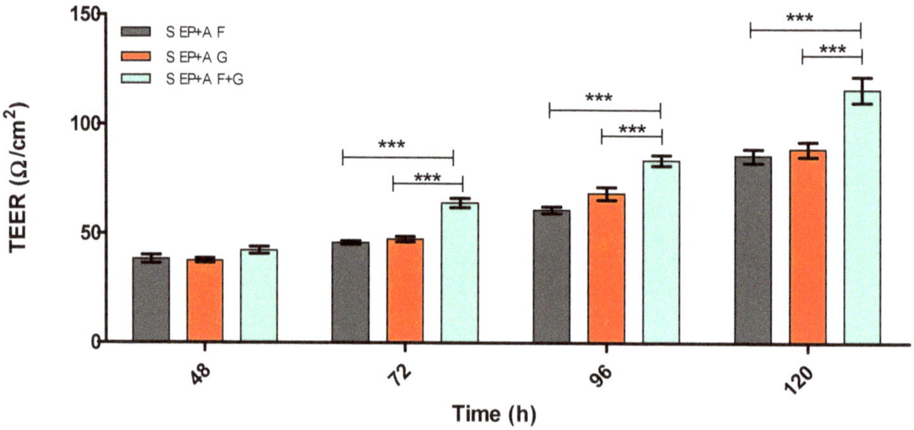


**Figure 3.** TEER ($\Omega/cm^2$) of static (S) EP + A in vitro BBB model over 120 h on different substrata. Endothelial cells (E), Pericytes (P) and Astrocytes (A), Fibronectin (F), Gelatin (G) Fibronectin + Collagen (F + C), Fibronectin + Gelatin (F + G), $n = 9 \pm$ SD, *** = $p < 0.001$; statistical analysis was performed using two-way ANOVA Bonferroni post hoc tests.

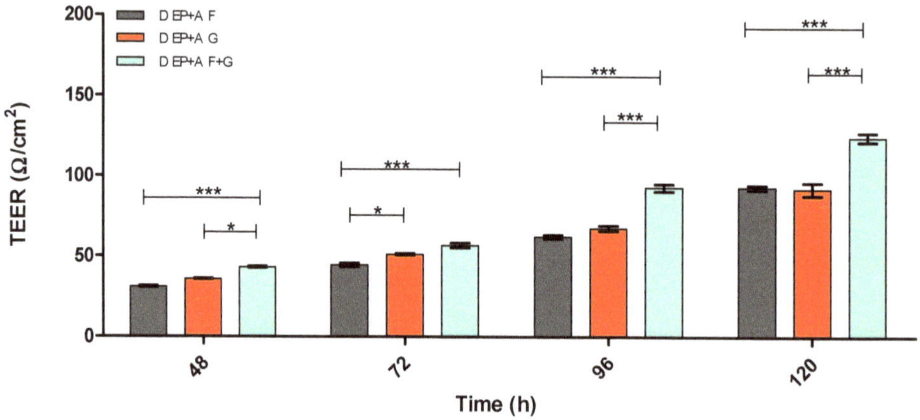


**Figure 4.** TEER ($\Omega/cm^2$) of dynamic (D) EP + A in vitro BBB model over 120 h on different substrata. Endothelial cells (E), Pericytes (P) and Astrocytes (A), Fibronectin (F), Gelatin (G) Fibronectin + Collagen (F + C), Fibronectin + Gelatin (F + G), $n = 9 \pm$ SD, * = $p < 0.05$, *** = $p < 0.001$; statistical analysis was performed using two-way ANOVA Bonferroni post hoc tests.

Figure 5 demonstrates how increasing cell concentration of IA and IP from $2 \times 10^4$ cells/mL to $4 \times 10^4$ cells/mL influences BBB integrity (TEER). It also demonstrates how adjusting substrata placement can influence BBB integrity of the monoculture model.

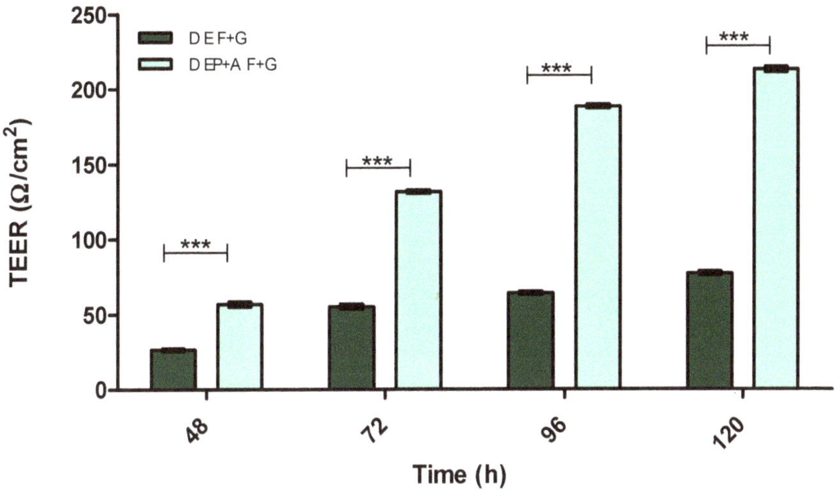


**Figure 5.** TEER ($\Omega/cm^2$) of dynamic (D) mono- and tri-culture in vitro BBB models over 120 h on Fibronectin + Gelatin (F + G) substratum combination, Endothelial cells (E), Pericytes (P) and Astrocytes (A), $n = 9 \pm$ SD, *** = $p < 0.001$; statistical analysis was performed using two-way ANOVA Bonferroni post hoc tests.

Figure 6 demonstrates the effect $Mg^{2+}$ has on BBB integrity of a mono- and triculture model using TEER measurement.

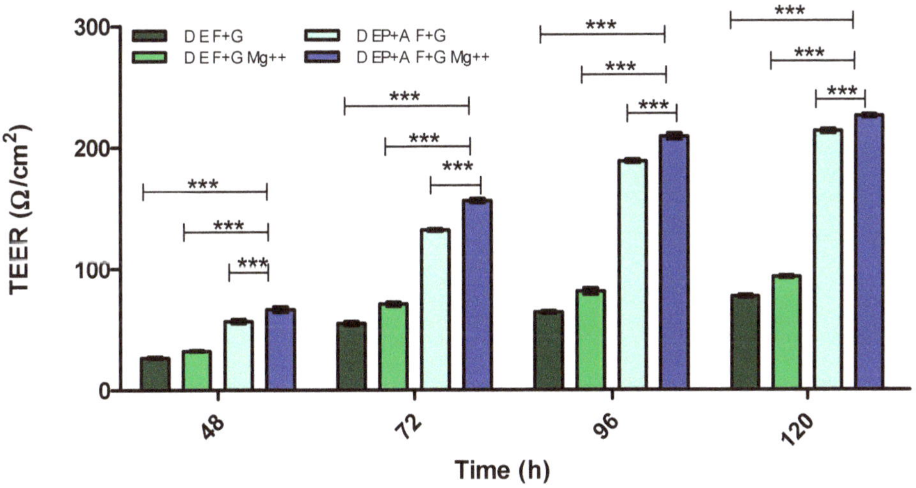


**Figure 6.** TEER ($\Omega/cm^2$) of two different dynamic (D) in vitro BBB models over 120 h with and without magnesium ($Mg^{2+}$). Fibronectin + Gelatin (F + G), Endothelial cells (E), Pericytes (P) and Astrocytes (A). $n = 9 \pm$ SD, *** = $p < 0.001$; statistical analysis was performed using two-way ANOVA Bonferroni post hoc tests.

Figure 7 demonstrates the distinct differences between a monolayer with no substratum, and a monolayer with combined substratum F + G and $Mg^{2+}$ to that of the optimal in vitro BBB model (D EP + A F + G $Mg^{2+}$) using TEER measurement.

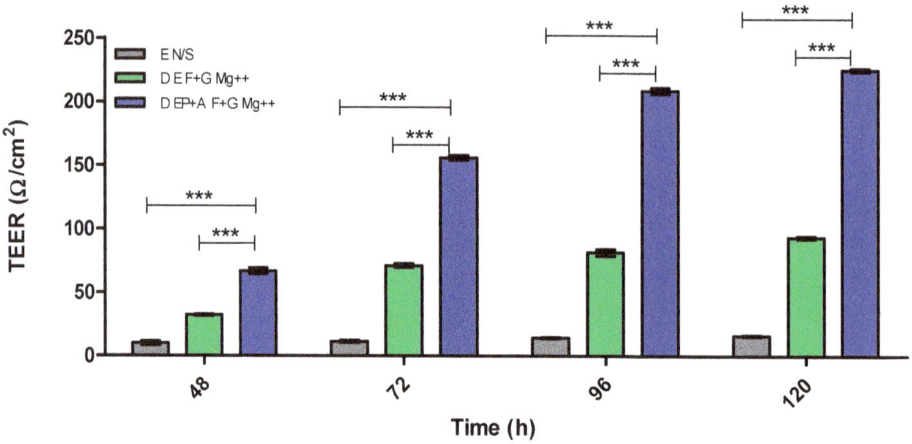


**Figure 7.** TEER ($\Omega/cm^2$) of dynamic (D) models: endothelial monolayer N/S, endothelial monolayer F + G $Mg^{2+}$ and EP + A F + G $Mg^{2+}$. N/S = no substratum, E = endothelial cells, P = pericyte, A = astrocyte, F + G = fibronectin + gelatin and Mg = magnesium. $n = 9 \pm$ SD, *** = $p < 0.001$; statistical analysis was performed using two-way ANOVA Bonferroni post hoc tests.

### *3.2. Evaluation of Barrier Integrity*

Figure 8 demonstrates the integrity of the optimal in vitro BBB model (D EP + A F + G $Mg^{2+}$) over 24 h. This was determined by measuring the percentage (%) of Fitc-CM-dextran versus DAS-Fitc-dextran, to traverse the in vitro BBB by fluorimetry (exc. 485 nm, em. 520 nm).

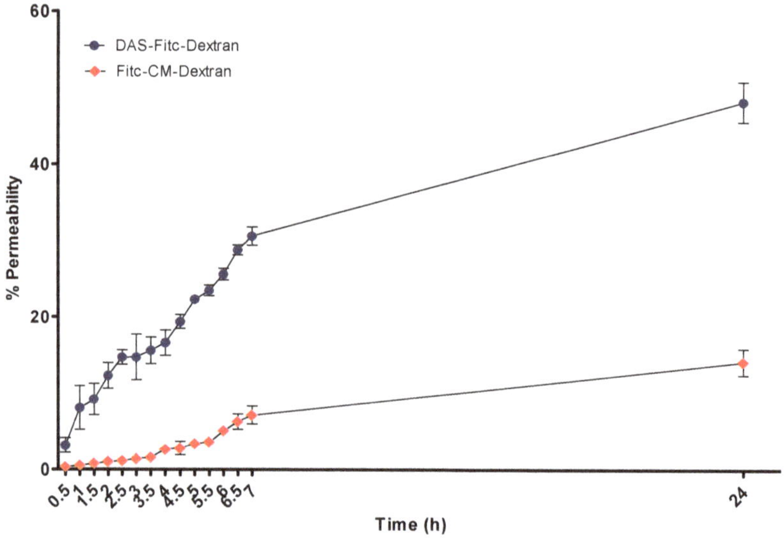


**Figure 8.** The percentage permeability of DAS-Fitc-dextran and Fitc-dextran on our in vitro BBB model, over 24 h (exc. 485 nm, em. 520 nm), $n = 9 \pm$ SD.

Figure 9 demonstrates the significant difference in permeability of Fitc-CM-dextran and DAS-Fitc-dextran, in the in vitro BBB at specific time points of (1 h, 2.5 h and 24 h). Statistical analysis was performed by two-way ANOVA.

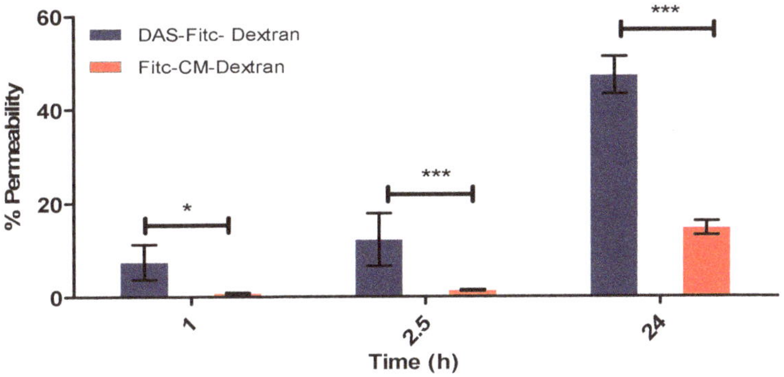


**Figure 9.** Graph demonstrating, permeability at specific time points between DAS-Fitc-dextran and Fitc-dextran using optimal in vitro BBB model. $n = 9$, 2-way ANOVA, * significant difference of $p < 0.05$, *** significant difference of $p < 0.001$ between permeability of fluorescent compounds at same time point.

### 3.3. Immunocytochemistry

Figure 10 shows IA (Figure 10A) and IP (Figure 10B) growing together, demonstrating the ability of the cells to co-localise (a necessity for our EP + A BBB model). Anti-α SMA primary antibody was used to detect IP (which are known to produce α SMA proteins) and a secondary goat anti-rabbit TRITC (exc. 547 nm, em. 572 nm) antibody conjugate, which produces a red signal that could be detected under a fluorescence microscope. An anti-GFAP antibody Alex fluor®488 (exc. 499 nm, em. 520 nm) conjugate was used to detect glial fibrillary acidic protein (GFAP) which is expressed exclusively by astrocytes to produce a green signal under a fluorescence microscope.

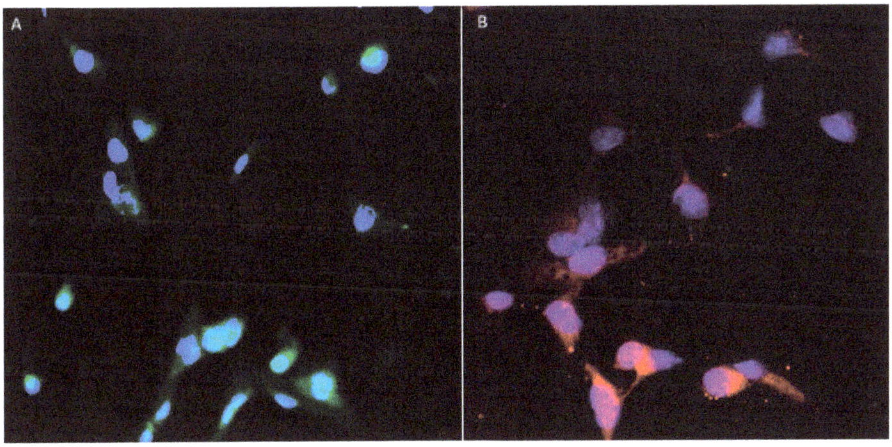


**Figure 10.** Immunocytochemistry imaging of (**A**) immunofluorescence of GFAP proteins expressed on IA (green signal) and (**B**) immunofluorescence of α SMA proteins expressed on IP (red signal). Both cells' nuclei were counter-stained with DAPI (blue signal).

### 3.4. Protein Expression

SDS-PAGE and Western Blotting

Figure 11 demonstrates BBB model integrity by detection of the TJ protein ZO1 in the different BBB models shown in Figures 1–6 (Section 3.1). Figure 12 shows the relative protein expression of ZO1 compared to endothelial cells grown on no substratum.

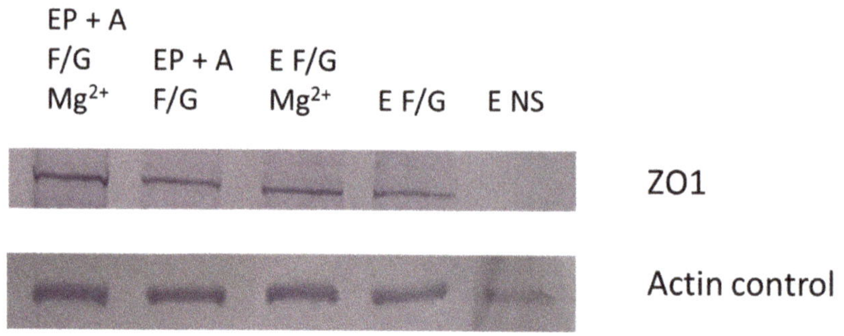


**Figure 11.** Image of Western blot membrane, detecting ZO1 TJ-protein (mw 195 kDA) in lysed cells from different in vitro BBB models. Endothelial cells (E), Pericytes (P), Astrocytes (A), Fibronectin + Gelatin (F + G), Fibronectin + Collagen (F + C), No substrata (NS) and Magnesium ($Mg^{2+}$), Dynamic mode.

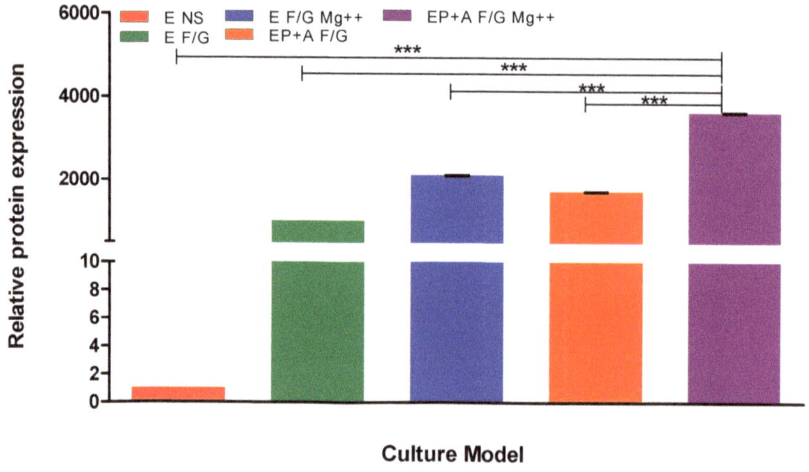


**Figure 12.** Quantitative analysis of relative protein expression of ZO1 in each BBB model. Endothelial cells (E), Pericytes (P), Astrocytes (A), Fibronectin + Gelatin (F + G), Fibronectin + Collagen (F + C), No substrata (NS) and Magnesium ($Mg^{2+}$). $n = 3$, *** = $p < 0.001$; statistical analysis was performed using one-way ANOVA Bonferroni post hoc tests.

### *3.5. Sizing and PDI*

Table 1 provides information on PDI and size of PLGA NP in comparison to Fitc-dextran PLGA NP.

**Table 1.** Sizing and PDI results gained from blank and Fitc-dextran encapsulated NP. $n = 3 \pm$ SD.

| PLGA NP | Size (nm) ± SD | PDI ± SD |
|---|---|---|
| Blank PLGA NP | 268.5 ± 36.63 | 0.22 ± 0.052 |
| Fitc-dextran-PLGA NP | 347.7 ± 62.48 | 0.35 ± 0.153 |
| DAS-Fitc-dextran-PLGA-NP | 386.50 ± 11.30 | 0.27 ± 0.08 |

### 3.6. Encapsulation Efficiency

Table 2 provides information on the encapsulation efficiency (EE) of Fitc-dextran encapsulated within the PLGA NP.

**Table 2.** Encapsulation efficiency (EE) of Fitc-dextran in PLGA NP and conjugation efficiency (CE) of DAS to Fitc-dextran-PLGA NP.

| Fitc-Dextran PLGA NP | EE% | CE% |
|---|---|---|
| Sample 1 | 64.49 | 62.50 |
| Sample 2 | 61.87 | 64.06 |
| Sample 3 | 64.94 | 56.80 |

### 3.7. Release

A release study was performed to determine cumulative release (%) of Fitc-dextran from the PLGA NP, as shown in Figure 13 where 1.5 mg of Fitc-dextran NP was dispersed in buffers of different pHs (DMGA pH 4.5, DPBS pH 7.1) to determine the influence of pH on the release of Fitc-dextran from PLGA NP over 24 h.

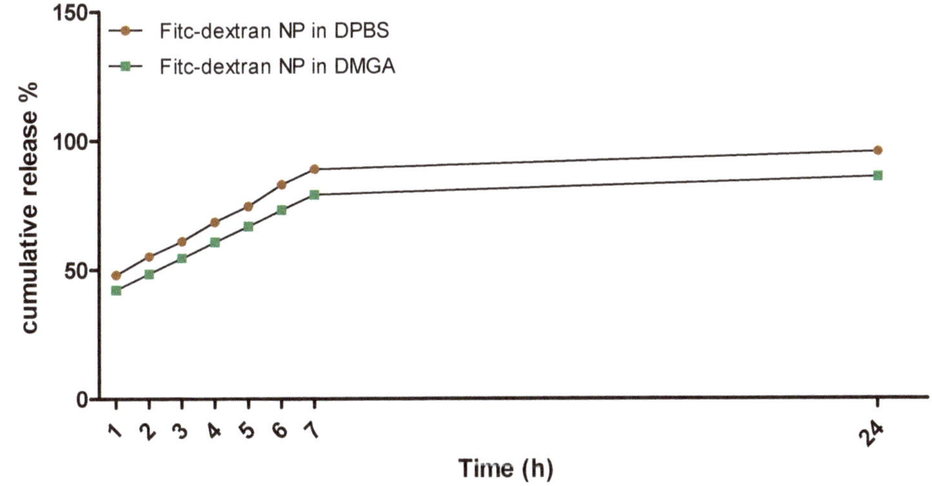


**Figure 13.** Cumulative release (%) of Fitc-dextran PLGA NP in DPBS and DMGA buffers over 24 h. $n = 3 \pm$ SD (exc. 485 nm, em. 520 nm). Statistical analysis was performed using two-way ANOVA Bonferroni post hoc tests, $p < 0.001$ comparing both buffers at each time point (error bars too small to be visualised on graph).

### 3.8. Delivery across BBB Model

Figure 14 demonstrates the ability of DAS-Fitc-dextran PLGA NP as a vehicle to successfully transport and release a large hydrophilic compound (Fitc-dextran) (70,000 Da) across the optimal BBB model compared to Fitc-dextran PLGA NP. The NP were dispersed in SFM and added to the apical layer of the BBB model. At the 24 h timepoint, samples were removed from the basolateral layer of the BBB model inserts and analysed by fluorimetry (exc. 485 nm, em. 520 nm). Fitc-dextran PLGA NP and DAS-Fitc-dextran PLGA NP were tested on the optimal BBB model (D EP + A F + G $Mg^{2+}$). Figure 14 also demonstrates that transport of the DAS-labelled NP across the BBB model can be blocked by the addition of α-7 nicotinic acetylcholine receptor antibody, mecamylamine and hexamethonium.

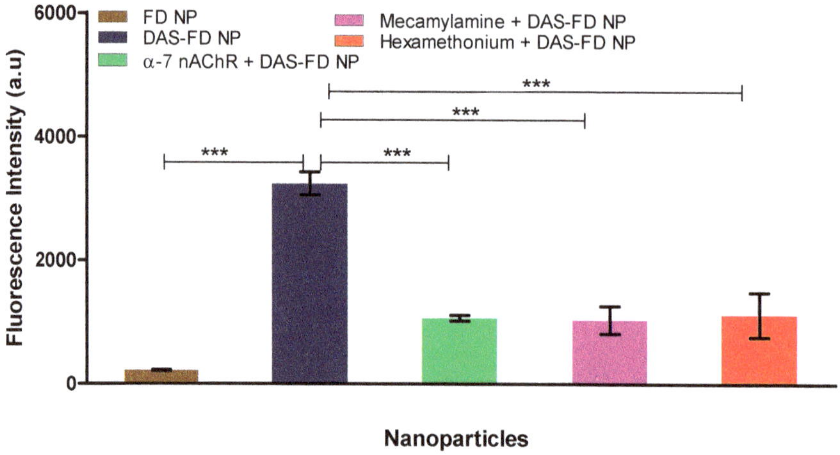


**Figure 14.** Fluorescence (a.u) intensity of the basolateral medium of the optimal BBB after delivery of Fitc-dextran NP and DAS-Fitc-dextran NP, after 24 h (exc. 485 nm, em. 520 nm), also in the presence of α-7 nicotinic acetylcholine receptor antibody, mecamylamine and hexamethonium. FITC NP = Fitc-dextran PLGA NP, DAS FITC NP = DAS conjugated to Fitc-dextran PLGA NP. $n = 3 \pm$ SD, *** = $p < 0.001$; statistical analysis was performed using one-way ANOVA Bonferroni post hoc tests.

## 4. Discussion

### 4.1. In Vitro BBB Construction

When developing novel therapeutics, delivery and efficacy of the drugs must be determined before going forward. For assessment of the efficacy of drug-encapsulated NP, such as a DDS, we developed a cost-effective, easily manipulated, human in vitro BBB model that closely mimics the in vivo BBB architecture. In vitro models are an indispensable aid for drug permeability and toxicity studies, ensuring only lead compounds are brought forward to preclinical studies, reducing the cost and time frame of in vivo studies [27]. When developing an in vitro BBB model, cell selection and placement, choice of substratum and inclusion of shear stress must be considered to ensure the model achieves suitable integrity, which is determined by TEER values in excess of 150 $\Omega/cm^2$ and TJ protein expression [38]. Transepithelial electrical resistance (TEER) of a cell monolayer is a widely accepted quantitative measure of in vitro barrier integrity. TEER measurement can be performed on real-time assays with no detrimental effects on cell viability. A high TEER value suggests that paracellular transport of molecules is severely limited, thereby reducing the non-specific permeability of the in vitro model [39]. Models producing TEER values below 150 $\Omega/cm^2$ are deemed to have deceased integrity and will be prone to paracellular transport [39–43]. The addition of fluid shear stress to in vitro models allows the model to mimic the in vivo BBB more accurately by promoting cell elongation, which encourages TJ protein expression, enhancing the in vitro BBB function [44–46]. In vivo, shear stress has been shown to vary between 5 and 23 dny/cm$^2$. In vitro models that apply shear stress above 5 dny/cm$^2$ may cause cell detachment, and the most effective shear stress applied to in vitro models has shown to be 1.5 dny/cm$^2$. Therefore, we utilised 1.5 dny/cm$^2$ shear stress for our in vitro model [44,47,48].

Immortalised cells were used for this model due to a reduced risk of contamination with other cell types (a problem when using primary and stem cells) and their cost-effectiveness. However, they have been deemed 'leaky' due to the low TEER values and low TJ protein expression obtained from monolayer in vitro BBB models [42,49]. Therefore, Figures 2–12 describe the process of developing and optimising the ideal in vitro model to test our drug-encapsulated NP, by mimicking the in vivo BBB more accurately to increase

TEER and TJ expression. Figure 2 shows how the addition of substratum compared to no substratum (N/S) influences TEER values. Substrata are used to mimic the basement membrane (BM) of the BBB. Substrata are forms of extracellular matrix (ECM) proteins which are found within the BM in vivo and are natural ligands for the BECs. They promote cell anchoring, give structural support, and promote signal transduction and are an important factor to consider when constructing an in vitro BBB model [50–52]. The optimal substrata chosen were a combination of fibronectin (F), an ECM protein found in vivo *and* gelatin (G), the denatured form of collagen, which has an exposed backbone allowing increased cell adhesion and increased BBB stability [50–53]. The addition of these substrata to the apical surface of the transwell inserts increased cell adhesion and therefore TEER. A study carried out by Maherally et al. (2018) explains the importance of ECM proteins and how certain ECM proteins stabilise TJ proteins and increase TJ expression, and this is in agreement with our results in Figure 2 [54]. The addition of shear stress on an endothelial cell monolayer did not increase TEER levels. Therefore, to mimic the in vivo BBB more accurately, we produced a tri-culture model utilising the substrata discussed previously (Figures 3 and 4). The cells used and cell placement in tri-cultures replicate the NVU configuration and proximity to BECs which occur in vivo. Astrocytes and pericytes interact with the BECs and promote TJ protein expression and cellular transportation [32,35,55–57]. To increase the promotion of TJ proteins and, in turn, increase TEER, the cells were placed in close proximity to one another, along with the substrata and applied shear stress. In Figures 3 and 4, substrata were pre-coated on the apical surface of the transwell insert, with IA and IP cell concentrations of $2 \times 10^4$ cells/mL seeded to the basolateral surface of the transwell inserts.

From the results shown in Figures 3 and 4, the dynamic (D) triculture model EP + A grown on fibronectin and gelatin substrata produced a higher TEER value but did not reach the gold standard of $\geq$150 $\Omega/cm^2$. The results show that the TEER is higher due to the application of shear stress, which is in agreement with Ferrell et al. (2019) and Elbakary et al. (2020). Their research has shown that shear stress on different cell types has increased protein expression, cell elongation and cell orientation, increasing TEER and barrier integrity [45,46]. Therefore, we kept the application of shear stress but altered the cell concentration of both the IA and IP (increased to $4 \times 10^4$ cells/mL) and pre-coated both apical surface and the basolateral surfaces of the inserts to mimic the basement membrane more accurately (Figure 5). Figure 5 compares the TEER of an endothelial cell (E) monolayer BBB to that of the dynamic EP + A F + G model which produces a TEER value almost three times higher (approx. 200 $\Omega/cm^2$) than that of the monolayer model (approx. 70 $\Omega/cm^2$). Zhu et al. (2018) and Leon et al. (2021) have suggested that elevated magnesium levels in the culture medium can enhance BBB activity by significantly reducing the permeability of the barrier by regulating its function in vitro [58,59]. Figure 6 shows that the addition of 10 mM $MgSO_4$ to the culture medium increases the TEER value of both the D EP + A F + G BBB model and on the endothelial cell monolayer. Because the addition of $Mg^{2+}$ to the medium increased the TEER of the D EP + A F + G BBB model (230 $\Omega/cm^2$); it was decided that to produce the optimal in vitro BBB model, the addition of $Mg^{2+}$ was required.

Figure 7 illustrates the difference in TEER of each model, to show how the adjustments made to mimic the architecture and physiology of in vivo BBB structure produce an optimal model (D EP + A F + G $Mg^{2+}$) to be utilised for the assessment of non-invasive drug delivery systems.

To test the permeability of the optimal BBB model, a large molecular weight compound was utilised, which would not permeate the BBB model via intercellular or paracellular routes, due to its hydrophilic nature. The compound used was Fitc-CM-dextran, which has a molecular weight of 70,000 Daltons. To test DAS's ability to transport a large hydrophilic compound across the BBB, DAS was conjugated to Fitc-CM-dextran and tested alongside Fitc-CM-dextran on our optimal model with results shown in Figures 8 and 9. DAS is an 18 amino acid ligand, which has an affinity for alpha 7 nicotinic acetylcholine receptors ($\alpha$-7 nAChR) [37] found on endothelial cells of the BBB. It allows NP conjugated to the peptide to be transported transcellularly by RMT and is, therefore, an ideal mode to transport large hydrophilic molecules (such as antibodies) into the brain [7,22–24]. Figure 8 demonstrates that our optimal model has high integrity and low paracellular permeability as only 10% Fitc-CM-dextran permeated the BBB after 24 h, which shows that paracellular transportation is severally restricted. The Fitc-CM-dextran conjugated with DAS showed a higher percentage of compound to traverse the BBB (approximately 50%) after 24 h, indicating that the DAS is facilitating the transportation of Fitc-CM-dextran. Huey et al. (2019) developed the DAS ligand, and their study indicated that DAS, which was designed around a 5-mer sequence from RDP, had an affinity for the α-7 nAChR, and showed good stability in human serum and enhanced transport across the BBB via RMT in in vitro models compared to previous ligands [37]. This also agrees with results shown in Figure 9, which shows the statistically significant difference in transport efficacy which started to occur after one hour, with a significant difference of $p < 0.05$, and after 2.5 h, the significant difference increases to $p < 0.001$. Overall, these results from TEER measurement (Figure 7) and permeability assays, demonstrate that our optimal model has high integrity and low paracellular permeability, and that by conjugating the DAS ligand to a large molecule, it can aid transcellular transportation via RMT.

Immunocytochemistry was carried out to confirm the presence of IA and IP grown together on a glass coverslip, after the visualisation of cells with GFAP and αSMA antibodies, respectively [60–63] (Figure 10). DAPI-stained nuclei are visible in both cell types (Figure 10A,B).

In Figure 10, both IA and IP are visible, clearly demonstrating that cells can be co-grown in the same space; an important factor for the construction of our optimal model (where both IA and IP are grown on the underside of the transwell insert).

The increased TEER in our optimal model is due to the increased expression of TJ protein. Isolated proteins were analysed by SDS PAGE and Western blotting to show the expression of the ZO1 (Figure 11). ZO1 is a cytoplasmic protein, which is crucial for increasing BBB integrity as every TJ protein must interact with it to reduce the permeability of the BBB [3,35,64]. The top image demonstrates that ZO1 is expressed by I-HBMECs and that, depending on the model, different concentrations of ZO1 are expressed in the models. Figure 11 clearly demonstrates that the highest ZO1 expression levels are seen in our optimal model. The ZO1 bands for each model were quantified using Image J (Figure 12) to show the relative expression of ZO1 in the different models compared to endothelial cells grown as a monolayer. It can be clearly seen that over 3500 times the amount of ZO1 is produced by our optimal model compared to monolayer endothelial cells. Research carried out by Eigenmann et al. (2013), compared TEER and TJ-protein expression in four immortalised endothelial cell lines. They showed that TJ proteins had been expressed such as ZO1, but in varying degrees depending on the cell line. They also mentioned that the inclusion of pericytes and astrocytes did not increase TJ protein expression in immortalised endothelial cells [49]. However, when comparing their findings to our results in Figures 11 and 12, we clearly demonstrate ZO1 levels increase with the presence of pericytes and astrocytes. This could be due to the presence of shear stress and substrata proteins that are found within the NVU, so our model more accurately resembles the in vivo NVU and, therefore, promotes TJ proteins expression due to cell anchoring and adhesion of pericytes and astrocytes in close proximity to BECs. Therefore, the results obtained in Figures 11 and 12 support the TEER results, and it was concluded that the D EP + A F + G $Mg^{2+}$ model was our optimal in vitro BBB model going forward.

### 4.2. Nanoparticle (NP) Development

NP were developed using poly (D, L-lactide-co-glycolide) (PLGA) and stabilised using 1.25% PVA solution. PLGA has been approved by the US FDA for sustained and controlled drug delivery systems as it is biodegradable, biocompatible and has low toxicity [65,66]. PLGA NP are not only ideal for encapsulating large hydrophilic molecules but the surface of PLGA NP can be chemically modified for the conjugation of ligands. Ligands on the surface of PLGA NP recognise and target the receptors found on the BECs and then traverse the BBB via RMT [67]. When developing PLGA NP for encapsulation of large molecules, the size of the PLGA NP should be in the range of 200–400 nm to have the ability to encapsulate the high mass of payloads. Chigumira et al. (2015) used PLGA NP to encapsulate pralidoxime and obtained size ranges between 300 and 400 nm [65]. Azizi et al. (2013) encapsulated bovine serum albumin (BSA) within PLGA NP of sizes 251.3 ± 8.5 nm [68]. BSA is a large globular protein with a molecular weight of 66 kDa, which is a similar molecular weight to that of Fitc-dextran which we encapsulate within our PLGA NP [69]. Our preferred size is between 200 and 400 nm to ensure high encapsulation of large MW compounds and more effective release. The polydispersity index (PDI) determines the uniformity of the NP in solution, with NP PDI ideally being close to zero as this indicates reduced size distribution and reduces particle aggregation [70,71].

Table 1 demonstrates the size and PDI of both blank PLGA NP and Fitc-dextran-encapsulated PLGA NP. Blank PLGA NP have a size of 268.5 nm (±36.63) with a PDI of 0.22 (±0.052), and the Fitc-dextran PLGA NP have a size of 347.7 nm (±62.48) with a PDI of 0.35 (±0.153), which is similar to PLGA NP sizes obtained by Chigumira et al. (2015). Fitc-dextran PLGA NP have a larger size than blank PLGA NP due to the encapsulation of Fitc-dextran. The PDI is slightly higher for Fitc-dextran PLGA NP, but a PDI below 0.5 is preferred, and we have obtained that for both NP. The size of both NP shown in Table 1 is within the 200–400 nm range with acceptable PDI. Table 2 shows the encapsulation efficiency (EE%) of Fitc-dextran within the PLGA NP was between 60 and 65%. This result is more stable than that of Chigumira et al. (2015), whose encapsulation range varied between 28 and 70% EE [65]. Fornaguera et al. (2015) had an EE% of over 90% of loperamide within PLGA NP. This molecule has a molecular weight of 477 Da and therefore the size of the payload may have affected EE% [72]. Huey et al. (2019) used PLGA NP to encapsulate Fitc-dextran and obtained similar sizes and encapsulation efficiency (286.5 ± 11.3 nm, EE 77%); therefore, from the results gained in this paper, it was determined that the next step was to carry out a release in different pH buffers to see if pH affected the NP release [37].

Figure 13 shows Fitc-dextran release from PLGA NP. At 1 h, Fitc-dextran released between 45 and 50% in both the DPBS buffer and DMGA buffer, with a gradual release up to 24 h. At 24 h, approximately 95% of Fitc-dextran has been released from the PLGA NP in DPBS and approximately 85% of Fitc-dextran has been released from the PLGA NP, proving that almost all the payload has released at 24 h irrespective of the pH of the release medium. This differs from the results of Patel et al. (2018), which show that pH does influence the release from PLGA NP [73]. They found that pH 5.5 buffer (after 48 h) had a higher release than pH 6.8 and pH 7.4 buffers; however, they only achieved a maximum release of 40% from PLGA NP at pH 5.5 [73]. When compared to our results in Figure 13, they also see an initial burst of release within the first couple of hours [73]. The variation between our release results and those of Patel et al. (2018) could be due to different PLGA NP formulation processes and payloads used. Therefore, it can be stated that the release results obtained within this paper demonstrate that PLGA NP are a suitable vehicle for sustained and controlled drug release of large hydrophilic compounds.

The NP-encapsulated Fitc-dextran payload will not be able to traverse the BBB unaided; therefore, the DAS ligand was attached to the NP to aid in the transportation via RMT. DAS was conjugated to the Fitc-dextran PLGA NP using a protocol developed by Huey et al. (2019). DAS was added in excess to the surface of the PLGA NP, which had been chemically modified by activating the free carboxyl groups on the surface of the PLGA NP using EDC/NHS in MES buffer [37]. As shown in Figure 8, DAS successfully aids in the transportation of large hydrophilic compounds across the BBB, which occurs via RMT utilising the α-7 nAChR found on the surface of BECs [37]. DAS Fitc-dextran PLGA NP and Fitc-dextran PLGA NP were tested on our optimal in vitro BBB model.

Figure 14 shows the DAS Fitc-dextran PLGA NP were able to traverse the in vitro BBB model more successfully than the unconjugated Fitc-dextran PLGA NP, as the DAS Fitc-dextran PLGA NP had 14 times higher fluorescence intensity (a.u) (3200 a.u) than that of the unconjugated NP (225 a.u). We have also demonstrated that delivery of the DAS-labelled NP occurs via RMT, as this process can be blocked by the addition of an anti-α-7 nAChR antibody, mecamylamine (a nAChR non-competitive antagonist) and by hexamethonium (a nAChR competitive antagonist). Huey et al. (2019) showed the ability of DAS to bind to the α-7 nAChR and release a payload of Fitc-dextran within a monolayer of SH-SY5Y neuroblastoma cells [37]. Our results substantiate what Huey et al. (2019) visualised, confirming that DAS does have the ability to transport loaded PLGA NP across the BBB by RMT targeting the α-7 nAChR.

## 5. Conclusions

In conclusion, the optimal in vitro BBB model D EP + A F + G $Mg^{2+}$, which utilises immortalised human cells, is an ideal, cheap, reproducible and effective method to test novel drug delivery systems for the CNS, such as ligand-targeted nanoparticulate systems. It has also been established that PLGA NP, which are easily developed, can successfully encapsulate and release large hydrophilic compounds. Finally, DAS-conjugated PLGA NP have been determined to be a suitable vehicle to successfully transport and release a large hydrophilic compound across the BBB by RMT. This targeted drug delivery system is a non-invasive effective method of transporting large hydrophilic payloads, such as therapeutic antibodies, to the CNS for the treatment of neurological disorders.

**Author Contributions:** Conceptualization, S.H.; methodology, S.K. and S.H.; validation, S.K., B.C. and S.H.; formal analysis, S.K. and S.H.; investigation, S.K.; resources, S.H.; data curation, S.K., B.C. and S.H.; writing—original draft preparation, S.K.; writing—review and editing, S.K., B.C. and S.H..; visualization, S.K., B.C. and S.H.; supervision, B.C. and S.H.; project administration, B.C. and S.H.; funding acquisition, S.H. All authors have read and agreed to the published version of the manuscript.

**Funding:** This research was funded by The Dowager Countess Eleanor Peel Trust #325 and S.K. was funded by DEL, NI.

**Institutional Review Board Statement:** Not applicable.

**Informed Consent Statement:** Not applicable.

**Data Availability Statement:** The data presented in this study are available on request from the corresponding author. The data are not publicly available due to privacy restrictions.

**Acknowledgments:** Special thanks to the Dowager Countess Eleanor Peel Trust and The Department of Employment and Learning (DEL) Northern Ireland for their financial support of this work and Rachel Huey for her input.

**Conflicts of Interest:** The authors declare no conflict of interest.

## References

1. Banks, W.A. Characteristics of compounds that cross the blood-brain barrier. *BMC Neurol.* **2009**, *9*, 1–5. [CrossRef] [PubMed]
2. Erdő, F.; Denes, L.; de Lange, E. Age-associated physiological and pathological changes at the blood–brain barrier: A review. *J. Cereb. Blood Flow Metab.* **2017**, *37*, 4–24. [CrossRef] [PubMed]
3. Pandit, R.; Chen, L.; Götz, J. The blood-brain barrier: Physiology and strategies for drug delivery. *Adv. Drug Deliv. Rev.* **2020**, *165*, 1–14. [CrossRef] [PubMed]
4. Segarra, M.; Aburto, M.R.; Acker-Palmer, A. Blood-brain barrier dynamics to maintain brain homeostasis. *Trends Neurosci.* **2021**, *44*, 393–405. [CrossRef]
5. Abbott, N.J.; Rönnbäck, L.; Hansson, E. Astrocyte-endothelial interactions at the blood-brain barrier. *Nat. Rev. Neurosci.* **2006**, *7*, 41–53. [CrossRef]
6. Engelhardt, B.; Liebner, S. Novel insights into the development and maintenance of the blood-brain barrier. *Cell Tissue Res.* **2014**, *355*, 687–699. [CrossRef]
7. Kadry, H.; Noorani, B.; Cucullo, L. A blood-brain barrier overview on structure, function, impairment, and biomarkers of integrity. *Fluids Barriers CNS* **2020**, *17*, 1–24. [CrossRef]
8. Lochhead, J.J.; Yang, J.; Ronaldson, P.T.; Davis, T.P. Structure, function, and regulation of the blood-brain barrier tight junction in central nervous system disorders. *Front. Physiol.* **2020**, *11*, 914. [CrossRef]

9. Galea, I. The blood-brain barrier in systemic infection and inflammation. *Cell Mol. Immunol.* **2021**, *18*, 2489–2501. [CrossRef]
10. Cohen-Pfeffer, J.L.; Gururangan, S.; Lester, T.; Lim, D.A.; Shaywitz, A.J.; Westphal, M.; Slavc, I. Intracerebroventricular delivery as a safe, long-term route of drug administration. *Pediatr. Neurol.* **2017**, *67*, 23–35. [CrossRef]
11. Tobinick, E.L. Perispinal delivery of CNS drugs. *CNS Drugs* **2016**, *30*, 469–480. [CrossRef]
12. Tobinick, E. Perispinal etanercept for neuroinflammatory disorders. *Drug Discov. Today* **2009**, *14*, 168–177. [CrossRef]
13. Tobinick, E. Perispinal etanercept advances as a neurotherapeutic. *Expert Rev. Neurother.* **2018**, *18*, 453–455. [CrossRef]
14. Tobinick, E.; Rodriguez-Romanacce, H.; Levine, A.; Ignatowski, T.A.; Spengler, R.N. Immediate neurological recovery following perispinal etanercept years after brain injury. *Clin. Drug Investig.* **2014**, *34*, 361–366. [CrossRef]
15. Ralph, S.J.; Weissenberger, A.; Bonev, V.; King, L.D.; Bonham, M.D.; Ferguson, S.; Smith, A.D.; Goodman-Jones, A.A.; Espinet, A.J. Phase I/II parallel double-blind randomized controlled clinical trial of perispinal etanercept for chronic stroke: Improved mobility and pain alleviation. *Expert Opin. Investig. Drugs* **2020**, *29*, 311–326. [CrossRef]
16. Manrique-Suárez, V.; Macaya, L.; Contreras, M.A.; Parra, N.; Maura, R.; González, A.; Toledo, J.R.; Sánchez, O. Design and characterization of a novel dimeric blood-brain barrier penetrating TNFα inhibitor. *Proteins* **2021**, *89*, 1508–1521. [CrossRef]
17. Kageyama, T.; Nakamura, M.; Matsuo, A.; Yamasaki, Y.; Takakura, Y.; Hashida, M.; Kanai, Y.; Naito, M.; Tsuruo, T.; Minato, N. The 4F2hc/LAT1 complex transports L-DOPA across the blood-brain barrier. *Brain Res.* **2000**, *879*, 115–121. [CrossRef]
18. Cornacchia, C.; Marinelli, L.; Di Rienzo, A.; Dimmito, M.P.; Serra, F.; Di Biase, G.; De Filippis, B.; Turkez, H.; Mardinoglu, A.; Bellezza, I. Development of l-Dopa-containing diketopiperazines as blood-brain barrier shuttle. *Eur. J. Med. Chem.* **2022**, *243*, 114746. [CrossRef]
19. Lane, E.L. L-DOPA for Parkinson's disease—A bittersweet pill. *Eur. J. Neurosci.* **2019**, *49*, 384–398. [CrossRef]
20. Chagraoui, A.; Boulain, M.; Juvin, L.; Anouar, Y.; Barrière, G.; De Deurwaerdère, P. L-DOPA in parkinson's disease: Looking at the "false" neurotransmitters and their meaning. *Int. J. Mol. Sci.* **2019**, *21*, 294. [CrossRef]
21. Bello, F.D.; Giannella, M.; Giorgioni, G.; Piergentili, A.; Quaglia, W. Receptor ligands as helping hands to L-DOPA in the treatment of Parkinson's disease. *Biomolecules* **2019**, *9*, 142. [CrossRef] [PubMed]
22. Jones, A.R.; Shusta, E.V. Blood–brain barrier transport of therapeutics via receptor-mediation. *Pharm. Res.* **2007**, *24*, 1759–1771. [CrossRef] [PubMed]
23. Pulgar, V.M. Transcytosis to cross the blood brain barrier, new advancements and challenges. *Front. Neurosci.* **2019**, *12*, 1019. [CrossRef] [PubMed]
24. Tashima, T. Smart strategies for therapeutic agent delivery into brain across the blood-brain barrier using receptor-mediated transcytosis. *Chem. Pharm. Bull.* **2020**, *68*, 316–325. [CrossRef]
25. Jain, A.; Jain, S.K. Ligand-appended BBB-targeted nanocarriers (LABTNs). *Crit. Rev. Ther. Drug Carr. Syst.* **2015**, *32*, 149–180. [CrossRef]
26. Kou, L.; Hou, Y.; Yao, Q.; Guo, W.; Wang, G.; Wang, M.; Fu, Q.; He, Z.; Ganapathy, V.; Sun, J. L-Carnitine-conjugated nanoparticles to promote permeation across blood-brain barrier and to target glioma cells for drug delivery via the novel organic cation/carnitine transporter OCTN2. *Artif. Cells Nanomed. Biotechnol.* **2018**, *46*, 1605–1616. [CrossRef]
27. Lee, S.W.L.; Campisi, M.; Osaki, T.; Possenti, L.; Mattu, C.; Adriani, G.; Kamm, R.D.; Chiono, V. Modeling nanocarrier transport across a 3D in vitro human blood-brain-barrier microvasculature. *Adv. Healthc. Mater.* **2020**, *9*, 1901486. [CrossRef]
28. Wilczewska, A.Z.; Niemirowicz, K.; Markiewicz, K.H.; Car, H. Nanoparticles as drug delivery systems. *Pharmacol. Rep.* **2012**, *64*, 1020–1037. [CrossRef]
29. Huey, R.; O'Hagan, B.; McCarron, P.; Hawthorne, S. Targeted drug delivery system to neural cells utilizes the nicotinic acetylcholine receptor. *Int. J. Pharm.* **2017**, *525*, 12–20. [CrossRef]
30. Bhalerao, A.; Sivandzade, F.; Archie, S.R.; Chowdhury, E.A.; Noorani, B.; Cucullo, L. In vitro modeling of the neurovascular unit: Advances in the field. *Fluids Barriers CNS* **2020**, *17*, 1–20. [CrossRef]
31. Logan, S.; Arzua, T.; Canfield, S.G.; Seminary, E.R.; Sison, S.L.; Ebert, A.D.; Bai, X. Studying human neurological disorders using induced pluripotent stem cells: From 2D monolayer to 3D organoid and blood brain barrier models. *Compr. Physiol.* **2019**, *9*, 565.
32. Sivandzade, F.; Cucullo, L. In-vitro blood-brain barrier modeling: A review of modern and fast-advancing technologies. *J. Cereb. Blood Flow Metab.* **2018**, *38*, 1667–1681. [CrossRef]
33. Cho, C.; Wolfe, J.M.; Fadzen, C.M.; Calligaris, D.; Hornburg, K.; Chiocca, E.A.; Agar, N.Y.; Pentelute, B.L.; Lawler, S.E. Blood-brain-barrier spheroids as an in vitro screening platform for brain-penetrating agents. *Nat. Commun.* **2017**, *8*, 15623. [CrossRef]
34. Naik, P.; Cucullo, L. In vitro blood-brain barrier models: Current and perspective technologies. *J. Pharm. Sci.* **2012**, *101*, 1337–1354. [CrossRef]
35. Jagtiani, E.; Yeolekar, M.; Naik, S.; Patravale, V. In vitro blood brain barrier models: An overview. *J. Control. Release* **2022**, *343*, 13–30. [CrossRef]
36. Jain, A.K.; Singh, D.; Dubey, K.; Maurya, R.; Mittal, S.; Pandey, A.K. Models and methods for in vitro toxicity. In *In Vitro Toxicology*; Elsevier: Amsterdam, The Netherlands, 2018; pp. 45–65.
37. Huey, R.; Rathbone, D.; McCarron, P.; Hawthorne, S. Design, stability and efficacy of a new targeting peptide for nanoparticulate drug delivery to SH-SY5Y neuroblastoma cells. *J. Drug Target.* **2019**, *27*, 959–970. [CrossRef]
38. Kaya, S.; Callan, B.; Hawthorne, S. Human in vitro blood brain barrier models—A review. *PLoS ONE* **2023**. *submitted*.
39. Srinivasan, B.; Kolli, A.R.; Esch, M.B.; Abaci, H.E.; Shuler, M.L.; Hickman, J.J. TEER measurement techniques for in vitro barrier model systems. *J. Lab. Autom.* **2015**, *20*, 107–126. [CrossRef]

40. Appelt-Menzel, A.; Cubukova, A.; Günther, K.; Edenhofer, F.; Piontek, J.; Krause, G.; Stüber, T.; Walles, H.; Neuhaus, W.; Metzger, M. Establishment of a human blood-brain barrier co-culture model mimicking the neurovascular unit using induced pluri-and multipotent stem cells. *Stem Cell Rep.* **2017**, *8*, 894–906. [CrossRef]
41. Gaillard, P.J.; de Boer, A.G. Relationship between permeability status of the blood–brain barrier and in vitro permeability coefficient of a drug. *Eur. J. Pharm. Sci.* **2000**, *12*, 95–102. [CrossRef]
42. Reichel, A.; Begley, D.J.; Abbott, N.J. An overview of in vitro techniques for blood-brain barrier studies. *Blood-Brain Barrier Biol. Res. Protoc.* **2003**, *89*, 307–324.
43. Deli, M.A.; Ábrahám, C.S.; Kataoka, Y.; Niwa, M. Permeability studies on in vitro blood–brain barrier models: Physiology, pathology, and pharmacology. *Cell Mol. Neurobiol.* **2005**, *25*, 59–127. [CrossRef] [PubMed]
44. Bagchi, S.; Chhibber, T.; Lahooti, B.; Verma, A.; Borse, V.; Jayant, R.D. In-vitro blood-brain barrier models for drug screening and permeation studies: An overview. *Drug Des. Dev. Ther.* **2019**, *13*, 3591–3605. [CrossRef] [PubMed]
45. Elbakary, B.; Badhan, R.K. A dynamic perfusion-based blood-brain barrier model for cytotoxicity testing and drug permeation. *Sci. Rep.* **2020**, *10*, 3788. [CrossRef]
46. Ferrell, N.; Cheng, J.; Miao, S.; Roy, S.; Fissell, W.H. Orbital shear stress regulates differentiation and barrier function of primary renal tubular epithelial cells. *ASAIO J.* **2018**, *64*, 766. [CrossRef]
47. Dardik, A.; Chen, L.; Frattini, J.; Asada, H.; Aziz, F.; Kudo, F.A.; Sumpio, B.E. Differential effects of orbital and laminar shear stress on endothelial cells. *J. Vasc. Surg.* **2005**, *41*, 869–880. [CrossRef]
48. Salvador, E.; Burek, M.; Löhr, M.; Nagai, M.; Hagemann, C.; Förster, C.Y. Senescence and associated blood-brain barrier alterations in vitro. *Histochem. Cell Biol.* **2021**, *156*, 283–292. [CrossRef]
49. Eigenmann, D.E.; Xue, G.; Kim, K.S.; Moses, A.V.; Hamburger, M.; Oufir, M. Comparative study of four immortalized human brain capillary endothelial cell lines, hCMEC/D3, hBMEC, TY10, and BB19, and optimization of culture conditions, for an in vitro blood-brain barrier model for drug permeability studies. *Fluids Barriers CNS* **2013**, *10*, 1–17. [CrossRef]
50. Xu, L.; Nirwane, A.; Yao, Y. Basement membrane and blood-brain barrier. *Stroke Vasc. Neurol.* **2019**, *4*, 78–82. [CrossRef]
51. Banerjee, J.; Shi, Y.; Azevedo, H.S. In vitro blood-brain barrier models for drug research: State-of-the-art and new perspectives on reconstituting these models on artificial basement membrane platforms. *Drug Discov. Today* **2016**, *21*, 1367–1386. [CrossRef]
52. Thomsen, M.S.; Routhe, L.J.; Moos, T. The vascular basement membrane in the healthy and pathological brain. *J. Cereb. Blood Flow Metab.* **2017**, *37*, 3300–3317. [CrossRef]
53. Seltzer, J.L.; Weingarten, H.; Akers, K.T.; Eschbach, M.L.; Grant, G.A.; Eisen, A.Z. Cleavage specificity of type IV collagenase (gelatinase) from human skin. Use of synthetic peptides as model substrates. *J. Biol. Chem.* **1989**, *264*, 19583–19586. [CrossRef]
54. Maherally, Z.; Fillmore, H.L.; Tan, S.L.; Tan, S.F.; Jassam, S.A.; Quack, F.I.; Hatherell, K.E.; Pilkington, G.J. Real-time acquisition of transendothelial electrical resistance in an all-human, in vitro, 3-dimensional, blood-brain barrier model exemplifies tight-junction integrity. *FASEB J. Off. Publ. Fed. Am. Soc. Exp. Biol.* **2018**, *32*, 168–182. [CrossRef]
55. Nakagawa, S.; Deli, M.A.; Kawaguchi, H.; Shimizudani, T.; Shimono, T.; Kittel, A.; Tanaka, K.; Niwa, M. A new blood–brain barrier model using primary rat brain endothelial cells, pericytes and astrocytes. *Neurochem. Int.* **2009**, *54*, 253–263. [CrossRef]
56. Malina, K.C.; Cooper, I.; Teichberg, V.I. Closing the gap between the in-vivo and in-vitro blood-brain barrier tightness. *Brain Res.* **2009**, *1284*, 12–21. [CrossRef]
57. Helms, H.C.; Abbott, N.J.; Burek, M.; Cecchelli, R.; Couraud, P.; Deli, M.A.; Förster, C.; Galla, H.J.; Romero, I.A.; Shusta, E.V. In vitro models of the blood-brain barrier: An overview of commonly used brain endothelial cell culture models and guidelines for their use. *J. Cereb. Blood Flow Metab.* **2016**, *36*, 862–890. [CrossRef]
58. Zhu, D.; Su, Y.; Fu, B.; Xu, H. Magnesium reduces blood-brain barrier permeability and regulates amyloid-β transcytosis. *Mol. Neurobiol.* **2018**, *55*, 7118–7131. [CrossRef]
59. León, J.; Acurio, J.; Bergman, L.; López, J.; Karin Wikström, A.; Torres-Vergara, P.; Troncoso, F.; Castro, F.O.; Vatish, M.; Escudero, C. Disruption of the blood-brain barrier by extracellular vesicles from preeclampsia plasma and hypoxic placentae: Attenuation by magnesium sulfate. *Hypertension* **2021**, *78*, 1423–1433. [CrossRef]
60. Alarcon-Martinez, L.; Yilmaz-Ozcan, S.; Yemisci, M.; Schallek, J.; Kılıç, K.; Can, A.; Di Polo, A.; Dalkara, T. Capillary pericytes express α-smooth muscle actin, which requires prevention of filamentous-actin depolymerization for detection. *eLife* **2018**, *7*, e34861. [CrossRef]
61. Su, X.; Huang, L.; Qu, Y.; Xiao, D.; Mu, D. Pericytes in Cerebrovascular Diseases: An Emerging Therapeutic Target. *Front. Cell Neurosci.* **2019**, *13*, 519. [CrossRef]
62. Reilly, J.F.; Maher, P.A.; Kumari, V.G. Regulation of astrocyte GFAP expression by TGF-β1 and FGF-2. *Glia* **1998**, *22*, 202–210. [CrossRef]
63. Baba, H.; Nakahira, K.; Morita, N.; Tanaka, F.; Akita, H.; Ikenaka, K. GFAP gene expression during development of astrocyte. *Dev. Neurosci.* **1997**, *19*, 49–57. [CrossRef] [PubMed]
64. Hajal, C.; Campisi, M.; Mattu, C.; Chiono, V.; Kamm, R.D. In vitro models of molecular and nano-particle transport across the blood-brain barrier. *Biomicrofluidics* **2018**, *12*, 042213. [CrossRef] [PubMed]
65. Chigumira, W.; Maposa, P.; Gadaga, L.L.; Dube, A.; Tagwireyi, D.; Maponga, C.C. Preparation and evaluation of pralidoxime-loaded PLGA nanoparticles as potential carriers of the drug across the blood brain barrier. *J. Nanomater.* **2015**, *2015*, 8. [CrossRef]

66. Sadat Tabatabaei Mirakabad, F.; Nejati-Koshki, K.; Akbarzadeh, A.; Yamchi, M.R.; Milani, M.; Zarghami, N.; Zeighamian, V.; Rahimzadeh, A.; Alimohammadi, S.; Hanifehpour, Y.; et al. PLGA-based nanoparticles as cancer drug delivery systems. *Asian Pac. J. Cancer Prev. APJCP* **2014**, *15*, 517–535. [CrossRef]
67. Monge, M.; Fornaguera, C.; Quero, C.; Dols-Perez, A.; Calderó, G.; Grijalvo, S.; García-Celma, M.J.; Rodríguez-Abreu, C.; Solans, C. Functionalized PLGA nanoparticles prepared by nano-emulsion templating interact selectively with proteins involved in the transport through the blood-brain barrier. *Eur. J. Pharm. Biopharm.* **2020**, *156*, 155–164. [CrossRef]
68. Azizi, M.; Farahmandghavi, F.; Joghataei, M.; Zandi, M.; Imani, M.; Bakhtiary, M.; Dorkoosh, F.A.; Ghazizadeh, F. Fabrication of protein-loaded PLGA nanoparticles: Effect of selected formulation variables on particle size and release profile. *J. Polym. Res.* **2013**, *20*, 1–14. [CrossRef]
69. Carter, D.C.; Ho, J.X. Structure of serum albumin. *Adv. Protein Chem.* **1994**, *45*, 153–203.
70. Hughes, J.M.; Budd, P.M.; Tiede, K.; Lewis, J. Polymerized high internal phase emulsion monoliths for the chromatographic separation of engineered nanoparticles. *J. Appl. Polym. Sci.* **2015**, *132*, 41229. [CrossRef]
71. Clayton, K.N.; Salameh, J.W.; Wereley, S.T.; Kinzer-Ursem, T.L. Physical characterization of nanoparticle size and surface modification using particle scattering diffusometry. *Biomicrofluidics* **2016**, *10*, 054107. [CrossRef]
72. Fornaguera, C.; Dols-Perez, A.; Calderó, G.; García-Celma, M.J.; Camarasa, J.; Solans, C. PLGA nanoparticles prepared by nano-emulsion templating using low-energy methods as efficient nanocarriers for drug delivery across the blood–brain barrier. *J. Control Release* **2015**, *211*, 134–143. [CrossRef]
73. Patel, J.; Amrutiya, J.; Bhatt, P.; Javia, A.; Jain, M.; Misra, A. Targeted delivery of monoclonal antibody conjugated docetaxel loaded PLGA nanoparticles into EGFR overexpressed lung tumour cells. *J. Microencapsul.* **2018**, *35*, 204–217. [CrossRef]

*pharmaceutics*

*Article*

# Molecular Imaging of Ultrasound-Mediated Blood-Brain Barrier Disruption in a Mouse Orthotopic Glioblastoma Model

**Chiara Bastiancich [1,†], Samantha Fernandez [2,†], Florian Correard [3], Anthony Novell [4], Benoit Larrat [5], Benjamin Guillet [2,6,*,‡] and Marie-Anne Estève [3,*,‡]**

1 CNRS, INP, Inst Neurophysiopathol, Aix-Marseille University, 13005 Marseille, France
2 Centre Européen de Recherche en Imagerie Médicale (CERIMED), CNRS, Aix-Marseille University, 13005 Marseille, France
3 APHM, CNRS, INP, Inst Neurophysiopathol, Hôpital Timone, Service Pharmacie, Aix-Marseille University, 13005 Marseille, France
4 CEA, CNRS, Inserm, BioMaps, Service Hospitalier Frédéric Joliot, Université Paris-Saclay, 91401 Orsay, France
5 CEA, CNRS, NeuroSpin/BAOBAB, Université Paris-Saclay, 91191 Gif-sur-Yvette, France
6 Centre de Recherche en Cardiovasculaire et Nutrition (C2VN), INSERM, INRAE, Aix-Marseille University, 13005 Marseille, France
* Correspondence: benjamin.guillet@univ-amu.fr (B.G.); marie-anne.esteve@univ-amu.fr (M.-A.E.)
† These authors contributed equally to this work.
‡ These authors contributed equally to this work.

**Abstract:** Glioblastoma (GBM) is an aggressive and malignant primary brain tumor. The blood-brain barrier (BBB) limits the therapeutic options available to tackle this incurable tumor. Transient disruption of the BBB by focused ultrasound (FUS) is a promising and safe approach to increase the brain and tumor concentration of drugs administered systemically. Non-invasive, sensitive, and reliable imaging approaches are required to better understand the impact of FUS on the BBB and brain microenvironment. In this study, nuclear imaging (SPECT/CT and PET/CT) was used to quantify neuroinflammation 48 h post-FUS and estimate the influence of FUS on BBB opening and tumor growth in vivo. BBB disruptions were performed on healthy and GBM-bearing mice (U-87 MG xenograft orthotopic model). The BBB recovery kinetics were followed and quantified by [99mTc]Tc-DTPA SPECT/CT imaging at 0.5 h, 3 h and 24 h post-FUS. The absence of neuroinflammation was confirmed by [18F]FDG PET/CT imaging 48 h post-FUS. The presence of the tumor and its growth were evaluated by [68Ga]Ga-RGD$_2$ PET/CT imaging and post-mortem histological analysis, showing that tumor growth was not influenced by FUS. In conclusion, molecular imaging can be used to evaluate the time frame for systemic treatment combined with transient BBB opening and to test its efficacy over time.

**Keywords:** glioblastoma; focused ultrasound; blood-brain barrier; PET; SPECT; drug delivery

**Citation:** Bastiancich, C.; Fernandez, S.; Correard, F.; Novell, A.; Larrat, B.; Guillet, B.; Estève, M.-A. Molecular Imaging of Ultrasound-Mediated Blood-Brain Barrier Disruption in a Mouse Orthotopic Glioblastoma Model. *Pharmaceutics* **2022**, *14*, 2227. https://doi.org/10.3390/pharmaceutics14102227

Academic Editor: Carlotta Marianecci

Received: 16 September 2022
Accepted: 17 October 2022
Published: 19 October 2022



## 1. Introduction

Glioblastoma (GBM) is the most aggressive and malignant primary brain tumor in adults. Today, GBM is still incurable and its effective treatment is hampered, among other factors, by the presence of the blood-brain barrier (BBB). The BBB limits the access of active agents at the tumor site and in proximity of the tumor, where it is intact but where infiltrating tumor cells reside and are responsible for recurrences [1]. The BBB is a physiological barrier protecting the central nervous system physically and biochemically from pathogens, toxins and hormones circulating in the blood. It is regulated by physical, transport, and metabolic properties of the endothelial cells surrounding the blood vessels, which are held together by tight junctions and reduce permeation of polar solutes from the blood to the brain extracellular compartment. The BBB permeability is also regulated by interactions with different vascular, immune, and neural cells [2]. Consequently, BBB is a highly selective filter through which nutrients needed by the brain are transmitted and waste products are removed. This protection of the brain complicates the treatment of many neurological diseases, such as GBM. Several strategies can be used to bypass the BBB to achieve enhanced delivery into the brain. Thus, for decades, intensive work has been done on methods to enable the transport of active substances into the brain by bypassing—or better still by selectively crossing—the BBB [3,4]. A range of strategies for overcoming the BBB have been developed for this purpose or are still under development [5–7]. Among these, the transient and local permeabilization induced by the application of focused ultrasound (FUS) to a selected region of the brain immediately following intravenous microbubbles administration is promising. The stable oscillation of microbubbles induced by FUS leads to biomechanical effects (cellular massage, microstreaming) on the endothelial cells composing the BBB wall causing a transient disruption of tight junction integrity and an increase of paracellular permeability. This leads to an increased extravasation of molecules that could not spontaneously cross the BBB (either free drugs or nanomedicines). The oscillating microbubbles can also induce an immune response by triggering the release of damage-associated molecular patterns [8]. This noninvasive technique has been shown to improve the brain delivery of therapeutic agents in several animal models [9], and to be safe and well-tolerated in clinical trials performed in patients with Alzheimer's disease [10] and GBM [11,12]. Currently, at least two clinical trials are ongoing, testing single or multiple BBB disruptions during standard temozolomide chemotherapy in newly diagnosed GBM patients (clinicaltrials.gov ID NCT04614493 and NCT03712293 [13]). Others are ongoing on recurrent GBM patients in combination with other treatments (e.g., clinicaltrials.gov NCT03744026, NCT03626896, NCT04446416) showing a high interest of the neuro-oncology community for FUS-mediated BBB permeabilization.

Most of the preclinical studies reporting the use of this technique are performed under magnetic resonance (MR) guidance and use MR contrast agents (e.g., gadoterate meglumine, Gd-DOTA; Dotarem®) that do not cross the intact BBB to assess its disruption [14]. Indeed, molecules that do not have the physicochemical properties required to bypass the BBB are excellent markers of BBB integrity. In case of disease, brain lesion or induced-BBB opening, changes in the expression of BBB transporters and cell-cell junction proteins allow the increased delivery of contrast agents into the brain tissue making the BBB defects visible. Following this approach, Marty et al. used a quantitative $T_1$ relaxometry method to follow BBB closure dynamics after FUS [15]. Unfortunately, the lack of sensitivity and rather low time resolution remains a limitation of MR based molecular imaging. By means of radioactively labelled tracers, which do not normally pass through the BBB, it is also possible to investigate the function of the BBB. This can be done using single photon emission computed tomography (SPECT) or positron emission tomography (PET). For example, in patients with acute stroke, increased uptake of 99mTc chelated with hexa-methyl-propylene-amine-oxime (HMPAO) [16,17] can be shown. A recent review by Arif et al. describes how PET can provide insights into the underlying mechanisms of FUS-mediated BBB permeabilization [18]. Despite its potential for this scope, the number of studies reporting the use of nuclear imaging techniques to evaluate the transient FUS-mediated BBB permeability, the enhanced intratumoral uptake of drug-loaded nanoparticles or the physiological effects induced by the transient BBB opening on the brain remains limited. A few studies have used nuclear imaging to establish optimal therapeutic windows for brain tumor chemotherapy following FUS-mediated BBB permeabilization and the systemic administration of theranostics nanoparticles or radiolabeled active agents in tumor-bearing or healthy animals ([111In]-labeled liposomal doxorubicin [19]; [89Zr]–cetuximab [20]).

In this study, we used nuclear imaging as an alternative to magnetic resonance imaging, which is not always available for preclinical studies. Our main objective was to use nuclear imaging to evaluate the effect of BBB opening on GBM-bearing mice. The secondary objectives were the evaluation the impact of BBB-opening on neuroinflammation and tumor growth. To do so, we evaluated the kinetics of transient FUS-mediated BBB opening via SPECT, together with computed tomography (CT) imaging using 99mTc-tagged diethylenetriamine pentaacetate acid ([99mTc]Tc-DTPA) [21] as a radiotracer. The neuroinflammation will be evaluated on GBM-bearing mice by PET/CT imaging using 18F-fluorodeoxyglucose ([18F]FDG) as a radiotracer [22,23] 48 h post-permeabilization. The tumor growth profile will be evaluated using 68Ga-labeled amino acid sequence arginine-glycine-aspartic ([68Ga]Ga $RGD_2$) via PET/CT [24]. A survival analysis will be performed to evaluate if BBB permeability in the early stages of tumor development (before day 10 post-grafting [25]) can induce a delay in tumor growth. To the best of our knowledge, we are the first to use these radiotracers sequentially and on the same GBM-bearing animal.

## 2. Materials and Methods

The in vivo experiments reported in this work have been approved by the institution's Animal Care and Use Committee (CE71, Aix-Marseille Université, reference n° 14713) and performed following the French national regulation guidelines in accordance with EU Directive 2010/63/EU. Mice were housed in enriched cages placed in a temperature- and hygrometry-controlled room, had free access to water and food and were monitored daily. The mice were six-week-old female athymic Nude-Foxn1nu mice (Envigo, Gannat, France). The animals were sacrificed at the end of the study (healthy animals) or when they reached the end-points ($\geq$20% body weight loss or 10% body weight loss plus clinical signs of distress e.g., paralysis, arched back, or lack of movement for glioma-bearing animals).

### *2.1. Pilot Study on Healthy Animals*

Ultrasound waves were produced using a spherically focused single element ultrasound transducer (central frequency 1.5 MHz, diameter 25 mm, focal depth 20 $\pm$ 2 mm, Imasonic, Voray sur I'Ognon, France) driven by a built-in signal generator connected via a 50 W power amplifier (Image Guided Therapy, Pessac, France). The output pressure of the transducer was measured in a degassed water tank, using a 0.2 mm lipstick hydrophone (HGL, ONDA Corporation, CA, USA) mounted on a positioning stage. The acquired signal from the calibrated hydrophone was sampled by the scope (Picoscope 5243A, Pico Technology, Eaton Socon, UK). Electrical power sent to the transducer was monitored in real-time during the sonication. The focal point size (e.g., 6 dB pressure focal region) of the transducer was $1.2 \times 1.2 \times 6$ mm$^3$.

Animals underwent the permeabilization protocol either for a single spot opening ($1.2 \times 1.2$ mm) or a large brain opening ($6 \times 6$ mm raster scan trajectory): in either case, they were anesthetized, placed on a temperature-monitored stereotactic device, and injected with microbubbles before launching the appropriate sequence.

Mice were anesthetized by ketamine/xylazine (100 and 10 mg/kg intraperitoneal injection, respectively) and placed in a dedicated temperature-controlled frame in a prone position under the set-up. The ultrasound transducer was coupled to the head via a water-filled latex balloon (Comed; Strasbourg, France) and degassed echographic gel (70% $v/v$ in water). A hundred µL of SonoVue® microbubbles (Bracco, Milan, Italy) were systemically administered via retro-orbital injection in the right eye using an insulin syringe (27G), and the ultrasound sequence was started immediately after. Depending on the experimental group, the transducer was still during the sonications or mechanically moved following programmed trajectories using a 2D-axis motorized positioning stage. Group A: single spot sonication (pulse length of 3 ms every 100 ms for 2 min) ($n$ = 3); Group B: a $6 \times 6$ mm raster scan mechanical trajectory was designed to cover most of the brain ($n$ = 3). As described in [20,26], ultrasonic waves were quasi-continuously transmitted at 1.5 MHz during transducer motion except during the changes of direction in the raster scan (duty cycle 69%). This avoided an excessive deposit of ultrasound energy at these locations. The sequence was repeated 25 times for a total exposure of 127 s. The transmitted in situ peak negative pressure in the mouse brain is estimated to be 430 kPa (520 kPa in deionized water) considering a skull attenuation of 18% (average value of the skull attenuation measured in [27]) at 1.5 MHz. One sham animal, undergoing the same procedure as the animals of group A and B (anesthesia, stereotactic fixing, microbubbles injections, SPECT imaging protocol) but without launching the mechanical scan and BBB permeabilization sequence was also included in the pilot study and imaged.

## 2.2. *Hemispheric Blood-Brain Barrier Permeabilization on Healthy and Tumor-Bearing Mice*

### 2.2.1. Glioma Cell Cultures

U-87 MG glioma cells (ATTC, Manassas, FL, USA) were cultured in Eagle's Minimum Essential Medium (EMEM; Gibco, Life Technologies, Carlsbad, CA, USA). Culture medias were supplemented with 10% Fetal Bovine Serum (FBS; Gibco, Life Technologies), 100 U/mL penicillin G sodium and 100 µg/mL streptomycin sulfate (Gibco, Life Technologies). Cells were subcultured in 75 $cm^2$ culture flasks (Corning® T-75, Sigma-Aldrich, Saint-Louis, MO, USA) and incubated at 37 °C and 5% $CO_2$.

### 2.2.2. Orthotopic U-87 MG Human Glioblastoma Tumor Model

Animals were anesthetized by ketamine/xylazine (100 and 10 mg/kg intraperitoneal injection, respectively) and fixed in a stereotactic frame. The skin surface on the head was disinfected by application of an antiseptic solution (Vétédine® solution, Vetoquinol, Lure, France). Lidocaine (10 mg/mL; Aguettant, Lyon, France) was injected subcutaneously at the site of incision, and the eyes were protected with an ophthalmic gel (Ocry-gel, TVM lab, Lempdes, France). To hydrate the animal, 200 µL of physiological solution (0.9% Sodium Chloride; Aguettant, France) were injected subcutaneously in the flank. An incision was made along the midline and a burr hole was drilled into the skull at the right frontal lobe, 0.5 mm anterior and 2 mm lateral to the bregma (high speed drill: Tack life Tools, New York, NY, USA; 0.8 mm diameter round end engraving burrs: Dremel, Breda, The Netherlands). A 10 µL 26 s gauge syringe with cemented 51 mm needle (Hamilton, Rungis, France) was used to inject $5 \times 10^4$ U-87 MG glioma cells suspended in EMEM (without FBS and antibiotics) at a depth of 3 mm from the outer border of the brain, using an automatic pump device at a speed of 0.7 µL/min. The wound was then closed using a tissue adhesive glue (3M Vetbond®, Sergy-Pontoise, France) and the animals recovered under an infrared heating lamp.

### 2.2.3. Blood-Brain Barrier Permeabilization Protocol

Eight days following tumor grafting, mice were anesthetized by the intraperitoneal injection of ketamine/xylazine (100 and 10 mg/kg, respectively) and placed in a dedicated stereotactic frame positioned below the BBB opening set up as previously explained. For this experiment the mice were divided in three groups ($n$ = 4–5 per group): Group "GBM + FUS": tumor-bearing animals undergoing FUS-mediated hemispheric BBB permeabilization (3.6 × 3.6 mm trajectory covering the whole right hemisphere; quasi-continuous sonication—duty cycle 71%—repeated 36 times and paused between each execution and a moving speed of 10 mm/s; the total sonication time of 115 s [28]); Group "GBM only": tumor-bearing animals undergoing the same procedure as group "GBM + FUS" (anesthesia, surgical procedure, microbubbles injections, SPECT/PET imaging protocols) but without launching the mechanical scan and BBB permeabilization sequence (tumor growth control); Group "FUS only": healthy animals undergoing FUS-mediated hemispheric BBB permeabilization (BBB opening control). Groups "GBM + FUS" and "GBM only" were imaged for [99mTc]Tc-DTPA, [18F]FDG and [68Ga]Ga-$RGD_2$. The animals of group "FUS only" received all the surgical procedures of the group "GBM + FUS" the day of the permeabilization and were imaged for [99mTc]Tc-DTPA and [18F]FDG. Figure 1 recapitulates the experimental plan used for the FUS-mediated hemispheric BBB permeabilization study on healthy and tumor-bearing animals.

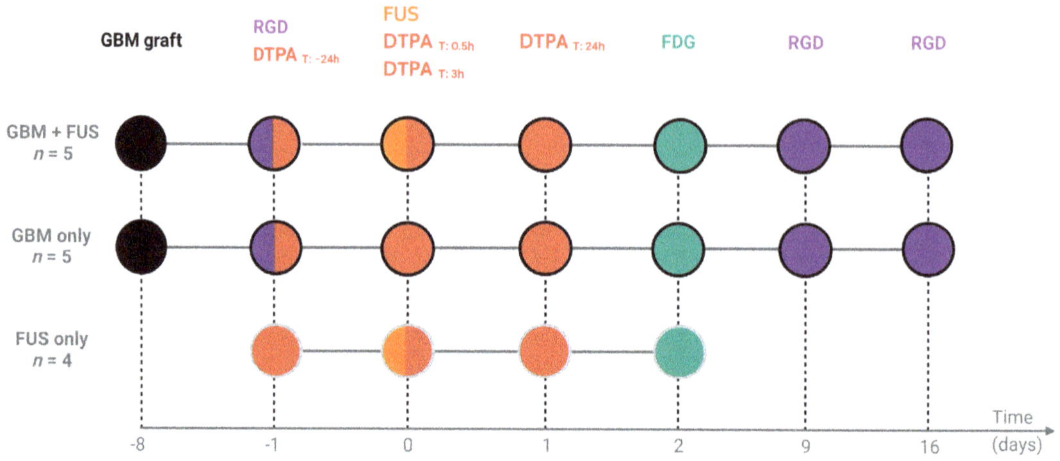


**Figure 1.** Schematic representation of the experimental plan used for the FUS-induced hemispheric BBB permeabilization and imaging study on healthy and tumor-bearing animals. Group "GBM + FUS": tumor-bearing animals undergoing FUS-mediated BBB permeabilization; Group "GBM only": tumor-bearing animals without BBB permeabilization (tumor growth control); Group "FUS only": healthy animals undergoing FUS-mediated BBB permeabilization (BBB opening control).

Mice were sacrificed when reaching the clinical end points (groups "GBM + FUS" and "GBM only") or after the last imaging session (group "FUS only"). For tumor-grafted animals, statistical analysis was estimated from comparison of Kaplan-Meier survival curves using the log-rank test (Mantel Cox test). The brains of these animals were extracted and fixed in 10% formalin solution (Merck, Darmstadt, Germany) for 24 h before being rinsed in PBS and kept at 4 °C until further use. Brains were then embedded in paraffin, sectioned at 4 µm thickness using a MICROM HM 335 E microtome (Thermo Fischer Scientific, Waltham, MA, USA), collected on Silane adhesive KF Frost slides (VWR, Amsterdam, The Netherlands) on a drop of glycerate albumin (DiaPath, Martinengo, Italy) mixed with distilled water and dried on a Leica HI1220 heating plate (Leica, Wetzlar, Germany). Slides were incubated at 37 °C overnight and then stored at room temperature until further use. For standard histology, the slides were deparaffinized and stained with hematoxylin and eosin (H&E) for tumor detection ($n$ = 3).

### 2.3. *Imaging*

#### 2.3.1. Single Photon Emission Computed Tomography (SPECT) Imaging

For mice included in the studies described in Sections 2.1 and 2.2, the BBB opening was evaluated by SPECT/CT imaging using [99mTc]Tc-DTPA as radiotracer 0.5 h, 3 h and 24 h post BBB permeabilization. For animals of the study described in Section 2.2, this procedure was also performed 24 h before BBB permeabilization.

[99mTc]Tc-DTPA was administered via an intravenous injection of 50 µL of radioactive tracer (20 MBq) in isotonic and pyrogen-free solution using an insulin syringe (27G). Thirty minutes after injection, the SPECT/CT acquisition was done for 20 min under anesthesia with 1.5% vol% isoflurane (IsoVet®, Laboratoire Osalia, Paris, France) using a NanoSPECT/CTplus® camera and the Nucline® 1.02 acquisition software (Mediso Medical Imaging System Ltd., Budapest, Hungary). SPECT and CT DICOM files were fused for reconstruction and image processing was carried out with VivoQuant® 3.5 and InvivoScope® 2.00 reconstruction software (InviCRO, Boston, MA, USA) to assess tracer uptake in the brain.

For the pilot study, statistical analysis was performed using two-way ANOVA (uncorrected Fisher's LSD test). For the hemispheric BBB permeabilization study, statistical analysis was performed using two-way ANOVA with Dunnett's multiple comparisons test of each time point vs. the basal value (−24 h).

2.3.2. Positron Emission Tomography (PET) Imaging

For the study described in Section 2.2, PET/CT imaging was also performed.

The presence, location and growth of the tumors were determined by PET/CT imaging using [68Ga]Ga-RGD$_2$ as a radiotracer. Imaging was performed for all tumor-bearing mice included in the study at 7-, 17- and 24-days post tumor cell implantations (day −1, 9 and 16 before/after BBB permeabilization). Neuroinflammation was estimated by PET/CT imaging 48 h following sonication using [18F]FDG as a radiotracer. Statistical analysis was performed using one-way ANOVA test.

[68Ga]Ga-RGD$_2$ or [18F]FDG were administered via an intravenous injection of 50 µL of radioactive tracer (5 MBq) in isotonic and pyrogen-free solution using an insulin syringe (27G). Forty-five minutes ([18F]FDG) or one hour ([68Ga]Ga-RGD$_2$) after injection, the PET/CT acquisition was done for 20 min under anesthesia with 1.5% vol% isoflurane using a NanoScanPET/CT® camera and the Nucline® 1.02 acquisition software (Mediso Medical Imaging System Ltd., Budapest, Hungary). PET and CT DICOM files were fused for reconstruction and image processing was carried out with VivoQuant® 3.5 and InvivoScope® 2.00 reconstruction software (InviCRO, Boston, MA, USA). A statistical analysis was performed using a two-way ANOVA (uncorrected Fisher's LSD test).

Quantitative analysis of the region of interest (ROI) of the PET or SPECT signal was performed on attenuation- and decay-corrected PET/SPECT images using InterviewFusion software (Mediso, Budapest, Hungary). Tissue uptake values for each mouse were expressed as an average ratio of the signal from each ipsilateral hemisphere to the contralateral signal ± SEM and in total brain as an average percentage of the injected dose per cubic millimetre of tissue (%ID/mm$^3$) ± SEM.

## 3. Results and Discussion

### *3.1. Pilot Study on Healthy Animals*

To understand the optimal permeabilization parameters and time frames for SPECT/CT imaging with [99mTc]Tc-DTPA, a FUS-mediated BBB-opening pilot study was performed on healthy animals. Animals underwent the permeabilization protocol either for a single spot opening (1.2 × 1.2 mm) or a large brain opening (6 × 6 mm raster scan trajectory); the sequences were selected based on previous results within our team of collaborators [15,29–31] and adapted to the characteristics of our transducer and animal species and strain (nude mice). For these experiments, a multi-functional preclinical device recently assembled for combined BBB permeabilization and photothermal therapy with photoacoustic temperature monitoring was used [32].

Immediately following sonication, animals were administered with [99mTc]Tc-DTPA and underwent SPECT/CT imaging 0.5 h later under isoflurane mild anesthesia (Figure 2). SPECT/CT imaging was also performed 3 h and 24 h later to evaluate the BBB closure kinetic.

For both sonication schemes (single spot and large brain opening), animals did not show any sign of pain or distress following BBB permeabilization. In both groups, an increase in the [99mTc]Tc-DTPA SPECT/CT signal was observed in the brain in the treated area and showed a peak 0.5 h following BBB disruption (0.5 h vs. 24 h: 3.9-fold increase in single spot scheme, $p = 0.0289$; 7-fold increase in the raster scan scheme, $p = 0.0003$), followed by a decrease of the signal at 3 h (3 h vs. 24 h: 3.1-fold increase in single spot scheme, $p = 0.0979$; 5.6-fold increase in the raster scan scheme, $p = 0.0016$) and returning to basal levels comparable to the sham animal at 24 h after FUS exposure. As expected, a higher increase (two-fold time at 0.5 h and 3 h) in the total amount of [99mTc]Tc-DTPA was observed in the raster scan scheme in comparison with the animals that underwent single spot sonication (single spot vs. raster scan trajectory: $p = 0.0144$ at 0.5 h; $p = 0.0379$ at 3 h; $p = 0.9290$ at 24 h) as the exposed volume in the latter is much lower.

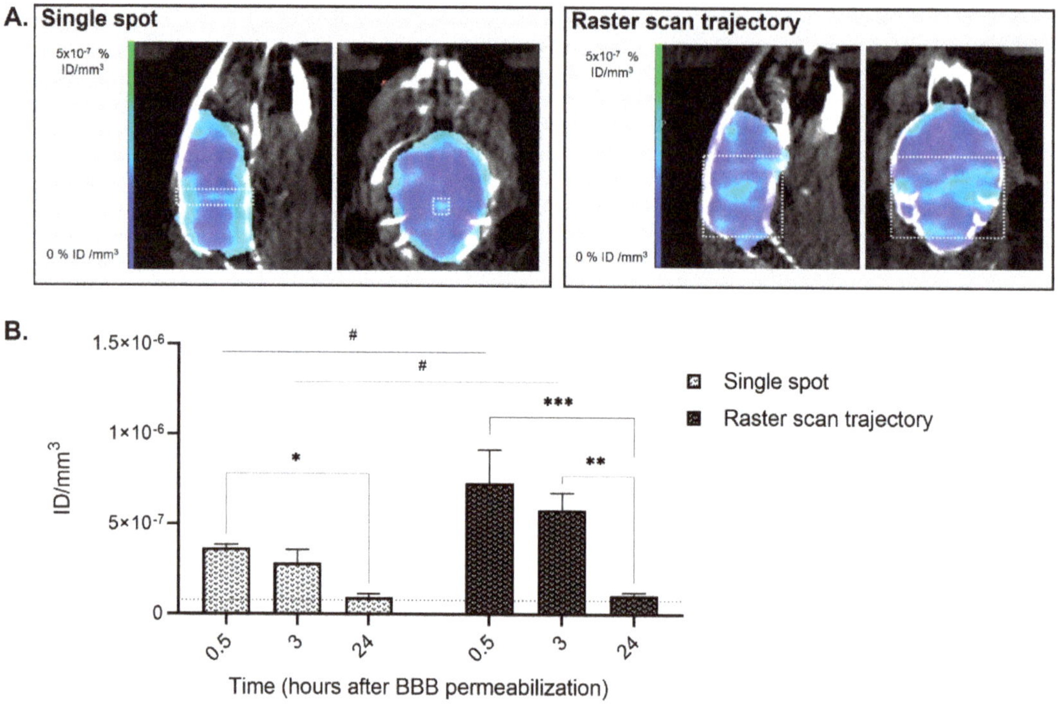


**Figure 2.** Imaging of the animal's brain following BBB disruption and [99mTc]Tc-DTPA intravenous injection in healthy mice 0.5 h later. (**A**) Brain representative SPECT/CT tomographic images of [99mTc]Tc-DTPA distribution in animals that received single-spot (group A, left panel) or raster scan trajectory (group B, right panel) focused ultrasound. The white square represents the approximate region were FUS were applied for both sonication schemes; (**B**) Quantification of [99mTc]Tc-DTPA activity 0.5 h, 3 h and 24 h following focused ultrasound. Results are expressed as injected dose per tissue volume (ID/mm$^3$; $n$ = 3; mean ± SEM). Statistical differences are reported as # for comparisons between single spot vs. raster scan trajectory and as * for comparisons between 0.5 h vs. 3 h vs. 24 h ($^{\#}$ $p < 0.05$; * $p < 0.05$; ** $p < 0.01$; *** $p < 0.001$). The black dotted line is a visual representation of the baseline of an animal that did not receive BBB permeabilization, obtained as an average of the 0.5 h, 3 h and 24 h [99mTc]Tc-DTPA quantifications of the sham animal ($7.8 \times 10^{-8} \pm 1.6 \times 10^{-8}$).

These results are in accordance with previous works showing that BBB closure following FUS permeabilization is gradual and depends on the size of the contrast agent injected [15]. As Dotarem® has a spherical hydrodynamic diameter similar to the one of [99mTc]Tc-DTPA (approximately 1 nm), a signal up to 24 h following sonication was expected as suggested in [15]. However, at 3 h, the amount of quantified [99mTc]Tc-DTPA was already decreasing, going back to basal values at 24 h. Variations in the experimental protocol (e.g., animal model, microbubbles concentration, FUS protocol and acoustic pressure) as well as physicochemical differences between the contrast agents could also explain the differences observed between previously reported studies. For example, one of the factors that could explain the different brain uptake between Dotarem® and [99mTc]Tc-DTPA is the different anesthetics used for our experiment compared to Marty et al. (ketamine/xylazine plus isoflurane in medical air only vs. isoflurane in a mixture of air and oxygen) [15]. Indeed, it has been previously demonstrated that the circulation time of the microbubbles in the presence of oxygen (used as carrier gas for inhalation anesthesia) and the different vasoactive effect of anesthetic protocols can modify BBB opening efficacy, limiting the comparison between experimental data obtained in different labs [33,34].

If the objective of BBB opening for GBM treatment is to increase the amount of drug reaching the tumor, the single spot scheme would be the most appropriate of the two, as it allows a localized BBB permeabilization around the tumor site, potentially increasing its efficacy while avoiding local side effects in other parts of the brain [15]. However, in our setup the animal is placed on the stereotactic frame but the control of the exact position of the transducer remains challenging. Indeed, contrarily to the MRI-guided BBB disruption protocol, where acoustic radiation force imaging (ARFI) can be performed before the injection of microbubbles to locate the ultrasound focal spot [35], our device does not allow such targeting accuracy. Only at the end of the experiment could signals obtained by [99mTc]Tc-DTPA-mediated SPECT be compared with the ones obtained by [68Ga]Ga-RGD$_2$-mediated PET/CT to evaluate if the opening was successfully performed around the tumor site. On the other side, the amount of drug (or tracer, in this case) that can reach the brain and then diffuse to the tumor site is much higher for the large brain sonication scheme. As in the configuration we used there is not enough brain left "untreated", quantification errors can be performed as the measures do not consider the interindividual heterogeneity. Indeed, each mouse presents a different basal value following the administration of contrast agents. Because of this inter-individual variability between different mice, the quantifications of radiolabeled tracer uptake for the whole brain experiments are challenging and can lead to errors, as no baseline can be acquired. To overcome these limitations and increase the amount of [99mTc]Tc-DTPA reaching the tumor, we decided to perform the next series of experiments using a one hemisphere only BBB permeabilization scheme. This would allow us to make sure to open the BBB around the tumor while using as an internal control the contralateral "untreated" hemisphere for the quantification of the imaging tracers.

### *3.2. Hemispheric Blood-Brain Barrier Permeabilization and Imaging Study on Healthy and Tumor-Bearing Animals*

Our purpose is to show the interest in using nuclear imaging to evaluate the efficacy and effect of an FUS-mediated BBB opening in healthy and tumor-bearing animals. To do so, we performed a study on animals with or without tumor grafting and exposed or not to hemispheric BBB permeabilization (see experimental plan in Figure 1). As for the pilot study, animals did not show any sign of pain or distress following the hemispheric permeabilization protocols. As shown in Figure 3, [99mTc]Tc-DTPA quantification confirmed the transient BBB opening on the hemisphere exposed to FUS on tumor-bearing animals (group "GBM + FUS") and healthy animals (group "FUS only"), with an increase in ipsilateral/contralateral ratio at times 0.5 and/or 3 h and a return to basal signal within 24 h (group "GBM + FUS": −24 h vs. 0.5 h $p = 0.0399$; −24 h vs. 3 h $p = 0.0301$; −24 h vs. 24 h $p = 0.1727$; group "FUS only": −24 h vs. 0.5 h $p = 0.0247$; −24 h vs. 3 h $p = 0.4162$; −24 h vs. 24 h $p = 0.5683$; raw quantification data Figure S1). These results also suggest that the tumor may have an impact on BBB permeabilization, which appears to be greater and longer in tumor-bearing animals than in healthy animals. The results of the "GBM only" group show that the BBB is not permeable to the tested tracer ([99mTc]Tc-DTPA) in GBM-bearing animals at the time of FUS-mediated opening (eight days post U-87 MG grafting). However, modifications in the composition and activation state of microglia and astrocytes and their interaction with pericytes and endothelial cells around the tumor lesion might lead to a prolonged effect of FUS-mediated BBB opening in the "GBM + FUS" group. Moreover, the increased mechanical stiffness of the tumor region as well as the cross-talk between healthy cells, tumor cells and other components of the tumor microenvironment (e.g., tumor associated macrophages) might also alter the extravasation of contrast agent after sonopermeabilization leading to a slower recovery following FUS-mediated BBB opening. Therefore, our results suggest that the consequences of tumor growth on its reaction to FUS-induced BBB stress will have to be investigated further.

Imaging techniques able to show the initiation and propagation of neuroinflammation (ex. BBB permeability, leukocyte infiltration, microglial activation, and upregulation of cell adhesion molecules) in real-time on living animals are useful to evaluate the consequences of BBB disruption on tumor growth and treatment outcomes. Immunocompetent CNS cells or peripheral immune cells can be used as neuroinflammatory targets [36]. For example, iron oxide nanoparticles that can be internalized by circulating monocytes or by macrophages following extravasation can be used as MRI contrast agents. This cell labelling technique should make it possible to monitor the evolution of the inflammatory reaction in the brain in real time in a non-invasive manner. The conjugation of the nanoparticles with ligands (ex. peptides, proteins, or antibodies) can increase the specificity of cellular uptake to target cells expressing cellular markers of neuroinflammation [37,38]. In this work, nuclear imaging of neuroinflammation was done with [18F]FDG, as this PET radiotracer is currently used in the clinics. The availability of compounds other than commercial radiopharmaceuticals is very limited in most PET centers. Other PET tracers are in preclinical development in our and other groups, but their use is costly and their clinical application still uncertain.

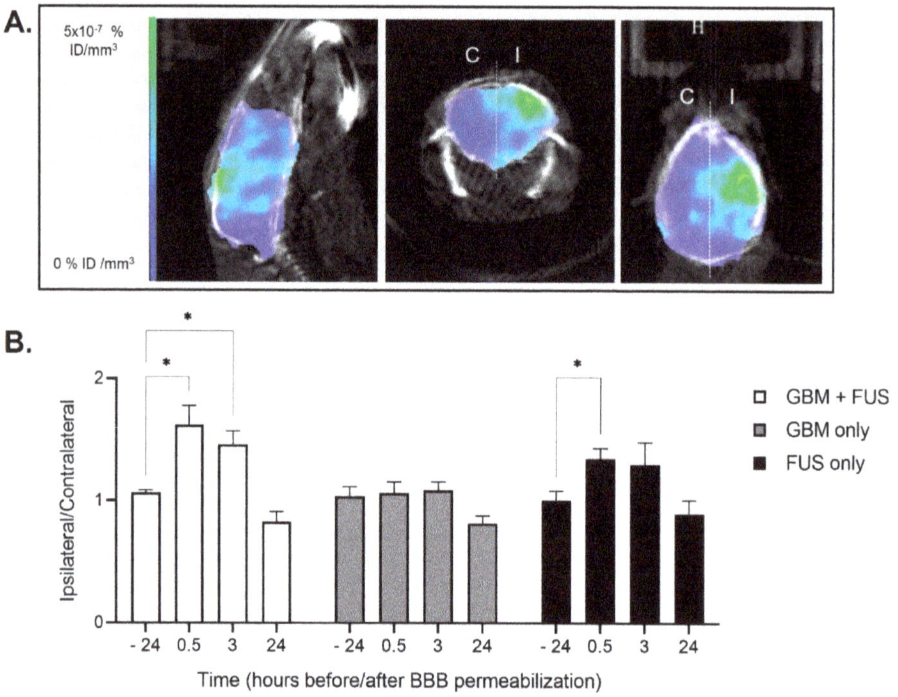


**Figure 3.** BBB permeabilization and [99mTc]Tc-DTPA SPECT/CT imaging on healthy and tumor-bearing animals. (**A**) Brain representative images obtained by [99mTc]Tc-DTPA-mediated SPECT/CT imaging in an animal of group "GBM + FUS" (tumor-bearing animals undergoing FUS-mediated BBB permeabilization) 0.5 h after hemispheric trajectory focused ultrasound. The white dotted line represents the separation between ipsilateral (I) and contralateral (C) brain hemispheres that was used for the quantifications; (**B**) Quantification of [99mTc]Tc-DTPA activity in animals of group "GBM + FUS" (tumor-bearing animals undergoing FUS-mediated BBB permeabilization, $n = 5$), group "GBM only" (tumor-bearing animals without FUS-mediated BBB permeabilization, $n = 5$) and group "FUS only" (healthy animals undergoing FUS-mediated BBB permeabilization, $n = 4$). Results are expressed as ipsilateral/contralateral ratio (mean ± SEM; * $p < 0.05$).

[18F]FDG is commonly used for oncologic imaging as tumor cells possess increased energy demand and elevated metabolism, but it also shows high uptake in inflammatory cells [39]. Brendel et al. correlated aging hypermetabolism and neuroinflammation using FDG and 18F-GE180 (a tracer for the 18-kDa translocator protein TSPO, which is highly expressed in activated microglia) PET imaging in conjunction with biochemical assessments of neuroinflammatory markers [40], thus validating this radiotracer for this use also in patients [41]. The physiologic uptake of FDG by cells is related to the rate of glucose metabolism and glucose transporters expression, varying in normal structures, inflammatory sites, and tumors. Several studies have shown that by modifying FDG-PET analysis methods or acquisition timings it is possible to differentiate inflammation from tumor malignancies. For example, Yang et al. have used dynamic FDG-PET in a mouse model of non-small cell lung carcinoma [42] for this purpose, while Hustinx et al. used dual time point FDG-PET in head and neck cancers as FDG uptake over time shows a different pattern in benign and malignant tissues [43]. Verhoeven et al. have used conventional (60 min post-injection) and delayed (240 min post-injection) FDG-PET in U-87 MG GBM tumors and turpentine-invoked flank inflammation to evaluate the ability of this tracer to differentiate tumor from necrosis. Their results showed that only delayed [18F]FDG PET was also able to discriminate GBM from radiation necrosis, while both conventional and delayed [18F]FDG display significant uptake in the turpentine-invoked lesion [44]. In our study, to assess inflammatory uptake and not the malignant lesion, we performed [18F]FDG PET/CT 45-min following tracer injection. Our results show that the BBB opening did not induce differences in brain metabolism in any of the groups as demonstrated by the [18F]FDG PET/CT imaging results 48 h post-permeabilization, suggesting the absence of neuroinflammation in this experimental protocol (Figures 4 and S2).

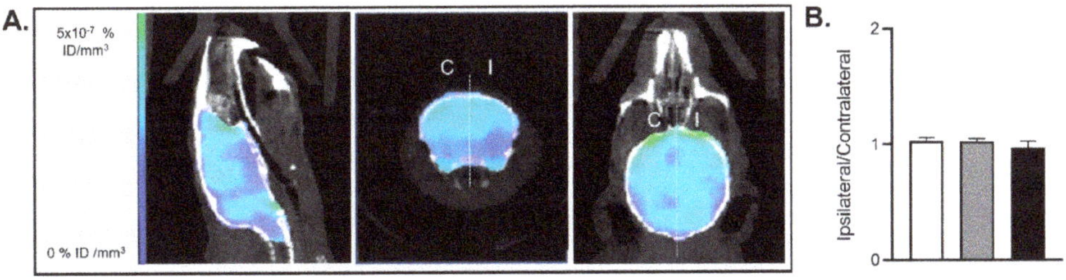


**Figure 4.** BBB permeabilization and [18F]FDG PET/CT imaging on healthy and tumor-bearing animals. (**A**) Brain representative images of [18F]FDG-mediated PET/CT two days after hemispheric trajectory focused ultrasound in an animal of group "GBM + FUS" (tumor-bearing animals undergoing FUS-mediated BBB permeabilization). The white dotted line represents the separation between ipsilateral (I) and contralateral (C) brain hemispheres that was used for the quantifications; (**B**) Quantification of [18F]FDG activity in animals of group "GBM + FUS" (tumor-bearing animals undergoing FUS-mediated BBB permeabilization, $n = 5$), group "GBM only" (tumor-bearing animals without FUS-mediated BBB permeabilization, $n = 5$) and group "FUS only" (healthy animals undergoing hemispheric FUS-mediated BBB permeabilization, $n = 4$). Results are expressed as ipsilateral/contralateral ratio (mean ± SEM).

Lastly, [68Ga]Ga-RGD$_2$ PET/CT imaging showed an increase over time for tumor-bearing animals, representing tumor growth, without significant differences between mice that were exposed to FUS-mediated BBB opening and control mice (day -1 $p = 0.3554$; day 9: $p = 0.2871$; day 16 $p = 0.8780$; Figure 5). Indeed, no direct RGD$_2$ brain uptake due to FUS was expected since RGD$_2$ imaging was performed late after BBB recovery. Thus, this confirms that a single session BBB opening does not seem to affect (negatively nor positively) $\alpha_v\beta_3$ integrin (the well-known target of RGD peptide) expression in our tumor model. No difference in the animals' survival was observed between groups "GBM + FUS" and "GBM only" (as shown in Figure 6A). The H&E staining shown in Figure 6B shows the presence of relatively low-enhancing glioblastoma tumor cells forming spheric tumor lesions neatly divided from the surrounding normal brain tissue both in the "GBM only" and "GBM + FUS" groups. In both cases, the tumor grows in one hemisphere suggesting that BBB-opening in early stages of tumor development does not induce a delay in tumor growth nor tumor cells infiltration in healthy regions of the brain.

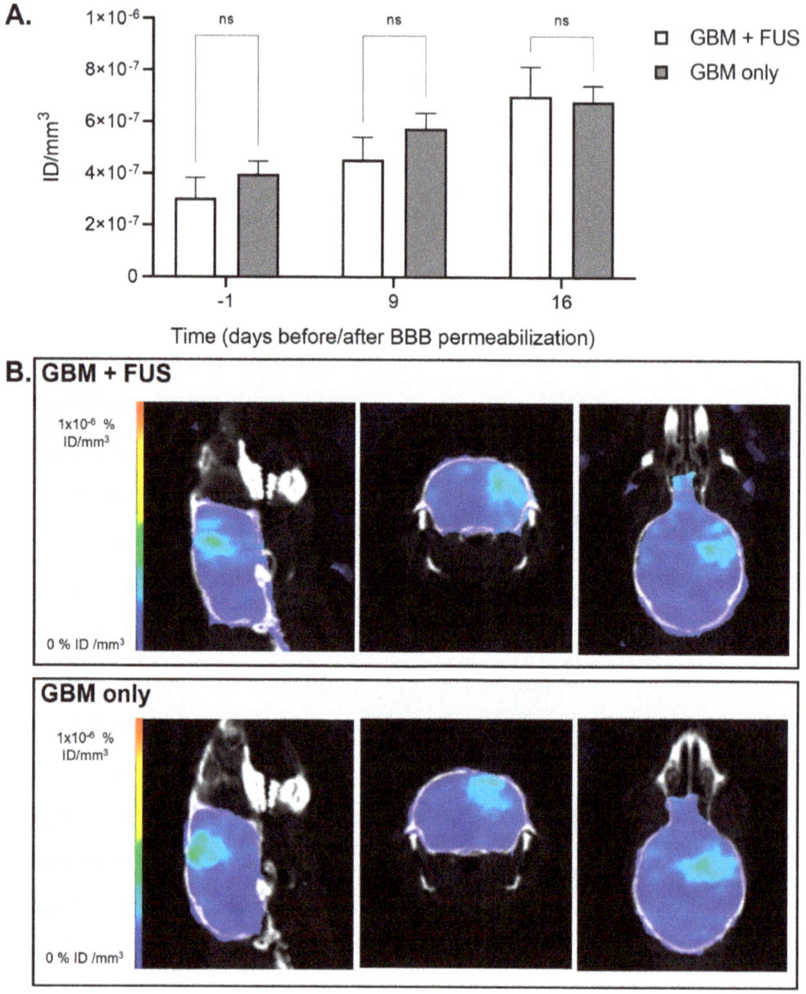


**Figure 5.** Tumor growth and [68Ga]Ga-RGD$_2$ PET/CT imaging following BBB permeabilization by focused ultrasound on tumor-bearing animals. (**A**) Quantification of [68Ga]Ga-RGD$_2$ activity in animals of group "GBM + FUS" (tumor-bearing animals undergoing FUS-mediated BBB permeabilization) and group "GBM only" (tumor-bearing animals without FUS-mediated BBB permeabilization) before and after BBB permeabilization. Results are expressed as injected dose per tissue volume (ID/mm$^3$; $n$ = 5 per group; mean ± SEM; ns: not significant); (**B**) Brain representative images obtained by [68Ga]Ga-RGD$_2$-mediated PET/CT imaging at day 16 after hemispheric trajectory focused ultrasound in an animal of group "GBM + FUS" (tumor-bearing animals undergoing FUS-mediated BBB permeabilization) and an animal of group "GBM only" (tumor-bearing animals without FUS-mediated BBB permeabilization).

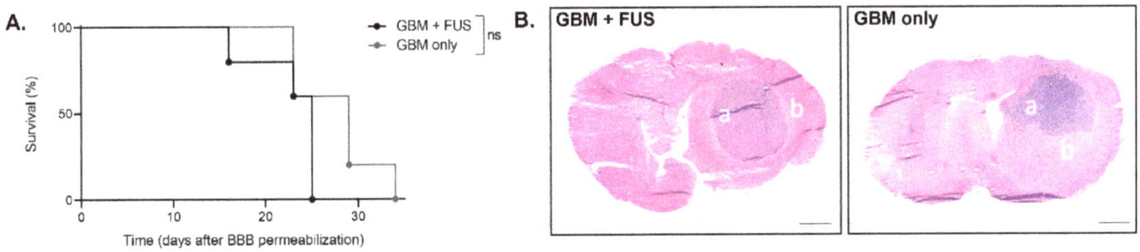


**Figure 6.** Survival and histological analyses following tumor grafting and BBB permeabilization by focused ultrasound. (**A**) Kaplan-Meier survival curves of the animals of group "GBM + FUS" (tumor-bearing animals undergoing BBB permeabilization) and group "GBM only" (tumor-bearing animals without FUS-mediated BBB permeabilization), $n = 5$ per group; ns: not significant; (**B**) Representative coronal section of Hematoxylin and Eosin staining of tumor-bearing animals that had been exposed or not to FUS-mediated BBB permeabilization (group "GBM + FUS" and "GBM only" respectively) at end point. The a represents relatively low-enhancing glioblastoma tumor cells forming a spheric tumor lesion and the b represents normal brain tissue surrounding the tumor (scale bar: 1 mm).

Lin et al. were the first to investigate the feasibility of micro-SPECT/CT and [99mTc]Tc-DTPA for identifying the disruption of the BBB induced by FUS in healthy Sprague-Dawley rats [21]. The sonication was performed after craniotomy (removing skull), directly on the brain to reduce the distortion of the ultrasonic focal beam. Static SPECT imaging showed a peak in [99mTc]Tc-DTPA signal 1.5 h post-sonication and injection of the tracer, and they compared the extent and intensity of radioactivity with autoradiography and histology. The authors reported that high acoustic powers allowed the delivery of higher amounts of radiotracer, but brain hemorrhage occurred at pression amplitudes higher than 1.9 MPa. Yang et al. evaluated the pharmacokinetics of [99mTc]Tc-DTPA after systemic administration in healthy or F98 glioma-bearing F344 rats with or without FUS-mediated BBB permeabilization of one hemisphere of the brain [45]. In both cases, animals were anesthetized by isoflurane (2% in 100% oxygen) and the tracer was co-injected with Evans Blue to quantify the BBB permeability by its extravasation rate. The maximum peak of radioactivity was observed within one hour from BBB permeabilization. To evaluate tissue damage, the authors performed histological analysis after sacrifice of the animals (about 4 h post-sonication) showing no significant differences in apoptosis between sonicated tumors and control tumors. This study demonstrated that [99mTc]Tc-DTPA microSPECT/CT can be used for pharmacokinetic analysis of FUS-induced BBB disruption. However, they did not evaluate the long-term consequences of the permeabilization on tumor growth, which is what we did in our study. The same authors evaluated the pharmacokinetics of [18F]FDG by dynamic PET and expression of glucose transporter 1 (GLUT1) protein by western blot analysis after FUS-mediated BBB disruption in healthy animals (0 h and 21 h post-sonication) [46]. Their results showed a decrease in glucose uptake and GLUT1 protein expression following transient BBB opening, which recovers after 24 h. In our study, we confirm the absence of difference in [18F]FDG uptake 48 h post-permeabilization. Okada et al. used 2-amino-[3-$^{11}$C]isobutyric acid ([3-$^{11}$C]AIB) as a PET probe to quantify BBB disruption (lipopolysaccharide-mediated or FUS-mediated) in healthy rats [47]. They compared their PET results with autoradiography and Evans Blue coloration ex vivo (for lipopolysaccharide-mediated BBB opening) and Gd-DTPA-enhanced MRI in vivo (for FUS-mediated BBB opening), showing the usefulness of this radiotracer for noninvasive BBB permeability measurement. The difference of kinetics observed between Gd-DTPA and [3-$^{11}$C]AIB in the brain can be explained by the difference in transport into the brain cells rather than a difference in the blood kinetics between the two agents. In addition, our collaborators recently reported the use of [18 F]-2-fluoro-2-deoxy-sorbitol ([18 F]-FDS) PET imaging to evaluate BBB integrity following FUS-induced permeabilization in healthy animals [28]. Brain distribution of [18 F]-FDS was consistent with ex vivo Evans Blue extravasation validating this tracer as a quantitative marker of BBB permeability. As previous studies have shown the accumulation of [18 F]-FDS in orthotopic GBM tumors in mice [48], we did not choose this radiotracer to evaluate the kinetic of BBB permeabilization in our work. Sultan et al. evaluated the effect of surface charges of $^{64}$Cu-integrated ultrasmall gold nanoclusters on brain distribution following FUS-mediated BBB permeabilization by PET/CT imaging [49]. They showed that neutrally charged nanocarriers perform the best in terms of theranostic delivery to the brain. Finally, Sinharay et al. used PET/CT imaging with [18F]-DPA714 (a biomarker of translocator protein), to assess neuroinflammatory changes in healthy animals 24 h or 1–2 weeks following single or multiple FUS-mediated BBB-permeabilization, respectively [50]. In this study performed on healthy rats, nuclear imaging was not used to evaluate BBB opening as the authors used MRI for this purpose. The neuroinflammation reported by PET/CT imaging was confirmed by histology (microglial activation by Iba1 staining; astrocytosis by GFAP staining) and seemed to persist for up to two weeks, with no evidence of cumulative inflammatory effect following multiple BBB-opening. In our study, we did not observe neuroinflammation 48 h after single BBB-opening with the [18F]FDG tracer. Immunophenotyping, morphological characterization, gene expression and phosphorylation levels of inflammatory proteins could be used in the future to confirm our results ex vivo (e.g., via flow cytometry, immunocytochemistry, quantitative RT-PCR and proteomics) [51].

## 4. Conclusions

In conclusion, molecular imaging using SPECT/CT and PET/CT allowed us to evaluate FUS-mediated BBB disruption and closure in mice bearing GBM tumors. By using three radiotracers ([99mTc]Tc-DTPA, [18F]FDG and [68Ga]Ga-RGD$_2$)sequentially and on the same GBM-bearing animal, we also demonstrated that our experimental protocol is safe (lack of neuroinflammation) and that tumor growth is not influenced by the BBB opening. This study could be relevant for future clinical applications as [99mTc]Tc-DTPA and [18F]FDG are currently used in patients and FUS-mediated BBB opening is tested in GBM clinical trials.

Our results show that rodent PET/SPECT imaging can be an efficient tool to evaluate the time frame for systemic treatment combined with transient BBB opening, and to test its efficacy over time. This versatile imaging modality allows us to follow the pathological processes and the opening efficiency with high sensitivity. Further characterization using more infiltrating GBM rodent models and assessing the impact of FUS-mediated BBB opening on the brain and tumor microenvironment could be of interest. Moreover, the use of nuclear imaging in combination with more commonly used imaging techniques such MRI could allow the optimization of drug delivery protocols.

**Supplementary Materials:** The following supporting information can be downloaded at: https://www.mdpi.com/article/10.3390/pharmaceutics14102227/s1, Figure S1: Quantification of [99mTc]Tc-DTPA activity in animals of group "GBM+FUS" (tu-mor-bearing animals undergoing FUS-mediated BBB permeabilization, $n$ = 5), group "GBM only" (tumor-bearing animals without FUS-mediated BBB permeabilization, $n$ = 5) and group "FUS only" (healthy animals undergoing FUS-mediated BBB permeabili-zation, $n$ = 4). Results are expressed as injected dose per tissue volume (ID/mm$^3$; mean ± SEM). Figure S2: Quantification of [18F]FDG activity in animals of group "GBM+FUS" (tumor-bearing animals undergoing FUS-mediated BBB permeabilization, $n$ = 5), group "GBM only" (tumor-bearing animals without FUS-mediated BBB permeabilization, $n$ = 5) and group "FUS only" (healthy animals undergoing hemispheric FUS-mediated BBB permeabili-zation, $n$ = 4). Results are expressed as injected dose per tissue volume (ID/mm$^3$; mean ± SEM).

**Author Contributions:** Conceptualization, C.B., S.F., M.-A.E. and B.G.; methodology, C.B., S.F., F.C., A.N. and B.L.; formal analysis, C.B. and S.F.; investigation, C.B.; resources, B.G.; data curation, C.B. and S.F.; writing—original draft preparation, C.B. and S.F.; writing—review and editing, all; funding acquisition, M.-A.E., B.L. and B.G. All authors have read and agreed to the published version of the manuscript.

**Funding:** This research was funded with financial support from ITMO Cancer AVIESAN (Alliance Nationale pour les Sciences de la Vie et de la Santé; National Alliance for Life Sciences & Health) within the framework of the Cancer Plan (GRAVITY Project).

**Institutional Review Board Statement:** Not applicable.

**Informed Consent Statement:** Not applicable.

**Data Availability Statement:** Not applicable.

**Conflicts of Interest:** The authors declare that they have no conflict of interest.

## References

1. Aldape, K.; Brindle, K.M.; Chesler, L.; Chopra, R.; Gajjar, A.; Gilbert, M.R.; Gottardo, N.; Gutmann, D.H.; Hargrave, D.; Holland, E.C.; et al. Challenges to curing primary brain tumours. *Nat. Rev. Clin. Oncol.* **2019**, *16*, 509–520. [CrossRef] [PubMed]
2. Daneman, R.; Prat, A. The blood-brain barrier. *Cold Spring Harb. Perspect. Biol.* **2015**, *7*, a020412. [CrossRef]
3. Begley, D.J. Delivery of therapeutic agents to the central nervous system: The problems and the possibilities. *Pharmacol. Ther.* **2004**, *104*, 29–45. [CrossRef]
4. Pardridge, W.M. Why is the global CNS pharmaceutical market so under-penetrated? *Drug Discov. Today* **2002**, *7*, 5–7. [CrossRef]
5. De Boer, A.G.; Gaillard, P.J. Strategies to improve drug delivery across the blood-brain barrier. *Clin. Pharmacokinet.* **2007**, *46*, 553–576. [CrossRef] [PubMed]
6. De Boer, A.G.; Gaillard, P.J. Drug targeting to the brain. *Annu. Rev. Pharmacol. Toxicol.* **2007**, *47*, 323–355. [CrossRef]
7. Paris-Robidas, S.; Brouard, D.; Emond, V.; Parent, M.; Calon, F. Internalization of targeted quantum dots by brain capillary endothelial cells in vivo. *J. Cereb. Blood Flow Metab. Off. J. Int. Soc. Cereb. Blood Flow Metab.* **2016**, *36*, 731–742. [CrossRef]
8. Snipstad, S.; Vikedal, K.; Maardalen, M.; Kurbatskaya, A.; Sulheim, E.; Davies, C.D.L. Ultrasound and microbubbles to beat barriers in tumors: Improving delivery of nanomedicine. *Adv. Drug Deliv. Rev.* **2021**, *177*, 113847. [CrossRef]
9. Meng, Y.; Suppiah, S.; Mithani, K.; Solomon, B.; Schwartz, M.L.; Lipsman, N. Current and emerging brain applications of MR-guided focused ultrasound. *J. Ther. Ultrasound* **2017**, *5*, 26. [CrossRef]
10. Lipsman, N.; Meng, Y.; Bethune, A.J.; Huang, Y.; Lam, B.; Masellis, M.; Herrmann, N.; Heyn, C.; Aubert, I.; Boutet, A.; et al. Blood-brain barrier opening in Alzheimer's disease using MR-guided focused ultrasound. *Nat. Commun.* **2018**, *9*, 2336. [CrossRef]
11. Idbaih, A.; Canney, M.; Belin, L.; Desseaux, C.; Vignot, A.; Bouchoux, G.; Asquier, N.; Law-Ye, B.; Leclercq, D.; Bissery, A.; et al. Safety and Feasibility of Repeated and Transient Blood-Brain Barrier Disruption by Pulsed Ultrasound in Patients with Recurrent Glioblastoma. *Clin. Cancer Res. Off. J. Am. Assoc. Cancer Res.* **2019**, *25*, 3793–3801. [CrossRef]
12. Mainprize, T.; Lipsman, N.; Huang, Y.; Meng, Y.; Bethune, A.; Ironside, S.; Heyn, C.; Alkins, R.; Trudeau, M.; Sahgal, A.; et al. Blood-Brain Barrier Opening in Primary Brain Tumors with Non-invasive MR-Guided Focused Ultrasound: A Clinical Safety and Feasibility Study. *Sci. Rep.* **2019**, *9*, 321. [CrossRef] [PubMed]
13. Park, S.H.; Kim, M.J.; Jung, H.H.; Chang, W.S.; Choi, H.S.; Rachmilevitch, I.; Zadicario, E.; Chang, J.W. One-Year Outcome of Multiple Blood-Brain Barrier Disruptions With Temozolomide for the Treatment of Glioblastoma. *Front. Oncol.* **2020**, *10*, 1663. [CrossRef]
14. Brighi, C.; Salimova, E.; de Veer, M.; Puttick, S.; Egan, G. Translation of focused ultrasound for blood-brain barrier opening in glioma. *J. Control. Release Off. J. Control. Release Soc.* **2022**, *345*, 443–463. [CrossRef]
15. Marty, B.; Larrat, B.; Van Landeghem, M.; Robic, C.; Robert, P.; Port, M.; Le Bihan, D.; Pernot, M.; Tanter, M.; Lethimonnier, F.; et al. Dynamic study of blood-brain barrier closure after its disruption using ultrasound: A quantitative analysis. *J. Cereb. Blood Flow Metab. Off. J. Int. Soc. Cereb. Blood Flow Metab.* **2012**, *32*, 1948–1958. [CrossRef]
16. Alexandrov, A.V.; Ehrlich, L.E.; Bladin, C.F.; Black, S.E. Clinical significance of increased uptake of HMPAO on brain SPECT scans in acute stroke. *J. Neuroimag. Off. J. Am. Soc. Neuroimag.* **1996**, *6*, 150–155. [CrossRef]
17. Masdeu, J.C.; Arbizu, J. Brain single photon emission computed tomography: Technological aspects and clinical applications. *Semin. Neurol.* **2008**, *28*, 423–434. [CrossRef]
18. Arif, W.M.; Elsinga, P.H.; Gasca-Salas, C.; Versluis, M.; Martínez-Fernández, R.; Dierckx, R.A.J.O.; Borra, R.J.H.; Luurtsema, G. Focused ultrasound for opening blood-brain barrier and drug delivery monitored with positron emission tomography. *J. Control Release* **2020**, *324*, 303–316. [CrossRef]
19. Yang, F.Y.; Wang, H.E.; Liu, R.S.; Teng, M.C.; Li, J.J.; Lu, M.; Wei, M.C.; Wong, T.T. Pharmacokinetic analysis of 111 in-labeled liposomal Doxorubicin in murine glioblastoma after blood-brain barrier disruption by focused ultrasound. *PLoS ONE* **2012**, *7*, e45468. [CrossRef]
20. Tran, V.L.; Novell, A.; Tournier, N.; Gerstenmayer, M.; Schweitzer-Chaput, A.; Mateos, C.; Jego, B.; Bouleau, A.; Nozach, H.; Winkeler, A.; et al. Impact of blood-brain barrier permeabilization induced by ultrasound associated to microbubbles on the brain delivery and kinetics of cetuximab: An immunoPET study using (89)Zr-cetuximab. *J. Control Release Off. J. Control Release Soc.* **2020**, *328*, 304–312. [CrossRef] [PubMed]
21. Lin, K.J.; Liu, H.L.; Hsu, P.H.; Chung, Y.H.; Huang, W.C.; Chen, J.C.; Wey, S.P.; Yen, T.C.; Hsiao, I.T. Quantitative micro-SPECT/CT for detecting focused ultrasound-induced blood-brain barrier opening in the rat. *Nucl. Med. Biol.* **2009**, *36*, 853–861. [CrossRef]

22. Bordonne, M.; Chawki, M.B.; Doyen, M.; Kas, A.; Guedj, E.; Tyvaert, L.; Verger, A. Brain (18)F-FDG PET for the diagnosis of autoimmune encephalitis: A systematic review and a meta-analysis. *Eur. J. Nucl. Med. Mol. Imag.* **2021**, *48*, 3847–3858. [CrossRef] [PubMed]
23. Crabbé, M.; Van der Perren, A.; Kounelis, S.; Lavreys, T.; Bormans, G.; Baekelandt, V.; Casteels, C.; Van Laere, K. Temporal changes in neuroinflammation and brain glucose metabolism in a rat model of viral vector-induced α-synucleinopathy. *Exp. Neurol.* **2019**, *320*, 112964. [CrossRef] [PubMed]
24. Zhao, Z.Q.; Ji, S.; Li, X.Y.; Fang, W.; Liu, S. (68)Ga-labeled dimeric and trimeric cyclic RGD peptides as potential PET radiotracers for imaging gliomas. *Appl. Radiat. Isot. Incl. Data Instrum. Methods Use Agric. Ind. Med.* **2019**, *148*, 168–177. [CrossRef]
25. Danhier, F.; Messaoudi, K.; Lemaire, L.; Benoit, J.P.; Lagarce, F. Combined anti-Galectin-1 and anti-EGFR siRNA-loaded chitosan-lipid nanocapsules decrease temozolomide resistance in glioblastoma: In vivo evaluation. *Int. J. Pharm.* **2015**, *481*, 154–161. [CrossRef]
26. Felix, M.S.; Borloz, E.; Metwally, K.; Dauba, A.; Larrat, B.; Matagne, V.; Ehinger, Y.; Villard, L.; Novell, A.; Mensah, S.; et al. Ultrasound-Mediated Blood-Brain Barrier Opening Improves Whole Brain Gene Delivery in Mice. *Pharmaceutics* **2021**, *13*, 1245. [CrossRef]
27. Choi, J.J.; Pernot, M.; Small, S.A.; Konofagou, E.E. Noninvasive, transcranial and localized opening of the blood-brain barrier using focused ultrasound in mice. *Ultrasound Med. Biol.* **2007**, *33*, 95–104. [CrossRef]
28. Hugon, G.; Goutal, S.; Dauba, A.; Breuil, L.; Larrat, B.; Winkeler, A.; Novell, A.; Tournier, N. [(18)F]2-Fluoro-2-deoxy-sorbitol PET Imaging for Quantitative Monitoring of Enhanced Blood-Brain Barrier Permeability Induced by Focused Ultrasound. *Pharmaceutics* **2021**, *13*, 1752. [CrossRef]
29. Gerstenmayer, M.; Fellah, B.; Magnin, R.; Selingue, E.; Larrat, B. Acoustic Transmission Factor through the Rat Skull as a Function of Body Mass, Frequency and Position. *Ultrasound Med. Biol.* **2018**, *44*, 2336–2344. [CrossRef] [PubMed]
30. Magnin, R.; Rabusseau, F.; Salabartan, F.; Mériaux, S.; Aubry, J.F.; Le Bihan, D.; Dumont, E.; Larrat, B. Magnetic resonance-guided motorized transcranial ultrasound system for blood-brain barrier permeabilization along arbitrary trajectories in rodents. *J. Ther. Ultrasound* **2015**, *3*, 22. [CrossRef]
31. Novell, A.; Kamimura, H.A.S.; Cafarelli, A.; Gerstenmayer, M.; Flament, J.; Valette, J.; Agou, P.; Conti, A.; Selingue, E.; Aron Badin, R.; et al. A new safety index based on intrapulse monitoring of ultra-harmonic cavitation during ultrasound-induced blood-brain barrier opening procedures. *Sci. Rep.* **2020**, *10*, 10088. [CrossRef] [PubMed]
32. Metwally, K.; Bastiancich, C.; Correard, F.; Novell, A.; Fernandez, S.; Guillet, B.; Larrat, B.; Mensah, S.; Estève, M.A.; Da Silva, A. Development of a multi-functional preclinical device for the treatment of glioblastoma. *Biomed. Opt. Express* **2021**, *12*, 2264–2279. [CrossRef]
33. McDannold, N.; Zhang, Y.; Vykhodtseva, N. Blood-brain barrier disruption and vascular damage induced by ultrasound bursts combined with microbubbles can be influenced by choice of anesthesia protocol. *Ultrasound Med. Biol.* **2011**, *37*, 1259–1270. [CrossRef] [PubMed]
34. McDannold, N.; Zhang, Y.; Vykhodtseva, N. The Effects of Oxygen on Ultrasound-Induced Blood-Brain Barrier Disruption in Mice. *Ultrasound Med. Biol.* **2017**, *43*, 469–475. [CrossRef] [PubMed]
35. Larrat, B.; Pernot, M.; Aubry, J.F.; Dervishi, E.; Sinkus, R.; Seilhean, D.; Marie, Y.; Boch, A.L.; Fink, M.; Tanter, M. MR-guided transcranial brain HIFU in small animal models. *Phys. Med. Biol.* **2010**, *55*, 365–388. [CrossRef]
36. Albrecht, D.S.; Granziera, C.; Hooker, J.M.; Loggia, M.L. In Vivo Imaging of Human Neuroinflammation. *ACS Chem. Neurosci.* **2016**, *7*, 470–483. [CrossRef]
37. Roesler, R.; Dini, S.A.; Isolan, G.R. Neuroinflammation and immunoregulation in glioblastoma and brain metastases: Recent developments in imaging approaches. *Clin. Exp. Immunol.* **2021**, *206*, 314–324. [CrossRef]
38. Candelario-Jalil, E.; Dijkhuizen, R.M.; Magnus, T. Neuroinflammation, Stroke, Blood-Brain Barrier Dysfunction, and Imaging Modalities. *Stroke* **2022**, *53*, 1473–1486. [CrossRef]
39. Wunder, A.; Klohs, J.; Dirnagl, U. Non-invasive visualization of CNS inflammation with nuclear and optical imaging. *Neuroscience* **2009**, *158*, 1161–1173. [CrossRef]
40. Brendel, M.; Focke, C.; Blume, T.; Peters, F.; Deussing, M.; Probst, F.; Jaworska, A.; Overhoff, F.; Albert, N.; Lindner, S.; et al. Time Courses of Cortical Glucose Metabolism and Microglial Activity Across the Life Span of Wild-Type Mice: A PET Study. *J. Nucl. Med. Off. Publ. Soc. Nucl. Med.* **2017**, *58*, 1984–1990. [CrossRef]
41. Doroudinia, A.; Safarpour Lima, B.; Bakhshayesh Karam, M.; Ghadimi, N.; Yousefi, F. Interesting Manifestation of Autoimmune Encephalitis on FDG PET Scan. *Clin. Nucl. Med.* **2022**, *47*, e190–e191. [CrossRef] [PubMed]
42. Yang, Z.; Zan, Y.; Zheng, X.; Hai, W.; Chen, K.; Huang, Q.; Xu, Y.; Peng, J. Dynamic FDG-PET Imaging to Differentiate Malignancies from Inflammation in Subcutaneous and In Situ Mouse Model for Non-Small Cell Lung Carcinoma (NSCLC). *PLoS ONE* **2015**, *10*, e0139089. [CrossRef]
43. Zhuang, H.; Pourdehnad, M.; Lambright, E.S.; Yamamoto, A.J.; Lanuti, M.; Li, P.; Mozley, P.D.; Rossman, M.D.; Albelda, S.M.; Alavi, A. Dual time point 18F-FDG PET imaging for differentiating malignant from inflammatory processes. *J. Nucl. Med. Off. Publ. Soc. Nucl. Med.* **2001**, *42*, 1412–1417.
44. Verhoeven, J.; Baguet, T.; Piron, S.; Pauwelyn, G.; Bouckaert, C.; Descamps, B.; Raedt, R.; Vanhove, C.; De Vos, F.; Goethals, I. 2-[18F]FELP, a novel LAT1-specific PET tracer, for the discrimination between glioblastoma, radiation necrosis and inflammation. *Nucl. Med. Biol.* **2020**, *82–83*, 9–16. [CrossRef] [PubMed]

45. Yang, F.Y.; Wang, H.E.; Lin, G.L.; Teng, M.C.; Lin, H.H.; Wong, T.T.; Liu, R.S. Micro-SPECT/CT-based pharmacokinetic analysis of 99mTc-diethylenetriaminepentaacetic acid in rats with blood-brain barrier disruption induced by focused ultrasound. *J. Nucl. Med. Off. Publ. Soc. Nucl. Med.* **2011**, *52*, 478–484. [CrossRef]
46. Yang, F.Y.; Chang, W.Y.; Chen, J.C.; Lee, L.C.; Hung, Y.S. Quantitative assessment of cerebral glucose metabolic rates after blood-brain barrier disruption induced by focused ultrasound using FDG-MicroPET. *NeuroImage* **2014**, *90*, 93–98. [CrossRef]
47. Okada, M.; Kikuchi, T.; Okamura, T.; Ikoma, Y.; Tsuji, A.B.; Wakizaka, H.; Kamakura, T.; Aoki, I.; Zhang, M.R.; Kato, K. In-vivo imaging of blood-brain barrier permeability using positron emission tomography with 2-amino-[3-11C]isobutyric acid. *Nucl. Med. Commun.* **2015**, *36*, 1239–1248. [CrossRef]
48. Li, Z.B.; Wu, Z.; Cao, Q.; Dick, D.W.; Tseng, J.R.; Gambhir, S.S.; Chen, X. The synthesis of 18F-FDS and its potential application in molecular imaging. *Mol. Imaging Biol.* **2008**, *10*, 92–98. [CrossRef]
49. Sultan, D.; Ye, D.; Heo, G.S.; Zhang, X.; Luehmann, H.; Yue, Y.; Detering, L.; Komarov, S.; Taylor, S.; Tai, Y.C.; et al. Focused Ultrasound Enabled Trans-Blood Brain Barrier Delivery of Gold Nanoclusters: Effect of Surface Charges and Quantification Using Positron Emission Tomography. *Small* **2018**, *14*, e1703115. [CrossRef]
50. Sinharay, S.; Tu, T.W.; Kovacs, Z.I.; Schreiber-Stainthorp, W.; Sundby, M.; Zhang, X.; Papadakis, G.Z.; Reid, W.C.; Frank, J.A.; Hammoud, D.A. In vivo imaging of sterile microglial activation in rat brain after disrupting the blood-brain barrier with pulsed focused ultrasound: [18F]DPA-714 PET study. *J. Neuroinflamm.* **2019**, *16*, 155. [CrossRef]
51. Monnet-Tschudi, F.; Defaux, A.; Braissant, O.; Cagnon, L.; Zurich, M.-G. Methods to Assess Neuroinflammation. *Curr. Protoc. Toxicol.* **2011**, *50*, 12.19.11–12.19.20. [CrossRef] [PubMed]

MDPI
St. Alban-Anlage 66
4052 Basel
Switzerland
www.mdpi.com

*Pharmaceutics* Editorial Office
E-mail: pharmaceutics@mdpi.com
www.mdpi.com/journal/pharmaceutics

www.ingramcontent.com/pod-product-compliance
Lightning Source LLC
LaVergne TN
LVHW070433100526
838202LV00014B/1591
* 9 7 8 3 7 2 5 8 0 6 8 0 5 *